THE PSYCHOSOCIAL A

GARLAND REFERENCE LIBRARY
OF SOCIAL SCIENCE
(VOL. 547)

THE PSYCHOSOCIAL ASPECTS OF AIDS
An Annotated Bibliography

Paula L. Levine
John G. Bruhn
Norma H. Turner

GARLAND PUBLISHING, INC. • NEW YORK & LONDON
1990

© 1990 Paula L. Levine, John G. Bruhn, and Norma H. Turner
All rights reserved

Library of Congress Cataloging-in-Publication Data

Levine, Paula L.
    The psychosocial aspects of AIDS: an annotated bibliography /
Paula L. Levine, John G. Bruhn, Norma H. Turner.
        p.   cm. — (Garland reference library of social science; vol.
547)
    ISBN 0–8240–5835–6 (alk. paper)
    1. AIDS (Disease)—Social aspects—Bibliography. 2. AIDS
(Disease)—Psychological aspects—Bibliography. I. Bruhn, John G.,
1934–   . II. Turner, Norma H. III. Title. IV. Title: Psychosocial aspects of AIDS. V. Series: Garland reference library of
social science; v. 547.
Z6664.A27L48   1990
[RC607.A26]
016.3621'9697'92—dc20   90–32919
                                                              CIP

Printed on acid-free, 250-year-life paper
Manufactured in the United States of America

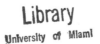

To Richard B. Pollard, M.D.,

whose extraordinary dedication to providing quality care to persons
with AIDS, in all its stages, provides an example to all his medical
colleagues

and

To Paul Curtis Hooks, Ph.D.,

a colleague who inspired others, through his struggle with AIDS, to
live life fully and with no regrets.

CONTENTS

vii

ACKNOWLEDGMENTS

A project of this scope cannot be undertaken without the help of dedicated library staff who willingly give the necessary time and effort to locate and verify references. Our sincere thanks go to members of the staff of Moody Medical Library at the University of Texas Medical Branch at Galveston, including Dierdre Becker, Alex Bienkowski, Laura Cambiano, Chris Foster, Maxine Franklin, Justin Gasper, Gonzo Gonzales, Jerry Gwinn II, Cindy Hanak, Renice Holt, Elaine Jones, Dianna Nixon, Carol Phillips, Marla Ryan, and Mary Vaughan of the Circulation, Interlibrary Loan, and Reference Departments. We thank Jeanetta James for her patience and skill in transferring our work to the word processor and for her determination to produce work of the highest quality. We also thank Patsy Marullo, who supervised the production of the final product on the word processor. Finally, we acknowledge the help of David James Taylor, who uncomplainingly obtained materials, xeroxed them, and assisted in the compiling of materials for inclusion in this book.

FOREWORD

On February 25, 1986, a little known, but significant, meeting was held at a Public Health Service building on the outskirts of Washington, D.C. Almost five years had passed since the first cases of the disease that came to be known as AIDS were identified. The Public Health Service had aimed its armada of agencies, including the National Institutes of Health and the Centers for Disease Control, at the disease. The virus had been identified and much was known about how the disease was spread. However, the American public and many of the country's political leaders did not understand AIDS. It was, therefore, appropriate that the Surgeon General of the United States preside over a meeting with four senior staff members to plan the development of the landmark document that, eight months later, would be released as *The Surgeon General's Report on AIDS*. They discussed the need to educate the general public and political leaders about the disease, the spread of the virus, the risk behaviors, destructive ignorance and prejudice, preventive education, and the service needs of people with AIDS. Before the report could be released, many months were spent on literature searches, discussions with affected individuals, testimony from groups and organizations, and policy reviews. Had a comprehensive, annotated bibliography on *The Psychosocial Aspects of AIDS* been available, the review and writing would have been far easier and more complete. Four more years of knowledge have not lessened the need for the early education, holistic understanding, and the compassion called for by Surgeon General C. Everett Koop in his controversial report. In a concise, complete, and organized manner, this bibliography reviews many of the dimensions of the disease covered in the Surgeon General's report.

The importance of this bibliography, and the impact that this disease is having and will continue to have on society, cannot be overemphasized. This compilation of information about the psychosocial aspects of a disease that has had devastating effects throughout society would have been useful in other times when other epidemics wrought havoc on uninformed societies. As this annotated bibliography documents, AIDS is causing us, as a society, to reexamine our views of many important issues. Human sexuality and sexual orientations are now more openly discussed, and the consequences of individual lifestyles and irresponsible behavior are more rationally debated. The inability of the health care system adequately to meet the physical and psychological needs of patients with HIV infection has also exposed the failures of the health care system to provide compassionate, quality care to patients suffering from other, less publicized diseases. AIDS has exposed societal intolerance and prejudice against the afflicted, the handicapped, and minorities, which festers in our schools and workplaces. The fact that we, as a society, allow ignorance about the contagion of a disease to engender fear and ignominious retribution in our supposedly scientifically literate communities lessens our confidence in our educational systems and information technology. We have become accustomed to the scientific development of cures for almost every malady. However, despite great advances in scientific knowledge about retroviruses and immunology during the last decade, no "magic bullet" against HIV has yet appeared.

The epidemiology of the acquired immunodeficiency syndrome will provide the textbook model for future generations of students. The first cases appeared in the homosexual communities, but subsequent spread among intravenous drug users and prostitutes may indicate that this epidemic, like others in history, will settle among inner-city dwellers, the indigent, the minorities, the homeless, and others on the periphery of mainstream society. High risk adolescents may become unwelcome statistics as the next manifestation of the epidemic affects runaway kids, who drop in and out of middle class neighborhoods. The runaways who survive in the cities by selling sex and dealing drugs may return to their suburban neighborhoods and unsuspecting heterosexual partners.

Medical services in many cities are overwhelmed by the impact of AIDS on their public health and medical care institutions, health manpower, and health care budgets. In the United States, the total cost of lost output and earnings due to premature illness and death, combined with the cost of providing care for a patient with AIDS, is estimated to be about $750,000. Third World countries are economically devastated by the financial burdens placed on their economies and scarce health care budgets. In these countries, AIDS mainly affects the age groups that encompass the wage earners, food producers, and mothers of young children, thus increasing the number of dependents each worker must support.

Political ideologies and elected officials have often avoided dealing with the imperatives of this disease. Public policies and governmental responses have suffered more from benign inaction than from outright opposition to strategies for the prevention of HIV and the care of people with HIV infection. Yet AIDS is a human problem, experienced by individual people. It affects families, friends, and loved ones. It affects all of us, directly or indirectly. Understanding AIDS requires knowledge of the clinical manifestations and prognosis, the psychological consequences, and the social impact of the disease. AIDS is a devastating experience that causes pain and grief for those affected, those who care, and those who provide services. It also provides opportunities to experience deeper compassion and sharing. In 1986, the Surgeon General wrote in his report to the nation:

> *At the beginning of the AIDS epidemic many Americans had little sympathy for people with AIDS. The feeling was that somehow people from certain groups "deserved" their illness. Let us put those feelings behind us. We are fighting a disease, not people. Those who are already afflicted are sick people and need our care as do all sick patients. The country must face this epidemic as a unified society. We must prevent the spread of AIDS while at the same time preserving our humanity and intimacy.*

The same exhortations apply today. This bibliography is a remarkable document in its comprehensive review of the psychosocial aspects of the HIV infection. The book brings together the copious literature on the disease and presents the current information with organization and clarity. Researchers, teachers, and students will now have available, in one place, a collection of important, up-to-date information about AIDS. The format also informs and guides the researcher to related topics and articles. *The Psychosocial Aspects of AIDS* is a rich store of excellent material that contributes to the base of knowledge necessary to human understanding so that, as a caring society, we can search for answers to reduce the spread of the infection and minimize the pain caused by the virus.

James F. McTigue, Ph.D.

Dr. McTigue was the Chief Scientist Officer, U.S. Public Health Service, where he worked on AIDS as an epidemiologist and was the principal scientific advisor for the Surgeon General's Report on AIDS. He is presently the Director of Clinical Research at Biospherics, Incorporated in Beltsville, Maryland.

PREFACE

Since 1981, when it first made its appearance on the printed page, the acquired immune deficiency syndrome (AIDS) has occupied an increasing portion of the scientific literature. The need for a guide through this burgeoning material, for students and researchers who are seeking reliable information in nontechnical language, soon became obvious and continued to grow with the published literature. We have attempted to serve that need by compiling a representative sample of the literature on AIDS in sociology, psychology, anthropology, health care, politics, law, medical economics, business, plus a limited number of background materials, and have provided an annotation for each source. This is not a comprehensive bibliography; because of the sheer volume of available material and because annotations, while they provide an additional resource for the reader as well as a form of peer review, also occupy space, we have had to be selective. However, many of the cited materials contain extensive bibliographies and should provide a good starting point for anyone who wishes to pursue the subject further.

We hope that this book will be useful to people in a wide variety of disciplines, including teachers, researchers, clinicians, and students in the social and behavioral sciences, the health professions, the social services, the humanities, business, law, religion, politics, and economics, as well as interested laypersons.

The bibliography includes books, book chapters, journal articles, and dissertations concerning AIDS published through June of 1989. Although we reviewed the literature from its beginnings in 1981, the majority of the cited works date from 1985, reflecting the scarcity of psychosocially oriented material on AIDS published prior to that time. The bibliography excludes letters, newsletters, and reports, as well as unpublished papers, which are not available to most readers. Although international in scope, the book only includes works written in English. The bibliography is organized into six chapters, each of which is broken down into subtopics. Books, journal articles, chapters, and dissertations are kept separate, and sources are alphabetized within each subtopic. Because of the complexity of the cited works, a number of them might be listed appropriately under several of the topics or subtopics; therefore, author and subject indices have been provided to aid the reader in searching for relevant materials.

We followed the thirteenth edition of the *Chicago Manual of Style* in compiling our references. Each reference contains a brief statement of purpose, a phrase noting what type of work it is (text, book of readings, editorial, review), a few sentences describing the main theme(s) or findings, and a list of suggested audiences who may find the work useful. Wherever possible, we used the authors' published statements with respect to purpose, themes, and findings, with some editing to shorten the statements and jargon. Therefore, we are responsible for possible misinterpretations resulting from our editing.

In any undertaking of this size, it is impossible not to overlook some of the published materials. Any offense caused by overlooking someone's work or minimizing the number of their citations is unintentional.

The incredible strides in knowledge made by the scientific world about the family of retroviruses responsible for AIDS, the mechanisms that transmit it, and the ways in which it affects the human body serve to point out how much is still unknown. The psychosocial impact of AIDS is so far reaching that almost no one remains untouched. Those who are most knowledgeable tell us our only effective weapon against the AIDS epidemic is education. We hope that our work will add some strength to that weapon.

Paula L. Levine
John G. Bruhn
Norma H. Turner
October 17, 1989

INTRODUCTION:
AIDS: The Plague of the 1980's

AIDS has had profound medical, political, and social ramifications. AIDS has become a political issue in both the public and private sectors and serious social problems have resulted, both from the fears of contagion and from the initial appearance of the syndrome among stigmatized minorities. Homophobia has increased at a time otherwise characterized by greater acceptance of homosexuality. Significant psychological concerns have arisen among health care workers, due to prejudice and fears of contagion. These issues have added to the psychological and social burdens of patients with AIDS who face a debilitating disease with a poor prognosis.

The psychological adaptation to any severe life-threatening disease depends upon factors derived from three major areas. These factors are medical (symptoms, clinical course, and complications, particularly of the central nervous system); psychological (personality and coping; interpersonal support); and sociocultural (social stigma attached to the disease and affected groups). The frequent complications of the central nervous system may impair the patient's ability to adapt to the stresses of this illness. The patient's behavior, especially risk reduction measures, may affect the clinical course. As evidence of the link between the central nervous and immune systems continues to grow, the implications for hypothesizing a relationship between stress and the clinical course of AIDS becomes more promising--as do the indications for using stress reduction strategies.

The medical or disease related factors are the primary determinants of adaptation because they constitute the altered physical state and medical circumstances to which the patient must adapt. These key factors in AIDS are the impact of diagnosis; common symptoms and events in the clinical course; nature of the frequent psychological distress and psychiatric disorders; central nervous system complications; and the responses of care givers.

The diagnosis of AIDS is a catastrophic event because it is known to have a rapid downhill course, no definitive treatment, and an extremely poor prognosis. The diagnosis is usually made over the course of weeks to months, as the patient fears that AIDS may be the cause of frequent infections, swollen nodes, and general malaise, with or without the diagnosis of a related complex. After a diagnosis of AIDS is made, each new symptom, infection, loss of weight, or fatigue is regarded as a sign of potential progression of disease. The characteristic skin lesions of Kaposi's sarcoma, when present, provide visible evidence of the diagnosis. Transmission of AIDS through sexual contact or body fluids often leads to self-imposed or physician-recommended limitation of social and intimate contacts. Guidelines for safe sex may require marked alteration of sexual behavior and the revelation of one's medical status to partners.

Pressure to accept a monogamous relationship or celibacy may be difficult.

The sociocultural burden of the diagnosis of AIDS results from several sources. The social stigma associated with the contagious aspect causes altered behavior in others, including avoidance of physical and social contact. Even children with AIDS have become subject to isolation from schools and from other children by frightened parents.

The diagnosis may force the patient's identification as a likely member of a stigmatized minority (homosexual, drug abuser, or recent immigrant). Families may abruptly learn of a lifestyle they find difficult to accept. In the largest risk group, homosexual and bisexual men, the diagnosis may create a crisis in which an otherwise private sexual preference is revealed. Drug abusers are already the objects of negative societal attitudes, and have little advocacy in society. Haitians, even long-term residents, have been the focus of prejudicial treatment. Hemophiliacs and recipients of blood trans-fusions receive the most sympathetic response due to the perceived random nature of the exposure. Although some persons have acquired AIDS through blood transfusions, the main tendency of the public is "to blame the victim" for having AIDS. Sexual transmission of AIDS by prostitutes has caused an association of the disease with this socially ostracized group.

Patients with AIDS are vulnerable to rejection and feelings of guilt, arising from concerns that their behavior, particularly sexual, may endanger others. The emotions associated with harboring a contagious agent may cause the patient to feel like an outcast.

Discrimination has occurred in housing, jobs, health care, and public assistance, due both to fear of contagion and to prejudice. These irrational fears and negative responses of the public are a problem confronted daily by patients, families, and advocacy groups. One of the most disruptive complications of AIDS is its impact on supportive relationships. Whether the family knows about and accepts a patient's homosexuality should be ascertained by the care giver. The onset of AIDS also may force disclosure of previously disguised drug use in drug-addicted patients, which may weaken familial support. The stigma attached to AIDS affects all patients, including children, women, and military service personnel.

Patients in the initial crisis stage of AIDS typically have difficulty retaining information and may distort what they are told regarding their illness. Contact with support services such as crisis counseling, legal, and financial assistance, and therapy should begin as early as possible.

The psychological and psychiatric sequelae of AIDS are modified by psychological factors that characterize the person's previous level of psychological adjustment and social (interpersonal) support. Presence of a personality disorder or of a previous major psychiatric disorder, is more apt to result in severe psychological symptoms and a maladaptive response to the stresses of illness. The availability of social support is especially crucial, due to the need for both physical and social assistance. Both homosexuals and drug abusers may have to face illness with inadequate support, especially from their estranged families. The drain on friends who accept their lifestyle can be great. As the illness progresses, the primary support of many patients may be the crisis-support groups that rapidly develop to meet the needs of these patients.

The major form of psychological distress is preoccupation with illness and with the potential for a rapidly declining course to death. The same issues raised by the diagnosis of cancer and of other diseases with high fatal outcomes are raised by AIDS. A normal stress response, characterized by disbelief, numbness, and denial, is seen at diagnosis and followed by anger and acute turmoil, with disruptive anxiety and depressive symptoms. The anxiety and uncertainty about the disease process, clinical course, possible treatment, and outcome continues. Patients are fearful when any new physical symptom develops because it may signal progression of the disease. Hypochondriacal concerns about body function also occur. Anxiety symptoms may take the form of panic attacks, agitation, insomnia, tension, anorexia, and tachycardia.

The symptoms of depression are also prominent. The patient's mood is characterized by sadness, hopelessness, and helplessness. Guilt, low self-esteem, worthlessness, and anticipatory grief are common, with social withdrawal and isolation. The idea of suicide if the disease progresses is common in most patients, especially those who have seen friends die of AIDS. Anger directed toward the illness, medical care, discrimination, and public response to the disease is often intense. Expectation of rejection by others, often the result of actual experiences, produces suspiciousness of the motivation of others.

A critical factor in quality of care is the attitude and responses of care givers (all persons providing direct care to patients). Several psychological issues that usually arise separately are combined in the treatment of AIDS, creating unusually difficult problems. Identification with and sense of personal vulnerability to disease and death is elicited by taking care of young healthy persons who face rapid physical deterioration and death. The fear of contagion was most frightening initially, when guidelines that assured protection from AIDS in large urban hospitals caused care givers to become overtaxed, stressed, fatigued, and fearful of being overwhelmed by the burden of the intensive complicated care. Negative social attitudes and personal prejudices, especially homophobia, can arise, as can negative attitudes toward drug abusers and Haitian immigrants.

Considerable information about these issues, which has been developed by consultation-liaison psychiatry in relation to other diseases, is applicable to AIDS. An understanding of care givers' responses to the care of patients with a potentially fatal disease comes largely from cancer care. Hospital staff need the opportunity to discuss their feelings about "special" patients with whom identification has occurred. These feelings are usually centered around anticipatory grieving for patients who will die; actual grief upon the death of patients; anger and frustration about the inability to alter the course of disease; and frustration with the negative responses of others. Care givers need instruction in how to recognize delirium and dementia, and how to adjust their expectations, in order to account for changes in these patients' ability to adhere to procedures and treatment.

The fear of contagion is best managed by providing up-to-date information about proper safety precautions. The panic among medical staff, with inappropriate behavior based on irrational fears, has diminished as institutions have promulgated Public Health Service guidelines similar to those for hepatitis B, and provided forums for clarifying misinformation from many sources. Meetings also serve to air concerns about institutional allocation of resources, organization of AIDS services, and the burden to care givers.

Personal interaction with AIDS patients may elicit otherwise masked attitudes of homophobia and negative views of drug abusers and patients from other cultures or different lifestyles. Care givers must be encouraged, through the consultation-liaison psychiatrist or a mental health consultant, to explore personal reactions, because it is important that patients feel free to discuss their lifestyles and sexual preferences and practices. Ability to discuss sexuality openly is clearly a factor in the relationship between staff and patients that provides emotional support and understanding. The need to discuss sexual precautions and answer questions of lovers and family requires that the staff member feel comfortable in these discussions. The same need applies to drug abusers. If negative attitudes preclude appropriate interaction, the care giver should ask to be replaced by another.

The facts outlined above suggest several guidelines for care givers to follow. Because psychological, social, psychiatric, and neurologic complications occur frequently, and early in the course of the disease, all patients should have early access to social workers for planning of physical and financial assistance and referral to local self-help AIDS crisis organizations, as well as psychiatric consultation for monitoring mental status and psychotherapeutic and psychopharmacologic treatment of psychiatric symptoms.

Psychological management requires attention to several key issues. Every health professional should be aware of his or her own negative attitudes toward patients with AIDS, fears of caring for the fatally ill, fears of contagion, and prejudices before undertaking patient care. The care giver should not let these attitudes interfere with care. Health professionals should maintain an active and updated file of information about AIDS, its mode of transmission, cause, and treatment, to provide facts and correct misinformation for other staff, friends, and family. New information emerges so rapidly that a poorly informed care giver may misinform a patient.

The care giver must feel comfortable discussing sexual matters with all patients and know enough about bisexuality and homosexuality to understand the issues and problems as they relate to AIDS transmission. The care giver should be able to evaluate a patient's mental status; identify altered memory, concentration, orientation, and abstraction; and monitor the patient for cognitive dysfunction at each visit. Otherwise, the care giver should have a referral resource regularly available to do the monitoring. Because the central nervous system dysfunction associated with encephalopathy and dementia may precede the definitive AIDS diagnosis, its presence must be assessed along with that of reactive depression and anxiety.

At time of diagnosis, the care giver must be able to assist the patient in understanding current information about the disease, cause, transmission, available treatment, and sources of care and social support. There must be recognition and discussion of the anxiety and panic associated with fears of progression of the disease, and realistic reassurance given in the context of the situation. Compassionate and sensitive discussion of current treatment and available research protocols must be provided. The range of depressive symptoms (such as sadness, helplessness, hopelessness, and poor self-esteem) should be explored, and questions should be asked about suicidal thoughts and plans. Referrals should be made for support and psychotherapy to deal with loneliness and depression through self-help crisis organizations.

Patients should be encouraged to explore feelings about sexual practices and the sense of guilt that accompanies the knowledge of being a source of contagion to others. Current understanding of precautions for partners, household members, and family, especially "safe sex" with partners, should be discussed, as well as precautions in the use of needles for drug abusers. Patients should be allowed to express anger toward discrimination, the behavior of others, and stigmatization; and to direct their anger in constructive ways. Help should be offered so they avoid acting in ways that would be self-destructive. Prejudice is likely to interfere with confidentiality and consideration of the patients' emotional well-being.

Fear, uncertainty, and a preoccupation with confidentiality are but a few of the many facets of the scientific and societal responses to AIDS. Many deeply troubling issues, particularly the use of the HIV antibody test, tax our abilities to balance the needs of the communities at risk for AIDS and the needs of society as a whole. Sensitivity and respect for the needs of all communities ensures us a responsible and valid solution to these problems. We must avoid simplistic solutions, such as quarantines, that some propose to protect society.

The acquired immunodeficiency syndrome causes two types of psychosocial crises, one among patients, the other in the general population; both yield opportunities and pitfalls. Medicine and its allied professions can help marshal intelligent responses to regressive societal forces unleashed by the AIDS dilemma, as well as help patients stave off senses of impending doom and hopelessness and accept the losses imposed on them by the disease. Persons with AIDS can serve as models of adjustment to progressive and devastating illness.

John G. Bruhn, Ph.D.

The Psychosocial Aspects of AIDS

Chapter 1

THE ACQUIRED IMMUNE DEFICIENCY SYNDROME

1. HISTORY OF THE EPIDEMIC

a. Books

1.   BAKER, Janet.   *AIDS: Everything You Must Know About Acquired Immune Deficiency Syndrome, The Killer Epidemic of the 80's.* Saratoga, CA: R & E Publishers, 1983.

Explores the facts that were known, at the time of publication, about AIDS.

Text

The 18 chapters cover the definition, symptoms, and groups at risk for AIDS and discuss the history of the outbreak; its epidemiology, etiology, and social consequences; efforts to combat, prevent, and control the disease; treatment and hospitalization of AIDS victims, mortality rate, and possible cures for AIDS; health insurance and welfare problems of AIDS victims and where they can go for help; and the future outlook for AIDS. The appendices contain reprints from the *Morbidity and Mortality Weekly Report* of the Center for Disease Control and an extensive scientific and clinical bibliography.

Intended for physicians, AIDS patients, and the general public.

2.   BLACK, David.   *The Plague Years: A Chronicle of AIDS, The Epidemic of Our Times.*   New York: Simon and Schuster, 1986.

A social history of the AIDS epidemic.

Monograph

Chronicles the history of AIDS from its early recognition, the investigation to discover its cause and method of transmission, its impact on the gay community and upon society in general, and the efforts of various groups to control the disease and help or isolate its victims.

Of interest to social and behavioral scientists and concerned laypersons.

3.   CAHILL, Kevin M. (Ed.).   *The AIDS Epidemic.*   New York: St. Martin's Press, 1983.

Based on a symposium on AIDS that was held in New York City in 1983.

Book of Readings

Papers by 11 noted clinicians and a member of the U.S. House of Representatives explore the epidemiology, immunology, clinical picture, implications, and future of the AIDS epidemic.

Of interest to epidemiologists, clinicians, public health professionals, and medical and scientific researchers.

4.   CANTWELL, Alan, Jr.   *AIDS and the Doctors of Death: An Inquiry into the Origin of the AIDS Epidemic.*   Los Angeles: Aries Rising Press, 1988.

A book on the origin of the AIDS epidemic.

Theoretical

In this exposé of AIDS and cancer research, the author links the outbreak of AIDS in the late 1970s in Manhattan, San Francisco, and Los Angeles to government-sponsored viral vaccine experiments that used gay men as human guinea pigs. AIDS may have also been introduced into Central Africa by vaccine programs sponsored by the World Health Organization. The author explains why scientific knowledge of the seriousness of the epidemic was withheld from the American public and why a cure for AIDS will not be forthcoming until the possible man-made origin of AIDS and the AIDS virus is fully understood.

Of interest to the general public.

5.   ———.   *AIDS: The Mystery and the Solution.*   Los Angeles: Aries Rising Press, 1983.

An attempt to promote a greater understanding of AIDS and its possible relationship to other diseases, such as cancer.

Monograph

Discusses the nature and origins of AIDS and hypothesizes about its most probable cause. Provides evidence to support the likelihood of a linkage between AIDS and cancer.

Should interest epidemiologists and medical researchers.

6. COLE, Helene M., and George D. Lundberg (Eds.). *AIDS From the Beginning*. Chicago: American Medical Association, 1986.

A collection of articles about AIDS from the *Journal of the American Medical Association*, which chronicles the growth of knowledge about acquired immune deficiency syndrome since its emergence, plus three introductory essays specifically written for this collection.

Book of Readings

Organized by type of article, with each section arranged chronologically. Following the introductory articles on the epidemiology, virology, and treatment of AIDS are: leads from the MMWR, medical news, letters, clinical and research reports, editorials, special reports, and questions and answers. Concludes with a selection of abstracts from other major journals and a concise bibliography.

Of interest to physicians and other health professionals, public health professionals, social scientists, and concerned laypersons.

7. CONNOR, Steve, and Sharon Kingman. *The Search for the Virus*. London: Penguin, 1988.

Tells how researchers discovered AIDS and examines the established links between AIDS, lifestyles, and the passing of blood.

Text

The 13 chapters trace the history of AIDS from its initial diagnosis; discuss its African connection, the nature of the virus, how it is spread, and the search for a cure; and appeal for the use of condoms to reduce the prevalence of AIDS. A glossary of terms is provided.

Of interest to the lay public as well as to health professionals.

8. FEE, Elizabeth, and Daniel M. Fox (Eds.). *AIDS: The Burdens of History*. Berkeley: University of California Press, 1986.

A beginning effort to take a historical approach to the AIDS epidemic.

Book of Readings

The authors offer a thorough reading of the history of infectious disease. The chapters exemplify some of the ways that the rigorous application of historical methods can contribute to public understanding of the AIDS epidemic.

Of interest to historians, especially medical historians, social scientists, ethicists, and social epidemiologists.

9.   FETTNER, Ann Guidici, and William A. Check.   *The Truth About AIDS: Evolution of an Epidemic.*   New York: Holt, Rinehart and Winston, 1984.

A detailed history of AIDS, incorporating its scientific, political, personal, and human aspects.

Text

Brings together, in chronological order, the medical, social, and psychological events of the AIDS epidemic and the struggles generated by them.   Presents different points of view and perspectives on every facet of AIDS.   Includes a glossary and a selected annotated bibliography of magazine and journal articles.

Classic reading for anyone interested in the AIDS epidemic.

10.   GREEN, John, and David Miller.   *AIDS: The Story of a Disease.* London: Grafton Books, 1986.

Tells the story of the emergence and recognition of AIDS, the discovery of the HIV virus, and the attempts to stop the spread of the disease and find a cure.

Monograph

Discusses, in non-technical language, the history, virology, epidemiology, possible origins, and transmission of AIDS; AIDS in Africa; the groups who are at risk, people who have been infected by the virus, and those who have AIDS; health care for victims of the HIV virus; the search for a cure; and speculations about the future.   Contains a list of useful addresses for members of high risk groups.

Intended for people who work in hospitals and others who want to know more about AIDS.

11.   KRAMER, Larry.   *The Normal Heart.*   New York: New American Library, 1985.

Intended to educate the public about the horror and impact of AIDS and the need for public policy to fight the epidemic.

Play/Social History

Personalizes the impact of the AIDS epidemic on the gay community in New York City, telling a story of love, loss, caring, and social support.   Tells the story of the organization of the Gay Men's Health Crisis and of the fight for public recognition of the societal threat posed by the "gay men's plague," public funds for research, and public education to help prevent the spread of AIDS.

An important book for everyone.

12.   KULSTAD, Ruth (Ed.).   *AIDS: Papers From Science,*
      1982-1985.   Washington, DC: American Association for the
      Advancement of Science, 1986.

A collection of 108 research papers and news stories on AIDS that
appeared in *Science* from 1982 to 1985.

Collection of Papers

Provides a brief history of the AIDS epidemic through September 1985,
a history that also has sociologic interest.   The research papers
reflect the interests of the authors and indicate the state-of-the-art
techniques applied to the study of AIDS.   The news stories focus on
some of the problems associated with investigating a disease occurring
predominantly, in the U.S., in homosexual men; on the early reluctance
of the federal government   to provide adequate funds for AIDS
research; and on problems that may be encountered in caring for large
numbers of sick and dying patients.

Of interest to health professionals, health policymakers, public
officials, and basic scientists.

13.   LEIBOWITCH, Jacques.   *A Strange Virus of Unknown Origin.*
      Translated from the French by Richard Howard.   New York:
      Ballantine Books, 1985.

A history of the AIDS epidemic, told by a clinical immunologist who
was among the first to point out the origin of the virus that causes
AIDS.

Text

Describes the events leading to the discovery of the AIDS virus;
discusses some of the reasoning processes that led to the discovery,
as well as some of the misleading hypotheses regarding the disease;
and draws attention to the disease itself, its pathological manifestations, and its unique social problems and stigmas.   The book is
divided into three sections--the history of AIDS and its virus, the
AIDS effect, and the clinical picture--and contains a bibliography.

Of interest to physicians, epidemiologists, and scientific researchers
concerned with AIDS, as well as social scientists, members of the
helping professions, and interested laypersons.

14.   McKIE, Robin.   *Panic: The Story of AIDS.*   Wellingborough:
      Thorsons, 1986.

A history of the AIDS epidemic.

Text

Tells the story of the recognition of the disease; its first victims;
how its cause was tracked down and the HTLV-III virus discovered; the
misinformation,   misunderstanding,   and   prejudice   that   further

victimized the afflicted; the clinical manifestations of AIDS; speculations regarding its origins; risk factors and transmission modes; methods of prevention; and current efforts to educate the public and combat the disease.

Of general interest.

15.   SIEGAL, Frederick P., and Marta Siegal.   *AIDS: The Medical Mystery.*   New York: Grove Press, 1983.

An accurate account of AIDS--what it is, who it affects, and how it manifests itself--and a description of research efforts, at the time of publication, to identify the disease's causative and contributing factors.

Text

The eight chapters provide information on the disease and how it manifests itself; the opportunistic infections that accompany and serve to identify AIDS; the immune system and how it is affected by AIDS; hypotheses, speculations, and predictions about AIDS; care and treatment of AIDS patients; the prevention of AIDS; and ongoing research and planning.   The book also includes a list of health resources, reprints of *Morbidity and Mortality Weekly Reports* on AIDS from 1981 to 1983, and a selected bibliography.

Of general interest.

b. Articles

16.   "FOLLOW-UP on Kaposi's sarcoma and *Pneumocystis* pneumonia." *Morbidity and Mortality Weekly Report* 30, no. 33 (August 28, 1981): 409-410.

Summarizes the sex, race, sexual preference, and mortality data of 108 persons with either Kaposi's sarcoma, *Pneumocystis carinii* pneumonia, or both without known underlying disease reported to the CDC between January 1976 and July 1981.

Report

The majority of cases occurred in white men, and most cases were reported from New York and California.   Patients ranged in age from 15 to 52, but over 95% were men between the ages of 25 and 49. Ninety-four percent of the men for whom sexual preference was known were homosexual or bisexual.   Of the 82 cases in which the month of diagnosis is known, 75 (91%) occurred since January 1980, and 55 (67%) were diagnosed from January through July 1981.   Forty percent of the reported cases were fatal.

Of particular interest to epidemiologists and public health officials.

17. GARRY, Robert F., Marlys H. Witte, A. Arthur Gottlieb, Memory Elvin-Lewis, Marise S. Gottlieb, Charles L. Witte, Steve S. Alexander, William R. Cole, William L. Drake, Jr. "Documentation of an AIDS virus infection in the United States in 1968." *Journal of the American Medical Association* 260 (1988): 2085-2087.

A case study of a 15 year old black male admitted to St. Louis Hospital in 1968.

Case Report

The patient had extreme lymphedema of genitalia and lower extremities. Chlamydial organisms were widely disseminated and isolated from numerous body fluids and organs. Over a 16 month clinical course, the patient's condition progressively deteriorated and, at autopsy, widespread Kaposi's sarcoma was found.

Of special interest to physicians and public health officials.

18. "KAPOSI'S sarcoma and *Pneumocystis* pneumonia among homosexual men--New York City and California." *Morbidity and Mortality Weekly Report* 30, no. 25 (July 3, 1981): 305-308.

Reports 26 recent cases of Kaposi's sarcoma in homosexual men in New York and California, and shows presenting complaints from 20.

Report

Twenty-six homosexual men, ranging from 26-51 years of age (mean age 39), were diagnosed, during the past 30 months, as having Kaposi's sarcoma. Twenty were in New York City and six in California; eight (seven in NYC, one in California) died within 24 months of diagnosis. Twenty-five of the patients were white and one was black. Seven KS patients had serious infections diagnosed after their initial physician visit; six had pneumonia (four confirmed by biopsy as *Pneumocystis carinii*), one had necrotizing toxoplasmosis of the central nervous system, and one with PC also experienced herpes simplex infection, candidiasis, and cryptococcal meningitis. Twelve patients tested for cytomegalovirus infection all had serological evidence of past or present CMV infection. Past infections of amebiasis and hepatitis were commonly reported. A review of the New York University Coordinated Cancer Registry for KS in men under 50 revealed no cases from 1970-1979 at Bellevue Hospital and three cases in this age group at the New York Hospital from 1961-1979.

Of interest to physicians, epidemiologists, and public health officials.

19. "PNEUMOCYSTIS pneumonia--Los Angeles." *Morbidity and Mortality Weekly Report* 30, no. 21 (June 5, 1981): 250-252.

Reports five cases of *Pneumocystis carinii* pneumonia in Los Angeles.

Report

Between October 1980 and May 1981, five young men, all active homosexuals, were treated for biopsy-confirmed *Pneumocystis carinii*
pneumonia at three different hospitals in Los Angeles.   All had
laboratory-confirmed previous or current CMV infection and previous or
current candidal mucosal infection.   Two of the patients died.   Case
reports of these patients are presented.

Of interest to physicians, epidemiologists, and public health
officials.

2. AIDS: GENERAL INFORMATION

a. Books

20.   ALYSON, Sasha (Ed.).   *You Can Do Something About AIDS.*
      Boston: The Stop AIDS Project, 1988.

Suggests concrete actions that individuals can take to slow the spread
of AIDS and to ease the suffering of the infected.

Book of Readings

Forty-three well-known Americans offer practical suggestions that
range from supporting an AIDS group to raising funds for AIDS
services.   Includes an annotated bibliography and lists of national,
state, and local AIDS-related organizations.

Of interest to health educators, social workers, nurses, and the
general public.

21.   AMERICAN Medical Association.   *AIDS: Information on AIDS for
      the Practicing Physician.*   Chicago: American Medical
      Association, 1987.

A concise review of the state-of-the-art information about selective
aspects of AIDS.

Book of Readings

The three sections or "volumes" contain chapters on the challenge of
AIDS for physicians today; classification of the clinical spectrum of
HIV infection in adults; pediatric AIDS; AIDS and the
obstetrician/gynecologist; blood transfusions and AIDS; serologic
tests for human immunodeficiency virus; the biology of HIV infection;
clinical trials of drugs for the treatment of AIDS; a brief overview
of the epidemiology of AIDS; and real and perceived risks of AIDS in
the health care and work environments and in the family and household.

Intended for all physicians and other health professionals.

22.   ANTONIO, Gene.   *The AIDS Cover-up? The Real and Alarming Facts About AIDS.*   Second Edition.   San Francisco: Ignatius Press, 1987.

Examines the underlying and legislative rationale that has fostered conditions encouraging the spread of the AIDS virus and undermined attempts to halt the epidemic's growth.   Designed to enable the discerning reader to determine which methods would be most effective in personally avoiding HIV infection and in preventing its continued widespread dissemination.

Text

Covers such information as: how the AIDS virus operates, how the epidemic is spreading into the general population, the real risks of casual transmission, the fading prospects of a cure or vaccine, and the major obstacles to stopping the spread of AIDS.

Of interest to the general public.

23.   BAKERMAN, Seymour.   *Understanding AIDS.*   Greenville, NC: Interpretive Laboratory Data, 1988.

An expansion of a series of lectures on AIDS given to second year medical students at East Carolina School of Medicine.

Textbook

Provides information on epidemiology, etiology, immunology, laboratory testing, clinical manifestations, control, prevention, treatment, and societal reactions.

Of interest to medical and other health professional students.

24.   BATESON, Mary Catherine, and Richard Goldsby.   *Thinking A.I.D.S.*   Reading, MA: Addison-Wesley, 1988.

An exploration of what it means to be a species shaped by both biology and culture.

Text

The ten chapters cover topics such as: the ecologies of disease, the human immune system, the AIDS viruses, a clinical view of AIDS, personal choices, and the epidemic and society.   A bibliography is provided.

Of general interest.

25.   BENZA, Joseph F., Jr., and Ralph D. Zumwalde.   *Preventing AIDS: A Practical Guide for Everyone.*   Cincinnati: Jalsco, 1986.

A compilation of data and recommendations from government reports about how AIDS is transmitted and how it can be prevented.

Text

Contains facts about AIDS, what causes AIDS, how it is diagnosed, how it is transmitted, and how it can be prevented.   Provides recommendations for general preventive measures for any persons who may unknowingly be exposed to HIV, and gives specific preventive measures for each of six potential risk groups.

Intended for a general audience.

Of general interest.

26.   BOGNER, Jerry L.   *Facts About AIDS and Other Sexually Transmitted Diseases: Sexual Decisions of Responsible Adults!*   Santa Barbara, CA: Vista International Press, 1987.

A synthesis of some of the most recent information available on the subject of AIDS and STD infections—not an exhaustive study of the topic.

Guidebook

Part I includes sections on AIDS, its history, transmission, symptoms, and prevention; the relationship between AIDS and alcohol and drugs; myths about AIDS; and AIDS treatment and research.   Part II covers sexually transmitted diseases including herpes, gonorrhea, syphilis, chlamydia, genital warts, and trichomoniasis.   An appendix and bibliography are provided.

Of general interest.

27.   CLARKE, Loren K., and Malcolm Potts (Eds.).   *The AIDS Reader.*   Boston: Branden, 1988.

Traces the path of the AIDS virus from its beginnings into the future, providing a picture of the epidemic through the first seven years of discovery.

Book of Readings

A compilation of significant articles covering the basic science of AIDS, its epidemiology, transmission characteristics, future projections, epidemiologic trends, therapy, and preventive strategies as well as the societal impact of the disease and its implications for our culture.

For the general public as well as for health professionals.

28.   COLMAN, Warren.   *Understanding and Preventing AIDS.*
      Chicago: Children's Press, 1988.

A book to assist teens in making intelligent decisions.

Text

Written in language understandable and relevant to teenagers. Covers the topic of AIDS from its origins, modes of transmission, effects of AIDS, and prevention.   Suggested readings and addresses and phone numbers for AIDS information are provided.

Written for teenagers.

29.   CORLESS, Inge B., and Mary Pittman-Lindeman (Eds.).   *AIDS: Principles, Practices, and Politics.*   New York: Hemisphere, 1988.

An abridged version of a comprehensive approach to the subject of AIDS to be published in 1988.   Addresses some of the most distressing issues confronting the general public.   These problems are examined by experts and specialists in each area.

Book of Readings

The 19 chapters deal with a wide range of topics including: children and AIDS, an ethic for AIDS, literature and AIDS, individual education programs for AIDS control, psychosocial considerations in the treatment of people with AIDS, the Surgeon General's Report on AIDS, and epidemic control measures for AIDS.

General readers will find the book helpful in dispelling some of the fears generated by AIDS, while professionals will gain valuable insights into how to develop practical strategies and programs to combat the disease.

30.   DANIELS, Victor G.   *AIDS: The Acquired Immune Deficiency Syndrome.*   Lancaster, England: MTP Press, 1985.

Provides practical and reliable information about AIDS for those who are concerned.

Text

Contains information on the epidemiology of AIDS, transmission of the virus, infection, early signs and symptoms, clinical aspects of AIDS, Kaposi's sarcoma, and treatment and management of AIDS.

Intended for members of the general public including those who are at risk, public health workers, and medical personnel.

31.   DOUGLAS, Paul Harding, and Laura Pinsky.   *The Essential AIDS Fact Book: What You Need to Know to Protect Yourself, Your Family, All Your Loved Ones.*   New York: Pocket Books, 1987.

Contains general facts about AIDS that everyone should know to protect themselves and others from this disease.

Text

Divided into sections on what you need to know about AIDS and what you can do about AIDS. Section one deals with causes and characteristics, treatment, transmission modes, and observed patterns of illness. Section two discusses safe and unsafe behavior, safe sexual practices, the HIV antibody test, monitoring physical and mental health, and harassment and discrimination. Hotline information is provided.

Of general interest.

32.   EAGLES, Douglas A.   *The Menace of AIDS: A Shadow on Our Land.*   New York: Franklin Watts, 1988.

A book about AIDS for young people.

Text

The seven chapters include: a puzzling new disease, the immune system, transmission, the AIDS virus, projections, cure and prevention, and social issues. The book is written in language that young people can understand.

Of interest to the general public.

33.   EBBESEN, Peter, Robert J. Biggar, Mads Melbye (Eds.).   *AIDS: A Basic Guide for Clinicians.*   Philadelphia: W.B. Saunders, 1984.

Presents a full picture of AIDS with greatest emphasis on the clinical and laboratory manifestations.

Book of Readings

The 15 chapters cover such topics as epidemiology of AIDS in the United States, epidemiology in Europe and Africa, risk factors, AIDS in clinical practice, treatment of opportunistic infections, Kaposi's sarcoma, histopathology of Kaposi's sarcoma and other neoplasms, cellular immunity, serology, role of viruses in the etiology, transfusion-associated AIDS, and the public health problem.

Of interest to health professionals, especially epidemiologists, virologists, and clinicians providing diagnostic and treatment services.

34. ECKERT, Ross D., and Edward L. Wallace. *Securing a Safer Blood Supply: Two Views.* Washington: American Enterprise Institute for Public Policy Research, 1985.

Two studies suggesting how the blood services system might be structured.

Theoretical

Discusses transfusion-related transmission of AIDS and hepatitis, and the need for public policy to ensure a safe blood supply. Eckert advocates a smaller, more tightly screened pool of donors who could receive cash payments to encourage regular donation, while Wallace defends the current volunteer donor system and supports the elimination of commercial services and paid donors.

Of interest to blood bank directors, public health officials, public policymakers, and legislators.

35. FISHER, Richard B. *AIDS: Your Questions Answered.* London: Gay Men's Press, 1984.

A short, easy to understand overview of the known facts and scientific hypotheses regarding AIDS.

Text

Contains current (January 1984) information regarding the AIDS epidemic, what AIDS is, who is at risk, the relationship of AIDS to herpes and other virus infections, how AIDS differs from other sexually transmitted diseases, infectivity, transmission modes, treatment, research, and prognosis. Three appendices provide information on the immune system, how viruses function, and viruses and cancer.

For the general public.

36. FROMER, Margot Joan. *AIDS: Acquired Immune Deficiency Syndrome.* New York: Pinnacle Books, 1983.

A general overview of the known facts about AIDS at the time of publication.

Text

Includes information on the AIDS epidemic, the definition of AIDS, the epidemiology of AIDS, progress of research, the link between blood and AIDS, politics and money, and homosexuality and AIDS patients. Written in language that the layperson can understand. Contains a glossary of medical and scientific terms.

Of interest to general audiences.

37.   FRUMKIN, Lyn Robert, and John Martin Leonard. *Questions and Answers on AIDS.* Oradell, NJ: Medical Economics Books, 1987.

Provides easy to read, general, but comprehensive information about AIDS.

Text

Uses a question and answer format to provide the following information: definitions and the origin of AIDS; the five principal manifestations of HIV infection; groups at risk; modes of transmission; the meaning of antibody positivity; protecting the individual and health care worker; the epidemiology of AIDS; research and funding for AIDS; resource centers for AIDS information and support; and ethical and social issues relating to the AIDS epidemic.

Although intended for health care workers, this volume provides an excellent reference for interested laypersons.

38.   GALEA, Robert P., Benjamin F. Lewis, Lori A. Baker (Eds.). *AIDS and IV Drug Abusers: Current Perspectives.* Owing Mills, MD: National Health Publishing, 1988.

Addresses the various social, psychological, medical, ethical, and epidemiological dimensions of HIV infection and AIDS among intravenous drug abusers.

Book of Readings

The five sections of this volume focus on the medical aspects of AIDS; AIDS epidemiology and drug abuse; psychiatric and psychosocial aspects of AIDS; the therapeutic community and health education; and social and ethical implications of AIDS. The editors emphasize the critical need for active educational intervention in the IV drug abuse population, which may have a profound impact on the spread of AIDS to other, non-drug-using heterosexuals.

Of particular interest to mental health professionals working with intravenous drug abusers, to health educators, and to public health public health officials.

39.   GALLIN, John I., and Anthony S. Fauci (Eds.). *Acquired Immunodeficiency Syndrome (AIDS).* *(Advances in Host Defense Mechanisms, Volume 5.).* New York: Raven Press, 1985.

Provides in-depth descriptions of the various aspects of AIDS from a broad range of perspectives.

Book of Readings

A state-of-the-art work that addresses the historical, epidemiologic, clinical, immunologic, etiologic, and potential therapeutic considerations in AIDS.

Should interest physicians working with AIDS patients, medical and scientific researchers engaged in researching this disease, and epidemiologists, anthropologists, and public health professionals.

40.   GIRALDO, G., E. Beth-Giraldo, N. Clumeck, Md-R. Gharbi, S.K. Kyalwazi, G. de Thé (Eds.). *AIDS and Associated Cancers in Africa.* Basel: Karger, 1988.

Based on the Second International Symposium on AIDS and Associated Cancers in Africa, which took place in Naples, Italy in October, 1987.

Symposium

Contains papers on the epidemiology of HIV infection in different parts of Africa, the natural history and clinical manifestations of HIV infections and Kaposi's sarcoma, laboratory diagnosis of HIV infection in Africa, virology and oncology, and prevention and control of HIV infection.

Of interest to epidemiologists, virologists, public health officials, and persons concerned with international health.

41.   GLUCKMAN, J. C., and E. Vilmer (Eds.). *Acquired Immunodeficiency Syndrome: International Conference on AIDS, Paris 1986--June 23-25.* Paris: Elsevier, 1986.

Contains the proceedings of the plenary session lectures and keynote communications of the International Conference on AIDS held in Paris, France in June 1986.

Conference Proceedings

Thirty-nine papers by international experts in their fields, which present up-to-date information about AIDS, have been divided into seven sections: virology, immunology, epidemiology, blood, clinical aspects, and psychosocial aspects.

Of interest to physicians, public health professionals, mental health professionals, social and behavioral scientists, and medical and scientific researchers.

42.   GONG, Victor. (Ed.). *Understanding AIDS: A Comprehensive Guide.* New Brunswick, NJ: Rutgers University Press, 1985.

An overview of the facts and issues surrounding the AIDS epidemic.

Book of Readings

Covers the definition of AIDS, its epidemiology, the clinical spectrum, implications of the epidemic, treating AIDS, and avoiding or coping with AIDS. The preface provides a summary of the most important new research findings and developments regarding AIDS in the time elapsed between the writing and publication of this book.

Of general interest.

43.   ————, and Norman Rudnick (Eds.). *AIDS: Facts and Issues.*
       New Brunswick: Rutgers University Press, 1986.

A revised, expanded, and up-dated version of *Understanding AIDS,* which was published in 1985.

Book of Readings

Offers a multidisciplinary perspective on the wide variety of complex issues surrounding AIDS. Divided into seven parts: an overview of AIDS, its epidemiology, and etiology; the clinical spectrum; groups at risk; society's response to AIDS; research on the prevention and cure of AIDS; avoiding or coping with AIDS; and AIDS information and resources.

Useful to health professionals, public health professionals, public policymakers; mental health professionals, health educators and counselors, and concerned laypersons.

44.   GOTTLIEB, M.S., D.J. Jeffries, D. Mildvan, A.J. Pinching,
       T.C. Quinn, R.A. Weiss (Eds.). *Current Topics in AIDS:
       Volume 1.* Chichester: John Wiley & Sons, 1987.

First in a series presenting authoritative, up-to-date review articles covering topics that are of particular current interest or have a vast accumulation of data.

Book of Readings

The 14 articles in this volume cover: social, scientific, and health policy perspectives on AIDS; current issues and trends concerning the epidemiology of AIDS; the spectrum of disease due to HIV infection; the natural history of HIV infection; HIV and related viruses; the immunopathogenesis of AIDS; serological tests for HIV; gastrointestinal manifestations of HIV; HIV infection in infants and children; T cell phenotyping in the diagnosis and management of AIDS and AIDS related diseases; HIV in the central nervous system; clinical observations; AIDS in Africa; and the psychosocial impact of AIDS and HIV.

Useful to a multidisciplinary audience of scientists, clinicians, and others working on AIDS or HIV or with those affected by it.

45.   GREENOUGH, Margaret. *Advances on the AIDS Horizon: 1986.*
       Sacramento, CA: Anderson Publishing, 1986.

An overview of current knowledge about the AIDS epidemic and the progress that has been made in dealing with it.

Text

This booklet covers the basic facts about the AIDS epidemic in clear, concise terms. Included are: epidemiology, definition, the relationship between generalized lymphadenopathy and AIDS, associated conditions, the virus, antibody tests, transmission, other issues in the workplace, treatment, and the psychology of AIDS. Concludes with a section on support for the AIDS patient that includes a list of AIDS support groups compiled by the news staff of the Journal of the American Medical Association and a list of references.

Of interest to the lay reader.

46.   HANCOCK, Graham and Enver Carim. *AIDS: The Deadly Epidemic.* London: Victor Gollancz, 1986.

An overview of AIDS as a global pandemic and a global threat of considerable magnitude.

Monograph

Discusses the scope of the problem created by AIDS--its devastating potential; biomedical, psychosocial, and economic consequences; and ethical and legal issues--and the urgent need for further research into vaccine development as well as wide-ranging public education.

Of interest to public health professionals, legislators, public policymakers, and health educators.

47.   HYDE, Margaret O., and Elizabeth H. Forsyth. *AIDS: What Does It Mean to You?* New York: Walker, 1986.

Reviews the basic facts and issues regarding the AIDS epidemic.

Text

The nine chapters discuss what AIDS means to the average person; living with AIDS; how AIDS is spread; medical progress; plagues in other times; AIDS: an epidemic of fear; international aspects of the AIDS epidemic; and efforts to halt the spread of AIDS. Includes the remarks made by Michael Callen, a gay man with AIDS discussing his personal experience with the disease, to the New York Congressional Delegation on May 10, 1983. Contains a glossary and a list of groups offering AIDS information and support.

An excellent text for young people.

48.   ———. *Know About AIDS.* New York: Walker, 1987.

A simple, straightforward account of the basic facts about AIDS.

Text

The ten chapters discuss the problem of AIDS, who gets AIDS, viruses and AIDS, where AIDS came from, the geography of AIDS, AIDS at home and in school, death in the family, the search for a cure, testing for AIDS, and high risk behavior. Written in language that even young children can understand.

An excellent text for teaching children about AIDS.

49.   JENNINGS, Chris.   *Understanding and Preventing AIDS: A Book for Everyone.*   Cambridge, MA: Health Alert Press, 1985.

This pamphlet, written by a Harvard-educated biologist for anyone of sexually active age, describes the known biological, medical, and social factors of AIDS and the AIDS epidemic.

Pamphlet

Covers topics such as: types of AIDS infections, the mechanisms of transmission, initial symptoms, treating AIDS, the hope for a vaccine, preventing AIDS, the origin of AIDS, and the magnitude of the AIDS epidemic.

A book for everyone.

50.   KOOP, C. Everett.   *Surgeon General's Report on Acquired Immune Deficiency Syndrome.*   Washington, DC: U.S. Department of Health and Human Services, 1986.

An informative report on AIDS to the people of the United States from the Surgeon General of the U.S. Public Health Service.

Report

Provides information about AIDS, its signs and symptoms, how it is transmitted, the relative risks of infection, and how to prevent it. Proposes educating children about AIDS in early elementary school and at home so that they will grow up knowing how to protect themselves from exposure to the virus by avoiding high risk behavior.

Intended for members of the general public.

51.   KURLAND, Morton L.   *Coping With AIDS: Facts and Fears.* New York: Rosen, 1988.

Describes AIDS, how it can be prevented and controlled.

Text

The 13 chapters include such topics as: what AIDS is, safe sex, how the virus kills, how the virus spreads, who can be infected, African origins, the severity of the epidemic, plagues of the past, coping with AIDS, prevention, future projections, and AIDS questions and answers. A glossary, bibliography, and list of crisis centers are included.

Useful for adolescents, their families, and friends.

52.   LANGONE, John.   *AIDS: The Facts*.   Boston: Little, Brown, 1988.

A factual, straightforward book on AIDS for the general public.

Text

The 14 chapters discuss the following questions: What is AIDS? What are the symptoms? What is the AIDS virus? Where did the virus originate? How does the virus cause infection? How contagious is AIDS? Can AIDS be conquered? Preventing AIDS and testing for AIDS are also discussed.

A book for laymen.

53.   LERNER, Ethan A.   *Understanding AIDS*.   Minneapolis: Lerner, 1987.

A book about AIDS for children.

Text

This book clearly explains the disease, including its medical and social effects, while promoting compassion. The author reassures the reader that his/her chances of getting AIDS are small. Good analogies help children understand the scientific complexities of AIDS.

For school children in the intermediate grades.

54.   LEVERT, Suzanne.   *AIDS: In Search of a Killer*.   New York: Julian Messner, 1987.

A general text, most of which is devoted to the various epidemiological aspects of AIDS.

Text

The 14 chapters cover a range of topics regarding AIDS, from its epidemiology to considerations about civil rights and health care for AIDS patients.

Of interest to the lay reader.

55.   LIEBMANN-SMITH, Richard.   *The Question of AIDS.*   New
       York: The New York Academy of Sciences, 1985.

Based primarily on a conference on Acquired Immune Deficiency
Syndrome, held in November 1983 by the New York Academy of Sciences,
this book provides a general overview of what is known about AIDS and
of the impact of the disease on our society.

Text

Traces the history of the AIDS epidemic from the report, in June 1981,
of *Pneumocystis* pneumonia in five young homosexual males in Los
Angeles hospitals to the present.   Discusses AIDS and the immune
system, clinical manifestations of AIDS, the epidemiology of AIDS, the
cause of AIDS, controlling AIDS, and the social impact of AIDS.

A good basic text for general audiences.

56.   LONG, Robert Emmett (Ed.).   *AIDS.   The Reference Shelf,*
       Volume 59, Number 3. New York: H.W. Wilson, 1987.

A collection of reprints of published materials, which provide clear
and concise information about the AIDS epidemic and its related
issues.

Book of Readings

Begins with accurate accounts of what AIDS is, how it evolved, the
manner in which it is transmitted, and precautions to prevent
infection. Part II focuses on the disease and its victims and reports
on medical efforts to conquer AIDS, and Part III discusses the
controversies that have arisen since AIDS was recognized in 1981. The
final section examines the outlook for the future and includes a
symposium of experts in AIDS-related fields.

Useful to laypersons.

57.   MADER, T.R. (Ed.).   *The Death Sentence of AIDS: Vital
       Information for You and Your Family's Health and Safety.*
       Gillette, WY: Ram Foundation, 1987.

Information and documentation about AIDS in all its aspects.

Sourcebook

A compilation of notes and quotes from doctors, researchers,
reporters, and others who have become familiar with AIDS. Features
topics that are both general and specific in nature, and provides
documented quotes from authorities on those topics. A plan of action
is suggested.

Intended for researchers and laypersons.

58.   MAYER, Ken, Hank Pizer.   *The AIDS Fact Book.*   New York:
      Bantam Books, 1983.

An accurate presention of the facts that were known about AIDS at the
time of publication.

Text

Defines and discusses the acquired immune deficiency syndrome, who is
at risk for the disease, its signs and symptoms, the ways it is
spread, its underlying effect upon the immune system, and the social
and emotional problems it creates.

Particularly useful for members of high risk groups.

59.   MIZEL, Steven B., and Peter Jaret.   *In Self-Defense.*   New
      York: Harcourt Brace Jovanovich, 1985.

Provides useful information on the breakthroughs in the coming years
that will expand our knowledge of the nature and function of the human
immune system.

Text

Examines the latest breakthroughs in our understanding of the form and
function of the human immune system and ways in which these breakthroughs offer new insight into physiologic processes that have long
baffled medical researchers.

Of interest to the general public.

60.   MOFFATT, BettyClare, Judith Spiegel, Steve Parrish, Michael
      Helquist (Eds.).   *AIDS: A Self-Care Manual.*   Los Angeles:
      AIDS Project Los Angeles, 1987.

Provides comprehensive coverage of many of the concerns and needs of
people touched, in a variety of ways, by the AIDS epidemic.

Manual

Begins with current basic information about AIDS. Deals with the
sociopsychological needs of persons with AIDS, the family, friends,
the workplace, social implications of youth and children at risk, and
the impact of AIDS as a terminal illness. Contains comprehensive
medical information for health care providers, information on alternative approaches to AIDS wellness, and general information on the
medical aspects of AIDS, and provides sexually explicit information
for sexually active people. Presents home care guidelines and
practical information regarding nutrition, hygiene, dental care, and
symptom management. Covers social services, benefits, the practical
aspects of making a will and power of attorney, and a comprehensive
guide to health, disability, and life insurance. Offers an assessment
of spiritual issues and needs by a clerical team from various denomi-
nations, as well as a perspective on life enhancing acceptance and

love in the face of death.   Concludes with useful information on self-care resources.

Of general interest.

61.   NICHOLS, Eva K.   *Mobilizing Against AIDS: The Unfinished Story of a Virus.* Cambridge, MA: Harvard University Press, 1986.

Based upon presentations made at the annual meeting of the Institute of Medicine held in Washington, D.C. in October 1985, this book provides an overview of the scientific facts and social implications of AIDS as they appeared in mid-1986.

Text

Control of the AIDS epidemic presently depends upon education and other public health measures to change high-risk sexual behavior and to reduce the spread of infection among intravenous drug abusers. Solving the problems created by the AIDS epidemic will require the cooperation of every segment of American society.

Of interest to physicians and other health care providers, public health professionals, scientific researchers, and public policymakers.

62.   NOURSE, Alan E.   *AIDS.*   New York: Franklin Watts, 1986.

A general overview of AIDS, with a special focus on viruses in general and the AIDS virus in particular--what it is, how it behaves, and how it kills.

Text

Discusses the history, nature, and etiology of AIDS; the unique nature and behavior of the AIDS virus, and its effect on the immune system; signs and symptoms of AIDS; truths and falsehoods about HIV infections; preventive behavior; and the outlook for the future.

Although specifically intended for teenagers and young adults, this would be helpful to any layperson interested in AIDS.

63.   O'MALLEY, Padraig (Ed.).   *The AIDS Epidemic: Private Rights and the Public Interest.* Boston: Beacon Press, 1989.

Handbook on the AIDS epidemic and its effects on private lives and public policy.

Book of Readings

Contains articles on the epidemiology of AIDS, public health issues, the testing debate, social and legal implications of the epidemic, and the impact on schools, hospitals, and communities. Addresses the needs of special populations including children, minorities, drug users, homosexual men, and families. Although some articles have a New England orientation, they raise questions that are not region-specific and cannot be resolved in a regional context.

Of interest to health professionals in general.

64. OSTROW, David G. (Ed.).   *Biobehavioral Control of AIDS*.
     New York: Irvington, 1987.

Contains papers presented at a workshop on the control of AIDS, held in conjunction with the First International AIDS Conference in Atlanta, Georgia in April 1985, plus several invited contributions addressing areas of concern that were not presented at the workshop.

Book of Readings

Addresses the issue of developing effective and appropriate AIDS control programs in the United States that take into account both the behavioral and biological perspectives. The papers cover HTLV-III and risk reduction guidelines; practical issues in AIDS risk reduction; examples of AIDS risk reduction education programs; and overviews of the crisis of AIDS. Fourteen appendices include lists of printed and audiovisual resources, lists of guidelines for high risk groups, and educational posters.

Of particular interest to public health professionals and health educators.

65. PRESIDENTIAL Commission on the Human Immunodeficiency
     Virus Epidemic. *Report of the Presidential Commission on the
     Human Immunodeficiency Virus Epidemic*. Washington, DC:
     June 24, 1988.

Reports on the investigation, by the presidential advisory committee, of the spread of HIV and AIDS and the public health dangers posed by the epidemic, and recommends measures that federal, state, and local officials can take to prevent its spread, assist in finding a cure, and care for those already ill.

Report

The 12 chapters of this document cover: incidence and prevalence; patient care; health care providers; basic research, vaccine and drug development; the public health system; prevention; education; societal issues; legal and ethical issues; financing health care; the international response; and guidance for the future.

Of particular interest to public health officials, health policymakers, and legislators.

66. ROGERS, David E., and Eli Ginzberg (Eds.).   *The AIDS
     Patient: An Action Agenda*. Boulder and London: Westview
     Press, 1988.

A collection of papers that address the societal, political, and health care value aspects of AIDS.

Conference Proceedings

The 18 papers cover a variety of topics including hospital, out-of-hospital, and nursing home care for people with AIDS; the relationship between IV drug use and AIDS; and financing the care of AIDS patients. The point is stressed that the greatest challenge is to put in place, strengthen, and implement comprehensive programs of AIDS prevention.

Of interest to health professionals in general.

67.   SELWYN, Peter A.   *AIDS: What is Now Known.*   New York: HP
       Publishing, 1986.

Contains four articles, originally published in *Hospital Practice* between May and October 1986, that provide an overview of the known facts about AIDS.

Monograph

Covers the history, immunovirology, epidemiology, clinical aspects, and psychosocial aspects of AIDS as well as prospects for treatment and prevention.

Of particular interest to health care providers, mental health professionals, and health educators and counselors.

68.   SIEGEL, Larry (Ed.).   *AIDS and Substance Abuse.*   New York:
       Harrington Park Press, 1988.

Papers presented at the first national conference on AIDS and chemical dependency, held in Ft. Lauderdale, Florida, February 1987.

Book of Readings

The 14 papers cover such topics as: to test or not to test; alcohol and drugs as co-factors for AIDS; heterosexual contacts of IV drug users; the response of state agencies to AIDS; treatment of substance abuse in patients with HIV infection; neurocognitive impairment in alcoholics; sterile needles and the epidemic of AIDS; and the role of substance abuse professionals in the AIDS epidemic.

Of interest to substance abuse counselors and public health officials.

69.   SILVERMAN, Benjamin K., and Anthony Waddell.   *The Surgeon
       General's Workshop on Children with HIV Infection and Their
       Families.*   Washington, D.C.: U.S. Department of Health and
       Human Services in conjunction with The Children's Hospital of
       Philadelphia, DHHS Publication No. HRS-D-MC 87-1,
       April 6-9, 1987.

Summarizes current knowledge about AIDS in children, and makes recommendations about future directions in research, prevention, and amelioration of the effects of pediatric AIDS.

Workshop Report

Contains excerpts from 15 papers, which, together, present an overview of the known facts and issues regarding pediatric AIDS, as well as summaries of the *Work Group Recommendations* for future action, and the response of the surgeon general. Included among the appendices are: guidelines for the management of HIV, a list of selected readings, and reprints from the *Morbidity and Mortality Weekly Report* of the "CDC Classification System" and "Education and foster care for children infected with HIV."

Of interest to physicians, nurses, economists, health educators, members of the helping professions, and concerned laypersons.

70.　SILVERSTEIN, Alvin, and Virginia Silverstein. *AIDS: Deadly Threat.* Hillside, NJ: Enslow, 1986.

Explains much of what is currently understood about AIDS.

Text

Explains and discusses, in accurate, straightforward terms, what AIDS is, who is at risk, and what is being done to conquer AIDS in the medical, social, and political arenas.

Intended primarily for young people, but helpful for any lay reader.

71.　SLAFF, James I., and John K. Brubaker. *The AIDS Epidemic: How You Can Protect Yourself and Your Family--Why You Must.* New York: Warner Books, 1985.

A practical guide for the layman about how to protect oneself and one's family from AIDS.

Paperback

Discusses the AIDS epidemic, its causes, past, present, and future; provides answers to 100 questions about AIDS; and discusses how to practice safe sex.

For the lay public.

72.　SMITH, Wm. Hovey (Ed.). *Plain Words About AIDS.* Second Edition. Sandersville, GA: Whitehall Press, 1986.

Largely based on the papers and posters presented at the Second International Conference on AIDS, held in Paris in June 1986.

Text

Chapters include: the body's defense systems; AIDS: what it is and is not; the AIDS epidemic; the AIDS virus; transmission of AIDS; prejudice and passion; precautions; and political and legal aspects. A glossary is provided.

Of interest to health professionals.

73.   TAYLOR, Barbara.   *Everything You Need to Know About AIDS.*
      New York: The Rosen Publishing Group, 1988.

A basic, straightforward book about AIDS for the layman.

Text

Brief chapters are presented on what AIDS is; why the AIDS virus is a killer; where AIDS came from; past plagues; how the AIDS virus is spread; how people can avoid AIDS; AIDS: the future is up to us; and questions and answers about AIDS.

Of interest to the general public.

74.   TSENG, C. Howard, T. Guilas Villanueva, Alvin Powell.
      *Sexually Transmitted Diseases: A Handbook of Protection,
      Prevention and Treatment.*   Saratoga, CA: R & E, 1987.

Compiles the results of a worldwide survey of commonly asked questions about sexually transmitted diseases.

Text

The eleven chapters include AIDS, herpes, gonorrhea, syphilis, chlamydia, trichomoniasis, candidiasis, toxic shock syndrome, pelvic inflammatory disease, and various others. The format is question and answer.

Written for the layperson.

75.   ULENE, Art.   *Safe Sex in a Dangerous World: Understanding
      and Coping with the Threat of AIDS.*   New York: Vintage
      Books, 1987.

A concise, factual book of essential information about AIDS written by a well-known physician.

Text

Chapter topics include: what AIDS is; how AIDS is spread; safe sex; almost safe sex; testing for AIDS; if your test is confirmed positive; counseling and support services.

Of interest to the general public.

76. WORMSER, Gary P., Rosalyn E. Stahl, Edward J. Bottone
     (Eds.).   *AIDS--Acquired Immune Deficiency Syndrome--and
     Other Manifestations of HIV Infection.*   Park Ridge, NJ:
     Noyes Publications, 1987.

A comprehensive overview of the HIV and AIDS.

Sourcebook

Fifty-four chapters cover the background and epidemiology of AIDS and
other manifestations of HIV infection; the etiologic agent; the
immunology of HIV infection; clinical manifestations; the pathology of
HIV infection; infection control; and treatment and prevention of HIV
infection.

Of primary interest to physicians and other health care workers.

b. Articles

77. "ACQUIRED immunodeficiency syndrome: Focus on the tri-state
     area."   *New York State Journal of Medicine* 88 (1988): Entire
     Issue.

A collection of current articles on AIDS covering a broad range of
topics.

Special Journal Issue

A variety of ethical, legal, epidemiological, educational, medical,
and psychosocial issues are discussed in this special journal issue on
AIDS, which focuses on the tri-state area comprised of New York, New
Jersey, and Connecticut.

Of interest to health professionals, educators, and public health
officials.

78. AMERICAN College of Legal Medicine. "Symposium."   *The
     Journal of Legal Medicine* 9 (1988): 489-635.

The first of a two-part series that addresses the medical, legal,
ethical, economic, and societal issues arising as a result of the AIDS
epidemic.

Special Journal Issue

The articles in this special issue cover: an overview of current
issues associated with AIDS; current medical and scientific aspects of
AIDS; AIDS dementia complex; formulating AIDS policy; AIDS public
health law; the case for quarantine; constitutional law as it applies
to AIDS; AIDS in the workplace; employer and employee rights; scientific, ethical, and legal issues associated with HIV screening; the
safety of the blood supply and liability for transfusion-associated
AIDS; and AIDS lab testing.

Of interest to physicians, health care administrators, management personnel, lawyers, and policymakers.

79. ———. "Symposium." *The Journal of Legal Medicine* 10 (1989): 1-210.

The second in a two-part series that addresses the medical, legal, ethical, economic, and societal issues arising as a result of the AIDS epidemic.

Special Journal Issue

The articles in this issue address: the medical profession and AIDS; AIDS and the response of organized medicine; AIDS and medical education; HIV infection and the ethics of clinical care; AIDS and the physician's duty to treat; outreach and counseling for high risk partners of HIV infected individuals; AIDS and institutional health policy development; AIDS and the insurance industry; financial problems inherent in the admission of AIDS patients to long-term care facilities; AIDS and the criminal justice system; AIDS and immigration policy; bases of liability for placement of children with AIDS in adoptive or foster homes; and the legal implications of AIDS.

Of interest to physicians, medical educators, ethicists, health economists, social workers, lawyers, and policymakers.

80. AMERICAN Medical Association Board of Trustees. "Prevention and control of AIDS: An interim report." *Journal of the American Medical Association* 258 (1987): 2097-2103.

An interim report of the AMA's recommendations regarding the prevention and control of AIDS.

Report and Recommendations

Education continues to be the major weapon against the spread of HIV infection. Physicians should assume the leadership role in educating themselves, their patients, and the public. Fifteen recommendations are offered dealing with testing, the role of health professionals, confidentiality, discrimination, etc.

Of interest to all physicians.

81. ANKRAH, E. Maxine. "AIDS: Methodological problems in studying its prevention and spread." *Social Science and Medicine* 29 (1989): 265-276.

Outlines some problems in conducting AIDS research in developing countries, discusses the impact of the sociocultural setting on study efforts, and emphasizes the need for adopting methodological approaches that are highly sensitive to the environment.

Theoretical

Considers the importance of seeing AIDS as a disease that affects humans, not merely biologically, but also socially, and stresses the potential of scientists to disregard this facet in the study of AIDS. Examines the imperatives for interdisciplinary collaboration between medical and social scientists, arguing that unless research agendas are combined, significant variables will be ignored in the search for ways to control AIDS. Gives special attention to the limitations of several methods employed by medical and social science researchers, and suggests that with AIDS research, these may be difficult to operationalize. Weighs the ethical implications of some research methods, and explores the interaction of economic and political conditions with research activity. Points out that it is human beings and Third World conditions, as well as the complexities of HIV and AIDS, that make AIDS research so problematic.

Of interest to medical and social science researchers.

82.   BLOOM, Arthur L.   "Acquired immune deficiency syndrome in childhood." *Public Health* 102 (1988): 97-106.

A survey of some of the features of HIV infections in childhood.

Descriptive

Discusses the HIV virus, serological response to the virus, epidemiological aspects of AIDS in childhood, mechanisms of perinatal AIDS, antenatal screening for HIV antibody, immunological and clinical features of AIDS in children, clinical presentation of AIDS, and prospects for treatment and prevention.

Of interest to pediatricians and epidemiologists.

83.   BOLTON, Ralph (Ed.).   "The AIDS pandemic: A global emergency." *Medical Anthropology* 10 (March 1989): Entire Issue.

A compilation of 10 papers by anthropologists who have studied AIDS.

Special Journal Issue

Topics include: the social classification of AIDS in American epidemiology; sexual behavior and the spread of AIDS in Mexico; dealing with AIDS: lessons from hepatitis B; human rights and public health; the legal status of AIDS at the workplace; the politics of AIDS; preventing AIDS contagion among IV drug users.

Of interest to social and behavioral scientists and public health professionals.

84.   BOWEN, Otis R.   "The war against AIDS." *Journal of Medical Education* 62 (1987): 543-548.

Describes the efforts of the United States Department of Health and Human Services to combat AIDS.

Review

Massive, comprehensive research efforts are under way and new drugs are rapidly being tested and made available for use. Although the war against AIDS may ultimately be won in the laboratories, education is presently the best available tool. The American public must be taught how to avoid or reduce the risks of catching the human immunodeficiency virus.

Of interest to medical educators and health educators.

85.   BROOKMEYER, Ron (Ed.).   "Special issue on statistics and mathematical modelling of the AIDS epidemic." *Statistics in Medicine* 8, no. 1 (1989): Entire Issue.

Explores a range of approaches to statistical and mathematical modelling of the AIDS epidemic and their underlying assumptions.

Special Journal Issue

Statistical and mathematical modeling of the AIDS epidemic have important roles to play in developing a coordinated approach for dealing with the epidemic, formulating public health policy, helping to provide an understanding of key factors which propagate the epidemic, and estimating its future course. The papers in this special issue focus on a variety of topics: the statistical analysis of AIDS incidence data; development of deterministic and stochastic models for the spread of HIV infection; approaches for evaluating the effects of intervention strategies; studies of the probability of viral transmission; and implications for public health policy.

Of interest to AIDS researchers and public health professionals.

86.   CHECK, William A.   "Beyond the political model of reporting: Nonspecific symptoms in media communication about AIDS." *Review of Infectious Diseases* 9 (1987): 987-1000.

A discussion of several ways in which communication to the public of medical and scientific information about AIDS and other complex public health problems can be improved.

Analytical

Analysis of news coverage of AIDS shows that mass media often respond to sensationalism rather than to important scientific developments. In addition, scientific disagreements are better adjudicated by evidence than by appeals to authority. As a result, media coverage often obscures the process of scientific deliberation.

Of interest to health professionals, public policymakers, and representatives of the mass media.

87.   CORLESS, Inge B., and Mary A. Pittman-Lindeman (Eds.).
      "AIDS: Principles, practices, and politics." *Death Studies* 12
      (1988): 371-615.

This double issue contains a selection of articles that have been
reprinted from the book, *AIDS: Principles, Practices, and Politics*,
edited by I.B. Corless and M. Pitman-Lindeman, which will be published
in unabridged form by Hemisphere in 1989. An abridged version of this
volume was published in 1988.

Special Journal Issue

The 16 articles deal with a wide variety of topics and are intended to
serve as the background information needed to appraise the rapid
developments in this pandemic. Included are articles that discuss the
retrovirus, treatment issues, public health measures, the needs of
persons with AIDS and of health care workers, policy issues, and
predictions for the future.

Of general interest.

88.   DESAI, Bindu T. "AIDS: Scourge of our times?" *Economic and
      Political Weekly* 22 (1987): 1179-1181.

A general review of the known facts about and public reaction to AIDS.

Review

A good concise overview of the disease, covering, in nontechnical
language, its history, epidemiology, virology, possible origins,
nature, mode of transmission, opportunistic infections, current
treatment, and future outlook. The author discusses public reactions
and public policy, illustrating the plight of AIDS victims in the face
of unreasonable fears.

A useful article for laypersons wanting to learn about AIDS.

89.   FICARRA, Bernard J. "Dynamics of AIDS--sociomedical
      aspects." *Journal of Medicine* 20 (1989): 1-50.

Provides an overview of numerous social, psychological, legal, ethical, and epidemiological aspects of AIDS.

Descriptive/Review

Discusses AIDS in the workplace, societal reflections and the prevention of AIDS, AIDS in the classroom, fear of AIDS in hospitals, nurses
and AIDS, screening donated blood, AIDS research, religion and AIDS,
prostitution and AIDS, prisons and AIDS, insurance ramifications of
AIDS, societal upheavals and AIDS, AIDS prevention, the cost of AIDS,
and medical-legal issues.

Of interest to laymen as well as health professionals in general.

90. IMPERATO, Pascal James (Ed.). "Acquired immunodeficiency syndrome." *New York State Journal of Medicine* 87 (May 1987): 251-312.

A collection of 20 articles on AIDS, encompassing a broad range of topics and opinions.

Special Journal Issue

The commentaries, research papers, review articles, and case reports that make up this special issue devoted to AIDS have been contributed by experts in a variety of fields, residing in different parts of the United States. They reflect the complexity of the challenge presented by AIDS, and demonstrate both the rapid advances in knowledge since AIDS was recognized in 1981 and the high degree of social commitment to dealing with the problems presented by this disease.

Of interest to medical and scientific researchers, educators, and clinicians.

91. "INTERNATIONAL Conference on Acquired Immunodeficiency Syndrome, 14-17 April 1985, Atlanta, Georgia." *Annals of Internal Medicine* 103, no. 5 (November 1985): 653-790.

Papers presented at the first International Conference on AIDS, including information from all major fields involved in the study of AIDS.

Special Journal Issue

Contains an introduction plus 25 multidisciplinary papers divided by subject matter into seven categories: epidemiology, virology, immunology, clinical aspects, psychosocial aspects, diagnosis and treatment, and perspective.

Of interest to physicians, scientists, mental health professionals, and others involved in patient care or research on AIDS.

92. KAPLAN, Howard B. "Methodological problems in the study of psychosocial influences on the AIDS process." *Social Science and Medicine* 29 (1989): 277-292.

Reviews recent psychosocial research on the onset and course of AIDS to determine major methodological problems in research.

Review

The major methodological problems identified in this review were related to guiding theoretical statements, sampling plans, validity of measurement models, and analytic strategies. Increased understanding of the onset and course of AIDS will depend on the speed and effectiveness with which methodological problems are addressed.

Of interest to social and behavioral scientists.

93.   ———, Robert J. Johnson, Carol A. Bailey, William Simon.
        "The sociological study of AIDS: A critical review of the
        literature and suggested research agenda." *Journal of Health
        and Social Behavior* 28 (1987): 140-157.

Reviews and critiques the sociologically relevant literature on the
onset and course of AIDS.

Literature Review

Points out two limitations in the existing literature: the limited
range of variables that are considered relevant, and the absence of
theoretical guides that specify the interrelationships among putative
explanatory factors. Offers methodological suggestions and outlines
of substantive factors that address these limitations.

Of interest to social scientists.

94.   LANDESMAN, Sheldon H., Harold M. Ginzburg, Stanley H.
        Weiss. "The AIDS epidemic." *New England Journal of
        Medicine* 312 (1985): 521-525.

Reviews the magnitude of HTLV-III exposure, the outcome of such
exposure, the economic burden of HTLV-III-related disease, and the
social, ethical, and public implications of the AIDS epidemic for the
future.

Review

Current estimates indicate that large numbers of persons are or will
become infected with the AIDS virus and tens of thousands will
contract AIDS and subsequently die. The need for a nationally
coordinated, locally managed health program has been recognized, and
the initial steps have been taken in a cooperative effort to minimize
morbidity and mortality from AIDS and to address the related social
and economic burdens. It is important to recognize that despite the
recent progress in understanding AIDS, much remains to be learned and
to be done about HTLV-III exposure and related diseases, and this will
require a continued commitment of resources.

Of general interest.

95.   LAYON, Joseph, Michael Warzynski, Ahamed Idris. "Acquired
        immunodeficiency syndrome in the United States: A selective
        review." *Critical Care Medicine* 14 (1986): 819-827.

Includes an analysis of immunologic data, means of preventing
transmission of the syndrome, and a discussion of the psychosocial and
ethical impact of the disorder.

Review

Discusses the epidemiology, etiology, clinical presentation, prevention, therapy, and psychosocial impact of AIDS.

Of interest to health professionals.

96.   LIFSON, Alan R., George W. Rutherford, Harold W. Jaffe.
      "The natural history of human immunodeficiency virus
      infection." *Journal of Infectious Diseases* 158 (1988):
      1360-1367.

Discusses current knowledge regarding the progression of HIV infection
and identifies specific areas that require further investigation.

Commentary

Discusses what happens after an individual is infected with HIV, the
number of individuals in whom infection will progress to clinical
disease, how long this takes and how the clinician can tell that
progression from asymptomatic infection to symptomatic disease is
beginning, what, if anything, can be done to slow progression, and how
the physician or other health care worker should evaluate, treat, and
counsel the HIV-infected patient. Delineates four major unresolved
issues regarding the natural history of HIV infection that are in need
of further investigation.

Of interest to clinicians and public health officials.

97.   OSBORN, June E. "AIDS and the world of the 1990s: Here to
      stay." *Aviation, Space, and Environmental Medicine* 57
      (1986): 1208-1214.

The 1986 Armstrong Lecture, delivered at Aerospace Medical Association's annual meeting in Nashville, Tennessee, April 20-24, 1986.

Lecture

The history of the onset of the AIDS epidemic was reviewed along with
pertinent aspects of the underlying biomedical science, which have
enabled precise recommendations concerning its control. The prospects
of drug treatment or vaccine interventions are remote, and, therefore,
health education and prevention are the chief weapons available to
combat the epidemic for years to come. Numerous impediments to those
effective strategies are discussed.

Of interest to public health officials, health educators, and
physicians.

98.   ———. "The AIDS epidemic: An overview of the science."
      Issues in Science and Technology 2, no. 2 (1986): 40-55.

Provides an overview of the AIDS epidemic.

Commentary

Describes the unraveling of AIDS and explains why countermeasures may
be elusive. Argues that the success of containment strategies rests

largely on the ability of public health officials to modify human behavior.

Of interest to health professionals and laymen.

99. ————. "The AIDS epidemic: Six years." *Annual Reviews of Public Health* 9 (1988): 551-583.

A review of the AIDS epidemic, focusing on selected data and concepts that have arisen or matured since the comprehensive study, detailed in the 1986 report of the Institute of Medicine/National Academy of Sciences, *Confronting AIDS*, was conducted.

Review

Reviews current information on the following facets of the AIDS epidemic: evolution of terminology and definitions; virology of the human immunodeficiency viruses; pathogenesis and modes of transmission; progress of the pandemic; clinical facets of HIV infection; strategies of care; and legal, ethical, and social issues.

Of interest to clinicians and researchers in the medical, social and behavioral, and life sciences as well as public health officials, legislators, and public policymakers.

100. RACHIN, Richard L. (Ed.). "Intravenous drug use and AIDS." *Journal of Drug Issues* 19 (Winter 1989): Entire Issue.

Draws together recent thought covering a range of issues pertinent to the HIV epidemic among IV drug users.

Special Journal Issue

Included are papers dealing with the epidemiology of AIDS and workable policy and program alternatives for the prevention of AIDS. The 10 papers cover topics such as: AIDS and IV drug use among ethnic minorities; women and IV drugs; AIDS in infants, children, and adolescents; the costs of caring for IV drug related cases; an overview of current AIDS prevention efforts.

Of interest to social and behavioral scientists, health educators, and public policy analysts.

101. RUBINSTEIN, Arye. "Pediatric AIDS." *Current Problems in Pediatrics* 16 (1986): 365-409.

An overview of pediatric AIDS.

Review

Discusses AIDS and ARC in children, the case definition for pediatric AIDS, differential diagnosis of pediatric AIDS, clinical manifestations, the immune system, the epidemiology of pediatric AIDS, school attendance of children with AIDS/ARC, recommendations for immunization, and treatment of infected children.

Of interest to pediatricians.

102. SCHMIDT, Kirsten, and Henrik Zoffmann. "AIDS and social medicine: Strategies for research." *Scandinavian Journal of Social Medicine* 15 (1987): 1-2.

An appeal for more systematic research and collaboration on "minimum protocols" in areas where collaboration is necessary or warranted.

Commentary

Cohorts of antibody negative persons will have to be followed in order to study the spread of AIDS and the social and psychological characteristics of those individuals who are infected and those who are not. Case-control studies and follow-up studies need to elucidate factors determining the different clinical outcomes of AIDS virus infection. The same type of studies will be needed to produce new knowledge about the social and psychological consequences of being infected with a virus. The success of preventive strategies will, to a large extent, depend on further research within the fields of social medicine, sociology, and sexology.

Of interest to social and behavioral scientists and mental health professionals.

103. SELIKOFF, Irving J., Alvin S. Teirstein, Shalom Z. Hirschman (Eds.). "Acquired immune deficiency syndrome." *Annals of the New York Academy of Sciences* 437 (1984): Entire volume.

Papers given at a conference titled Acquired Immune Deficiency Syndrome, held on November 14-17, 1983 by the New York Academy of Sciences.

Book of Readings

The six sections include the biology of immunodeficiency, immunological defects in AIDS, biological modifiers of the immune response in AIDS, viruses: possible etiologic agents, AIDS experiences in countries outside the United States, the epidemiology of AIDS, clinical symptoms in AIDS, treatment and management, blood and blood products, and brief communications.

Of interest to health professionals.

104. SIEGEL, Larry (Ed.). "The acquired immunodeficiency syndrome (AIDS) and substance abuse." *Advances in Alcohol and Substance Abuse* 7, no. 2 (1987): Entire issue.

Addresses the relationship between HIV infection and chemical dependency.

Special Journal Issue

The 13 papers in this issue explore: the impact of AIDS on the chemical dependency field; whether there should be HIV testing in chemical treatment programs; the value of routine testing for antibodies to HIV; current knowledge about the epidemiology, virology, and clinical manifestations of HIV infection and AIDS; alcohol and drugs as co-factors for AIDS; the prevention of HIV infection associated with drug and alcohol use during sexual activity; the implications of heterosexual contacts of IV drug abusers for the spread of the AIDS epidemic; sterile needles and AIDS as issues in drug abuse treatment and public health; a comparison of neurocognitive impairment in alcoholism with cognitive impairment due to AIDS; the response of state agencies to AIDS, addiction, and alcohol; treatment of substance abuse in patients with HIV infection; current and future trends in AIDS in New York City; and the role of substance abuse professionals in the AIDS epidemic. Also included is a selective guide to reference sources on AIDS and chemical dependency.

Of particular interest to substance abuse counselors and public health professionals.

105. "SYMPOSIUM on Controversies in Infectious Disease." *Bulletin of the New York Academy of Medicine* 64 (1988): Entire Issue.

This symposium, held at Laguna Niguel, California on November 14-16, 1987, devoted two of its sessions to AIDS. The first dealt with the epidemiology of AIDS, while the second focused on the ethical, social, political, and psychological issues.

Special Journal Issue

Session One, "AIDS: The Scientific Dilemma," focuses on two important epidemiologic questions: What is the risk of health care workers for acquiring HIV infection by caring for patients with AIDS? How important is heterosexual transmission of HIV in Africa and the Western World, and why does transmission in each of these areas appear to be different? Session Two, "AIDS: The Social Dilemma," covers: AIDS and the duty to treat: risk, responsibility, and health care workers; political and social issues surrounding AIDS; the expertise of the behavioral sciences in preventing and treating AIDS; and the press and AIDS.

Of interest to physicians, other health professionals, and social and behavioral scientists.

106. TASK Force on Pediatric AIDS. "Perinatal human immunodeficiency virus infection." *Pediatrics* 82 (1988): 941-944.

Presents an overview of perinatal HIV infection in the United States and recommendations for risk reduction in health care workers.

Review

Primary risk factors for perinatal HIV are prenatal exposure and transfusions of blood or blood products. Sexual distribution is relatively even, but prevalence is higher among blacks and Hispanics than among whites. Seroprevalence rates vary from 0.7/1000 in New Mexico to 20/1000 in New York City. The definitive means of diagnosis is a positive viral culture of blood or tissue. Clinical features include failure to thrive, generalized lymphadenopathy, developmental and neurologic dysfunctions, and bacterial infections. Health care workers should take precautions against exposure during delivery and initial care of infants. The prevalence of HIV infection among pregnant women does not warrant the cost of universal screening, but serologic testing should be offered to pregnant women at increased risk for HIV infection.

Of interest to physicians, nurses, health care workers, and family planning counselors.

107. THERIAULT, Richard L. "Acquired immune deficiency syndrome: An overview." *Journal of the American Osteopathic Association* 88 (1988): 109-113.

Presents current information on the clinical aspects of AIDS, HIV classification, transmission, testing, and therapy.

Review

Gives a concise, non-technical overview of the status of the AIDS epidemic in the United States. Points out that it is risk behavior, not a risk group, that is responsible for the spread of the virus. The 1987 revision of the CDC case definition for AIDS is included.

A useful update for medical, health, educational, and human service professionals.

108. WATTERS, John K., Ron Stall, Patricia Case (Eds.). "Intravenous drug use and AIDS." *Journal of Drug Issues* 19 (1989): 1-162.

Draws together recent thoughts covering a range of issues pertinent to the HIV epidemic among intravenous drug users.

Special Journal Issue

Intravenous drug use and the act of sharing needles now carry a risk far greater than ever before, even endangering individuals who may never have used drugs, such as the sexual partners and unborn children of IV drug users. The effects of HIV among IV drug users may come to touch all residents of some localities if state and local governments are forced to increase taxes or costs for medical and social services and/or curtail valuable government services to meet the medical costs created by IV drug users with AIDS. The behaviors which transmit HIV are beyond the effective regulatory reach of governments. Specific prevention measures are controversial, and debate continues regarding effective prevention strategies. These issues and others are discussed in the 10 articles in this special journal issue, which is divided into three sections: overview and epidemiology, special populations, and policy options.

Of interest to health educators, substance abuse counselors, public health officials, and public policymakers.

109. "WHAT science knows about AIDS." *Scientific American* 259 (1988): 41-134.

Provides an overview of all salient aspects of AIDS.

Special Journal Issue

Ten articles cover the following topics: AIDS in 1988; the molecular biology of the AIDS virus; the origins of the AIDS virus; the epidemiology of AIDS in the U.S.; the international epidemiology of AIDS; HIV infection: the clinical picture; HIV infection: the cellular picture; AIDS therapies; AIDS vaccines; and the social dimensions of AIDS.

Of interest to the general public, educators, and scientists.

c. Chapter

110. CURRAN, James W., Jonathan Gold, Harold W. Jaffe. "The acquired immunodeficiency syndrome (AIDS)." *In* King K. Holmes, Per-Anders Mardh, P. Frederick Sperling, Paul J. Wiesner (Eds.). *Sexually Transmitted Diseases.* New York: McGraw-Hill, 1984.

A general review of the known facts about AIDS.

Review

Briefly reviews the history of the AIDS epidemic. Discusses its epidemiologic and clinical aspects--including related diseases, opportunistic infections, other conditions associated with AIDS, and immunologic abnormalities found in AIDS patients and in individuals at high risk of developing AIDS--and discusses the etiology and prevention of the disease.

Useful to physicians, medical students, and other health professionals interested in learning about AIDS.

3. BIBLIOGRAPHIES

111. *AIDS (Acquired Immunodeficiency Syndrome): A Bibliography From All Fields of Periodical Literature, 1982 - 1986.* Madison, WI: Lincoln Associates, 1987.

A bibliography of articles on AIDS, published between 1982 and 1986.

Bibliography

Cites a selection of articles from magazines, journals, newsletters, and newspaper supplements.   Includes an alphabetical list of source publications and one that is arranged according to subject area. Citations are listed according to source, providing the title of each article, last name and first initial of the first author, page number, and date of publication.   Concludes with a list of books about AIDS.

Of general interest to persons wanting to learn about AIDS.

112. ABRAMS, Estelle.   *Acquired   Immunodeficiency   Syndrome (AIDS): Eleventh Update, July 1986 through September 1986.* Bethesda,   MD: U.S.   Department   of   Health   and   Human Services, Public Health Service, National Institute of Health, 1986.

One of a continuing series of literature searches put out by the National Library of Medicine, which contain citations to journal articles and monographs selected from a variety of online databases.

Bibliography

Contains 680 citations to the preclinical, clinical, epidemiologic, diagnostic, and prevention areas of AIDS.   Updates and supplements Literature Searches Nos. 83-1, 83-5, 83-25, 86-3, and 86-9, covering January 1980 through June 1986.

Of particular interest to AIDS researchers.

113. ABRAMS, Estelle J.   *AIDS Bibliography.*   Bethesda, MD: U.S. Department   of   Health   and   Human   Services,   Public   Health Service, National Institutes of Health, 1988.

A bibliographic series, beginning in January 1988 and continuing the National Library of Medicine's Literature Search Series, which contains seventeen bibliographies titled, *Acquired Immunodeficiency Syndrome (AIDS).*

Bibliography

This new series from the National Library of Medicine, which is published on a quarterly basis, consists of citations from the library's Medline and Catline databases.   The first section lists journal articles categorized by subject.   Subject headings are: clinical aspects; virology; epidemiology; blood and blood products; health policy, public health, ethics, legislation; preventive medicine; psychosocial aspects; pediatrics, including maternal transmission; dentistry, nursing; occupational exposure; and other. The following sections list monographs and audiovisuals.

Helpful to anyone doing research on HIV or AIDS.

114. DESSAINT, Alain Y., Jody L. Kirby, Barbara E. McLean (Eds.). *AIDS: Abstracts of the Psychological and Behavioral Literature, 1983-1988.* Washington, DC: American Psychological Association, 1988.

A collection of citations from the psychological, social, and behavioral sciences literature on AIDS.

Annotated Bibliography

Contains 340 abstracted and indexed references from journals, serials, and the dissertation literature on AIDS, covering the entire history of the AIDS epidemic from 1983 to June 1988, plus an additional listing of 64 recent citations, which have not been abstracted or indexed. References and abstracts are arranged alphabetically by author. Each has been given a unique number and indexed, using terms from the *Thesaurus of Psychological Index Terms*. A separate subject index based on these terms is provided. Six broad categories pertinent to the psychological and behavioral literature have been identified, and each article has been classified according to category and listed alphabetically, followed by its citation number, in the Title Index. An appendix describes the search strategy that was used in compiling the bibliography.

A useful resource for social, behavioral, and psychological researchers, clinicians, and students.

115. GAROOGIAN, Rhoda. *AIDS, 1981-1983: An Annotated Bibliography.* Brooklyn, NY: CompuBibs, 1984.

Presents sources of non-technical information regarding AIDS for members of the general public who wish to develop a better understanding of a major health problem.

Annotated Bibliography

Cites books, newspapers, magazines, the gay press, and non-technical articles from scientific and health-related journals written during the years 1981-1983. Arranged in chronological order for readers who may wish to trace the historic evolution of AIDS in print. Appendices include sources of additional information about AIDS and a list of groups that are fighting AIDS-related discrimination.

Intended for members of the general public.

116. HAUBRICH, Dennis J., and Donald W. McLeod. *Psychosocial Dimensions of HIV and AIDS: A Selected Annotated Bibliography.* Ottawa: Health and Welfare Canada, Federal Centre for AIDS, 1988.

Cites the work of social and health care researchers as well as others who appreciate the psychosocial impact of HIV/AIDS on individuals, families, and society at large.

Annotated Bibliography

Identifies and organizes English-language literature on the psychosocial dimensions of HIV and AIDS, focusing on the period from June 1981 to September 1987, with additional selected references to March 1988. Examines a range of personal, social, and ethical issues generated by the AIDS epidemic, which affect professionals and caregivers as well as people at risk for AIDS or infected with HIV.

Of interest to health professionals, mental health professionals, educators, public health officials, and public policymakers.

117. KELLY, Joyce V., and Judy K. Ball. *Selected Bibliography on AIDS for Health Sciences Research.* Rockville, MD: U.S. Department of Health and Humasn Services, Public Health Service, National Center for Health Services Research and Health Care Technology Assessment, 1987.

A selected annotated bibliography, covering a broad range of published articles on the costs and utilization of health services by AIDS patients.

Annotated Bibliography

Cites a selection of books and articles from scholarly, scientific, and other major publications on the following topics: bibliographies, classification and definition of AIDS, community services, costs, drug treatment and vaccines, epidemiology, federal policy, health insurance and medicaid coverage, hospital use, international, patient care and treatment, prevention, projections and trends, state activities on AIDS, and testing. Following each list of annotated references is an alphabetical list of additional references, many of them from nontechnical periodicals.

Intended primarily for health services researchers, but useful to all concerned individuals.

118. KORDA, Holly, Deborah Guiher, Raymond Glazier, Andrea Hassol. *An Annotated Bibliography of Scientific Articles on AIDS for Policymakers.* Cambridge, MA: Abt Associates for Office of the Assistant Secretary for Health, Health Planning and Evaluation, U.S. Department of Health and Human Services, Public Health Service, July 1987.

Provides a cross section of policy-relevant studies on AIDS and a listing of resources available through federal and state agencies and public, voluntary, and private organizations.

Annotated Bibliography

Cited articles include a broad range of biomedical, epidemiological, educational, and economic topics from the published literature, which appear in journals from January 1983 through December 1986. Divided into sections on: prevalence and spread of AIDS, transmission modes, characteristics of the disease, treatments for AIDS, risk reduction, related policy issues, and related scientific issues. An extensive glossary is included.

Intended for policymakers, but also useful to researchers and interested laypersons.

119. MILLER, Alan V. *Gays and Acquired Immune Deficiency Syndrome (AIDS): A Bibliography.* Second Edition. Toronto: Canadian Gay Archives, 1983.

An attempt to inform the general public about what has been written about AIDS and what is contained in the collection of the Gay Archives.

Bibliography

Divided by source into three sections: the medical press, the gay press, and the mainstream press. Entries in each section are listed alphabetically. Cited are articles from journals, newsletters, newspapers, and magazines. A few entries are briefly annotated.

Of interest to medical and social science researchers as well as members of the general public.

120. NATIONAL Library of Medicine. *AIDS Bibliography: 1986-1987.* Washington, DC: U.S. Department of Health and Human Services Public Health Service, National Institutes of Health, 1987.

Contains 2697 citations drawn from the bibliographic databases of the National Library of Medicine from January 1986 through April 1987.

Bibliography

Covers recent books and articles dealing with preclinical, clinical, epidemiologic, diagnosis, and prevention issues, ethical concerns, educational strategies, public health administration, and other related issues. Arranged alphabetically by author, and formatted according to the rules established for Index Medicus. Copies may be obtained from the National Technical Information Service.

Useful to all researchers concerned with AIDS.

121. NORDQUIST, Joan. *AIDS: Political, Social, International Aspects. Contemporary Social Issues: A Bibliographic Series,* No. 10. Santa Cruz, CA: Reference and Research Services, 1988.

Cites works from the social, political, legal, business, philosophical, scientific, and feminist literature representing various viewpoints on the topic of AIDS.

Bibliography

The 14 sections cover: social and political issues, AIDS and public policy, legal aspects, AIDS testing, AIDS and the insurance industry, the safety of the blood supply, AIDS in the workplace, AIDS drug research, AIDS and minorities, AIDS and women, AIDS and children, AIDS and drug users, AIDS in the prisons, international aspects, bibliographies, resources, organizations, and periodicals. Each section is arranged alphabetically by author or title. Most entries, particularly those from the periodical literature, date from the three years preceding publication.

Useful to anyone seeking information on the social, political, and international aspects of the AIDS epidemic.

122. POLINSKI, Roth. *Psychology and AIDS: Index of Modern Information*. Washington, DC: Abbe, 1988.

A reference guide to journals and books dealing with psychology and AIDS.

Reference Guide

Subject and research categories are indexed to a 228 item bibliography.

Useful to health professionals, laymen, and anyone interested in psychology and AIDS.

123. REED, Robert D. *A.I.D.S.: A Bibliography*. Saratoga, CA: R & E, 1987.

A paperback compilation on information about AIDS.

Bibliography

This 64 page bibliography includes magazine articles, newspaper articles, books, and a scientific and clinical bibliography. It is selected and dated, but would be valuable to laymen wanting an introduction to the AIDS epidemic.

Of interest to laymen and health personnel.

124. TYCKOSON, David A. *AIDS (Acquired Immune Deficiency Syndrome)*. (Volume 1 of the Oryx Science Bibliographies.) Phoenix, AZ: Oryx Press, 1985.

Cites 231 articles, written through 1984, selected from the literature on AIDS.

Annotated Bibliography

Begins with a brief research review and cites articles in the following categories: reports of a deadly new disease; AIDS in hemophiliacs and blood transfusions; AIDS and the Haitian connection; victims other than those primarily at risk; animal studies of AIDS; precursors, indicators, and relationships with other diseases; the human T-cell leukemia virus (HTLV) and AIDS; the possible cause and search for a cure; role of interferon in AIDS; psychological aspects of AIDS; risks to medical staff; funding for AIDS research; AIDS hysteria; and AIDS outside the United States.

Useful to students and researchers interested in AIDS.

125. ———. *AIDS (Acquired Immune Deficiency Syndrome)*. Second Edition. (Volume 7 of the Oryx Science Bibliographies.) Phoenix, AZ: Oryx Press, 1985.

A selective bibliography, citing 435 articles about AIDS.

Annotated Bibliography

Reflects the influx of AIDS into the scientific and popular literature during 1985 and the first half of 1986. Contains a research review and cites materials in 14 categories: medical aspects of AIDS; high risk groups; AIDS outside the high risk groups; transmission of the AIDS virus; the AIDS blood test; patent rights to the AIDS virus; the search for a cure; psychological aspects of AIDS; health care workers and AIDS; ethical and legal problems of AIDS; AIDS hysteria; sexual behavior changes due to AIDS; Rock Hudson: AIDS strikes a star; and the future of AIDS. All cited materials are understandable at the undergraduate level. Important articles are highlighted.

A useful bibliography for students and researchers interested in AIDS.

126. WEISSBERG, Nancy C. *AIDS (Acquired Immune Deficiency Syndrome) Bibliography for 1981-86.* Troy, NY: Whitston, 1988.

A complete bibliography of world-wide literature surrounding AIDS. This is the first in a series which will be updated annually.

Bibliography

Divided into three sections: a list of books, government publications, and monographs; periodical literature arranged alphabetically by title; and periodical literature listed by subject. The subject heads have been derived from the nature of the material indexed rather than imposed from Library of Congress subject heads. A list of journals, a subject heading index, and an author index to the periodical litera-ture all enhance the usefulness of this volume.

Of general use.

4. AGENCIES, ORGANIZATIONS, AND RESOURCES

a. Books

127. *AIDS: Reference Guide for Medical Professionals.* Los Angeles:
      UCLA School of Medicine, CIRID Outreach and Education
      Program, 1985.

A quick reference guide for medical professionals seeking information
relating to AIDS.

Sourcebook

Contains a brief overview of AIDS followed by information regarding
case definitions, psychosocial aspects, terminology, referral centers,
Los Angeles County services, other Southern California counties'
services, precautions, AIDS hot lines, financial assistance programs,
newsletters, and bibliographies. Reference tabs make this guide
extremely easy to use. Prepared specifically for use in Southern
California, but could easily be adapted for other localities.

Useful to all health professionals and to HIV-infected individuals
seeking information on where to find help.

128. *AIDS: Reference Guide for Medical Professionals.* Second
      Edition. Los Angeles: UCLA School of Medicine, CIRID
      Outreach and Education Program, 1986.

Builds on the first edition to provide a quick reference to recent
developments in immunologic laboratory and clinical research on AIDS.

Sourcebook

Provides general information about AIDS; case definitions; HTLV-III;
terminology; precautions; experimental therapies; national resources;
educational materials; and California County Resources. Text comes in
a loose leaf binder divided by subject tabs.

A useful reference guide for physicians and other health
professionals.

129. LINGLE, Virginia, and M. Sandra Wood. *How to Find Informa-*
      tion About AIDS. New York: Haworth Press, 1988.

Provides help in tapping into the vastly increasing flow of information about AIDS.

Reference

A selective listing of such key information access points as government agencies, community hotlines, organizational resources, funding
sources, major publications, and informational databases. Excluded

from the listings are national organizations that do not either provide service to AIDS patients and their loved ones or distribute information about the AIDS crisis and most popular works of literature.

Useful to health professionals and to members of the general public.

130. MALINOWSKY, H. Robert, and Gerald J. Perry. *AIDS Information Sourcebook*. Phoenix: Oryx Press, 1988.

A directory of educational resources about AIDS.

Sourcebook

Directs users to sources of information about AIDS, how AIDS is contracted, who is at risk, how to lessen one's chances of contracting AIDS, and what is being done to combat the AIDS virus. Brings together a wide variety of information sources, such as agencies, facilities, and organizations. Provides a chronology of the history of the AIDS epidemic as well as a select bibliography. The directory of organizations is arranged first by state, then alphabetically by name of facility. The bibliography, which lists publications that have appeared in the last five years, is divided into sections according to type of publication. A subject index is provided.

Intended for the general public.

131. THOMAS, Constance. *AIDS, A Public Health Challenge: State Issues, Policies and Programs*. Volume 3: Resource Guide. Washington DC: U.S. Department of Health and Human Services, Public Health Service, October 1987.

The third of three volumes, which provide a comprehensive review, for public policymakers, of the policy issues with which AIDS confronts the states, provides a directory of AIDS-related resources, information, and materials.

Sourcebook

Contains a bibliography, glossary, and directory to community, state, and national AIDS organizations, programs, education and training centers, and sources of information, as well as a summary of AIDS-related legislation from 1985-1987.

A useful reference for anyone seeking help or information regarding AIDS as well as for public policymakers.

132. UNITED States Conference of Mayors. *Local Responses to Acquired Immune Deficiency Syndrome: A Report of 55 Cities*. Washington, DC: United States Conference of Mayors, November 1984.

Documents the significant involvement of local government in responding to AIDS.

Report

The AIDS Information Exchange Program, established by the United States Conference of Mayors, sent questionnaires, in August 1984, to cities, counties, and community-based organizations that had expressed interest in exchanging information. Fifty-five questionnaires were returned. The results reveal a variety of local government and community involvement, often displaying effective collaboration among various levels of government and community-based organizations in providing services to people with AIDS. Innovative health education techniques are being employed for groups at risk, government employees, and the general public. Although the incidence of AIDS cases continues to rise despite education efforts, the rate of increase appears to have diminished in some areas. Because of the uncertainty regarding the eventual spread of the disease, some communities are beginning to organize against AIDS despite a low or nonexistent number of confirmed cases.

Of interest to public health professionals, government officials, members of community organizations, social scientists.

b. Articles

133. ARNO, Peter S. "The nonprofit sector's response to the AIDS epidemic: Community-based services in San Francisco." *American Journal of Public Health* 76 (1986): 1325-1330.

Examines the role of nonprofit community-based services in response to the epidemic in San Francisco, which has experienced the second largest caseload in the world.

Descriptive

During fiscal year 1984-85, the three largest community-based groups in San Francisco provided more than 80,000 hours of social support and counseling services, responded to over 30,000 telephone inquiries and letters, and distributed nearly 250,000 pieces of literature. Home-based hospice care was provided to 165 AIDS patients at an average cost per day of $94 per patient. Volunteers donated more than 130,000 hours.

Of interest to community leaders, health professionals, public health officials, social and behavioral scientists, and laymen.

134. CHANEY, Richard W., Ronald N. Bennett, R. James Kellogg, Rue Morrison, John Ognibene, V.J. Shorty. "AIDS: Community concerns, support services and resources." *Journal of the Louisiana State Medical Society* 137, no. 9 (1985): 62-63.

A description of what volunteer and community organizations in New Orleans and Louisiana are doing to assist in the AIDS crisis.

Descriptive

Volunteers from the New Orleans AIDS Task Force offer emotional, human, and financial support to persons with AIDS. Clerical and social service groups provide counseling and care. Legal assistance is available through the Legal Defense Fund. The Louisiana Medicaid program assists with medical expenses.

Of interest to health professionals, social service workers, volunteer organizations, and the lay public.

135. "RESOURCES." *Journal of School Health* 58 (1988): 162-166.

An annotated list of materials devoted to AIDS education.

Resource List

Lists curricula, books, pamphlets, video programs, and other products that could prove useful to educators. Grouped by categories.

Of interest to school health educators.

136. "The WORKPLACE and AIDS: A guide to services and information. *Personnel Journal* 66, no. 10 (October 1987): 65-80.

The first phase of an ongoing information clearinghouse on AIDS in the workplace.

Resource Guide

An annotated directory of organizations, education programs, consultants, books, articles, audiovisual, and other educational materials focusing on AIDS in the workplace. Services and information are listed under seven categories: company policy, directories, employee education, health care workers, insurance coverage, legal issues, and public policy.

Useful to employers, managers, administrators, human resource directors, and persons with AIDS.

137. "The WORKPLACE and AIDS: A guide to services and information, Part II." *Personnel Journal* 67, no. 2 (1988): 101-111.

Part two of an ongoing AIDS in the Workplace Clearinghouse--a directory of organizations, education programs, consultants, and articles focusing on AIDS in the workplace.

Resource Guide

Lists information sources for company policy regarding AIDS, employee education, general education, legal issues, medical coverage, testing, worker protection, and public policy.

Of interest to employers and large organizations and businesses.

138. The WORKPLACE Issues and AIDS; January 1989 Update. *Personnel Journal* 68, no. 1 (1989): 91-112.

A directory of organizations, education programs, consultants, and publications focusing on the impact of AIDS in the workplace.

Resource Directory

Twenty pages of a wide variety of resources regarding AIDS for employers update two previous directories.

Of interest to employers in all sizes and types of businesses and services.

Chapter 2

EPIDEMIOLOGICAL ASPECTS OF HIV INFECTION AND AIDS

1. EPIDEMIOLOGY

a. Books

139. DeVITA, Vincent T., Jr., Samuel Hellman, Steven A. Rosenberg (Eds.). *AIDS: Etiology, Diagnosis, Treatment, and Prevention.* Philadelphia: J.B. Lippincott, 1985.

Deals with the scientific issues that are crucial to the elimination of AIDS.

Book of Readings

Brings together information from experts in the fields of AIDS care and research on the epidemiology of AIDS; recent developments concerning the identification of its viral etiology; immunologic defects and pathologic findings in patients with AIDS and ARC; clinical findings in AIDS patients, including infectious complications and malignant tumors; psychosocial aspects of AIDS; and implications of recent findings for hospital management, patient and equipment isolation, and other treatment related issues.

Useful to health professionals, medical and scientific researchers, and social and behavioral scientists.

140. GUNN, Albert E., Nancy K. Hansel, George O. Zenner, Jr., Greta Harper. *AIDS in Africa.* Washington, DC: Foundation for Africa's Future, 1988.

Addresses the AIDS crisis on the African continent, recognizing that any presentation must include references to facts worldwide.

Monograph

Divided into four broad topics. The opening section is concerned with definition. Emphasis has been placed on the virology of the causative viral agent and clinical manifestations of the opportunistic infections associated with the virus. The succeeding section deals with the origin of AIDS on the African continent, and includes the epidemiology of the disease. The third section addresses the nature of the disease and the segments of the populations at greatest risk.

The characteristics of transmission in Africa are also presented. Finally, the authors present methods to identify and control AIDS.

Of interest to epidemiologists, public health professionals, and international health experts.

141. KOCH-WESER, Dieter, and Hannelore Vanderschmidt (Eds.). *The Heterosexual Transmission of AIDS in Africa.* Cambridge, MA: Abt Books, 1988.

A collection of selected articles demonstrate the differences between HIV infection and AIDS in Africa and in other parts of the world.

Book of Readings

The articles in chapter I describe the general dimensions of the AIDS epidemic, specifically in Africa. Chapter II looks at the historical perspective and estimates of how long the HIV was silently present in various populations. Chapter III deals with heterosexual transmission in African populations and the role of prostitution in that transmission. Chapter IV gives some background of the epidemiological, serological, and virological investigations in various African countries. Relationships to other diseases and conditions possibly acting as co-factors are dealt with in Chapter V. Finally, some of the social and cultural factors in the Sub-Saharan areas of Africa are discussed in Chapter VI.

Of interest to a broad audience of people in the health professions.

142. MENITOVE, Jay E., and Jerry Kolins (Eds.). *AIDS.* Arlington, VA: American Association of Blood Banks, 1986.

Papers presented at the AIDS Technical Workshop held in San Francisco in November 1986 as part of the 39th Annual Meeting of the American Association of Blood Banks.

Book of Readings

Addresses the epidemiology, natural history, and etiology of AIDS, and discusses the clinical aspects of the illness, including a description of the associated immunologic abnormalities and their effect on the patient. Describes a test for identifying HIV infected individuals and discusses predictions for future improvements. Concludes with a discussion of the important issues involved in notification of donors found to be HIV antibody positive.

Intended primarily for clinicians involved in blood banking, but should interest all clinicians.

143. TURNER, Charles F., Heather G. Miller, Lincoln E. Moses (Eds.). *AIDS: Sexual Behavior and Intravenous Drug Use.* Washington, DC: National Academy Press, 1989.

A special national committee was asked to: describe what is known about the spread of HIV and AIDS in the U.S.; identify critical populations and indicate tasks related to them; describe existing research findings in the behavioral and social sciences; describe existing research on interventions and ways to evaluate their effectiveness; and identify new research that should be undertaken.

Committee Report

The Committee on AIDS Research frankly discusses the health, social, and political issues that shape people's attitudes and the nation's policies in the fight against AIDS. Chapters examine the available data about the prevalence of HIV infection; patterns of sexual behavior in America; the relationship between AIDS and IV drug use; methods to persuade people to modify health-related behavior; and social barriers to effective AIDS prevention.

For policymakers, researchers, public health officials, and educators.

b. Articles

144. ABRAMSON, Paul R. "Sexual assessment and the epidemiology of AIDS." *Journal of Sex Research* 25 (1988): 323-346.

Isolates sexual parameters that are crucial to the epidemiology of AIDS.

Discussion/Review

Several representative mathematical models of HIV proliferation are described. From these models, three consistent sexual parameters emerge: sexual orientation, anal intercourse, and selection of sexual partners. Consequently, each parameter is examined for the feasibility of assessment and the reliability of existing data. However, relevant data on sexual parameters are either marginal or nonexistent. Therefore, alternatives are described, and the broader implications of measurement error on epidemiological predictions is developed.

Of interest to epidemiologists and sex researchers.

145. ALLEN, James R. "Epidemiology of the acquired immunodeficiency syndrome (AIDS) in the United States." *Seminars in Oncology* 11 (1984): 4-11.

Summarizes data from the Center for Disease Control surveillance of AIDS from 1981 to 1983.

Descriptive

Presents population characteristics and trends, geographic distribution, complicating diseases, and risk groups, and discusses AIDS as an infectious disease.

Of general interest to health professionals.

146. BERKELMAN, Ruth L., William L. Heyward, Jeanette K.
      Stehr-Green, and James W. Curran. "Epidemiology of human
      immunodeficiency virus infection and acquired immunodefi-
      ciency syndrome." *American Journal of Medicine* 86 (1989):
      761-770.

Provides an overview of the AIDS epidemic up to 1989.

Review

As of December 31, 1988, 82,764 cases of AIDS and more than 46,000
AIDS-related deaths had been reported in the U.S. In 1987, AIDS
accounted for nine percent of the total mortality among men, 25 to 34
years of age. Projections suggest that the impact of HIV infection on
morbidity and mortality in young adults and children will continue to
increase, with an estimated 50,000 cases projected to be diagnosed in
1989. The mean latency period between infection and diagnosis of AIDS
is estimated to be more than 7 years, and 78% to 100% of persons
infected with HIV are predicted to develop AIDS within 15 years of
onset of infection. Worldwide differences in the epidemiology of HIV
and AIDS are primarily due to differences in the proportions of the
modes of transmission and in the time at which HIV infection was
introduced.

Of interest to epidemiologists, infectious disease specialists, and
public health officials.

147. BIGGAR, Robert J. "AIDS and HIV infection: Estimates of the
      magnitude of the problem worldwide in 1985/1986." *Clinical
      Immunology and Immunopathology* 45 (1987): 297-309.

Summarizes observations about the distribution of AIDS and HIV
infection throughout the world.

Review

Data regarding the number of cases of AIDS and HIV infection in many
areas are lacking or incomplete, and even data from the United States,
which has reported the greatest number of cases to the World Health
Organization, are difficult to interpret. Little information is
available outside of the United States, Europe, and Australia. Almost
every country in South America has reported cases of AIDS to the WHO,
but the numbers are small. Countries in Asia have reported few or no
cases, and many countries in Africa have not yet reported any cases
despite the fact that regional studies show AIDS and HIV infecton to
be a major public health problem. Using admittedly questionable data,
the author estimates that between two and three million people
worldwide were infected with HIV in 1985/1986. Although there is no
effective therapy or vaccine, much can and is being done to limit the
global spread of HIV infection and AIDS.

Of interest to epidemiologists and public health professionals.

148. BURKE, Donald S., John F. Brundage, John R. Herbold, William Berner, Lytt I. Gardner, Jeffrey D. Gunzenhauser, James Voskovitch, Robert R. Redfield. "Human immunodeficiency virus infections among civilian applicants for United States military service, October 1985 to March 1986: Demographic factors associated with seropositivity." *New England Journal of Medicine* 317 (1987): 131-136.

Blood samples from 306,061 civilian applicants to military service from the U.S. were tested for antibody to HIV during the six month period between October 1985 and March 1986.

Research

Western blot reactivity determined 460 subjects from this population of teenagers and young adults to be positive for the antibody, showing the mean prevalence of HIV infection to be 1.50 per 1000. According to multivariate analysis the following demographic factors were found to be significant independent predictors of a positive HIV-antibody test: age, black race, male sex, residence in a densely populated county, and residence in a metropolitan area with a high incidence of AIDS. Antibody-positive applicants were from 43 of the 50 states, and counties with high prevalence rates for HIV were located in New York, New Jersey, California, Maryland, Texas, Colorado, and Washington, D.C.

Of interest to epidemiologists and public health officials.

149. CHAMBERLAND, Mary E., and Timothy J. Dondero, Jr. "Heterosexually acquired infection with human immunodeficiency virus (HIV): A view from the III International Conference on AIDS." *Annals of Internal Medicine* 107 (1987): 763-766.

An overview of the Third International Conference on AIDS.

Overview and Summary

Concern about widespread heterosexual transmission of HIV persists. Epidemiologic data suggest that the risk for acquiring HIV through heterosexual contact is far from uniform and differs widely by geographic region, race or ethnicity, sex, and age. Heterosexual men and women who abuse intravenous drugs are currently the primary source of heterosexual transmission. As of September 14, 1987, 41,250 cases of AIDS in adults had been reported to the Center for Disease Control; 74% in homosexual and bisexual men and 26% in heterosexual persons, most of whom were intravenous drug abusers. The risk for HIV infection for heterosexuals will continue to be greatest for those who abuse intravenous drugs and for their steady sex partners. Urban populations with consistently high rates of intravenous drug abuse, sexually transmitted diseases, and teenage pregnancies can be expected to become epicenters for heterosexual transmission of HIV as well.

Of interest to health professionals and laymen.

150.   CURRAN, James W., Harold W. Jaffe, Ann M. Hardy, W. Meade
       Morgan,   Richard   M.   Selik,   Timothy   J.   Dondero.
       "Epidemiology of HIV infection and AIDS in the United
       States." *Science* 239 (1988): 610-616.

An overview of HIV infection and AIDS in the U.S.

Discussion

Morbidity and mortality will continue to increase in the next few
years and remain particularly high in young and middle-aged men and in
black and Hispanic minorities where large numbers of IV drug abusers
are already infected with HIV.   More information is needed on the
incidence and prevalence of HIV infection, particularly at the local
level where prevention efforts must be targeted, implemented, and
evaluated.   The problem of HIV transmission through blood and blood
products in the U.S. is largely solved.   The major modes of transmission are known.   Progress in prevention efforts and control of HIV
infection will require a long-term commitment of both science and
society.

Of interest to laymen and health professionals.

151.   CURRAN, James W., W. Meade Morgan, Ann M. Hardy, Harold
       W. Jaffe, William W. Darrow, Walter R. Dowdle.   "The
       epidemiology of AIDS: Current status and future prospects."
       Science 229 (1985): 1352-1357.

The current status, in the U.S., of infection with HTLV-III/LAV and
projections for the future are discussed.

Review

AIDS has continued to increase throughout the world.   The cumulative
number of cases diagnosed and reported in the United States between
1981 and 1985 is expected to double in the following year; over 12,000
cases are projected by July 1986.   Single men in Manhattan and San
Francisco, IV drug users in New York City and New Jersey, and persons
with hemophilia A had an annual incidence rate of 261 to 350 per
100,000 population during 1984.   In 1984, AIDS was the leading cause
of premature mortality for single men, aged 25-44, in Manhattan and
San Francisco.   Infection with HTLV-III is considerably more common
than AIDS in high risk populations.   The screening of donated blood
and plasma and the use of safer clotting factor should reduce
transmission through blood and blood products.   Most infections occur
through sexual transmission, use of contaminated needles, and
transmission to newborns from their infected mothers.   Continued
research is needed to develop a vaccine and therapy, and widespread
community efforts are needed to minimize transmission.

Of particular interest to public health officials.

152. De GRUTTOLA, Victor, and Kenneth H. Mayer. "Assessing and modeling heterosexual spread of the human immunodeficiency virus in the United States." *Reviews of Infectious Diseases* 10 (1988): 138-150.

Presents and evaluates a model for the spread of HIV infection in heterogeneous populations, with an emphasis on the spread of infection from high to low risk populations.

Theoretical

No precise predictions concerning the AIDS epidemic among heterosexuals are possible now, but current epidemiologic findings neither predict nor preclude a major heterosexual epidemic. Projections depend strongly on the delay between infection and infectivity. The model can be used to demonstrate how interpretation of results of case-control studies of HIV infection depends on underlying assumptions about the dynamics of the epidemic.

Of interest to epidemiologists, infectious disease specialists, and public health officials.

153. DENNING, Peter J. "Computer models of AIDS epidemiology." *American Scientist* 75 (1987): 347-352.

Mathematical models of HIV disease are explained, and the use of computers to evaluate them is discussed.

Theoretical

Mathematical models of HIV disease will probably be accurate enough to produce realistic estimates of the spread of AIDS, the effects on the economy, and the transmission factors that can be efficaciously controlled as soon as parameter values are known. Early studies will concentrate on discovering parameter sensitivities. Even though they are not yet accurate enough for forecasting, the models are already producing insights into the epidemiology of HIV infection, helping to focus the inquiry of the research team, and influencing data collection. New tools, based on computer technology, that are being produced by researchers will be useful in analyzing other epidemics and may shorten the time needed to control them.

Useful to epidemiologists and other scientists engaged in research on AIDS.

154. DUTT, Ashok K., Charles B. Monroe, Hiran M. Dutta, Barbara Prince. "Geographical patterns of AIDS in the United States." *Geographical Review* 77 (1987): 456-474.

Data on incidence of AIDS between 1981 and 1986 from the U.S. Centers for Disease Control are analyzed geographically.

Research

Nationwide and regional patterns by source groups, gender, race, age cohorts, and survival rates in the U.S. are emphasized. Some elements, like association of AIDS incidence by source, display distinct regional variations, while others, like incidence by age cohort, have uniform patterns.

Of interest to public health officials, epidemiologists, and health educators.

155. EPSTEIN, Paul, and Randall Packard. "Ecology and immunology: The social context of AIDS in Africa." *Science for the People* 19 (1987): 10-17.

Details several facets of ecology that are necessary to a better understanding of the etiology and epidemiology of the AIDS pandemic.

Review

Focuses on Africa, giving examples of the importance of other illnesses, nutritional status, migration patterns, and cultural practices that may help explain the global distribution of AIDS. Specific recommendations for controlling the pandemic are listed.

Of interest to a general audience.

156. GARDNER, Lytt I., Jr., John F. Brundage, Donald S. Burke, John G. McNeil, Robert Visintine, Richard N. Miller. "Spatial diffusion of the human immunodeficiency virus infection epidemic in the United States, 1985-87." *Annals of the Association of American Geographers* 79 (1989): 25-43.

A geographical analysis of the first 22 months of the Department of Defense's HIV screening program for military applicants.

Research

The cartographic analysis highlights the diffusion of the HIV epidemic from areas with relatively high prevalence to areas with relatively low prevalence of antibody to HIV. While there are particularities specific to each region, the diffusion patterns are remarkably consistent; areas closer to an endemic experience a slight decline over time, while more distant areas show an increase. The data presented from California, Florida, and Texas strongly support the conclusion that diffusion of the HIV epidemic into low prevalence counties is occurring throughout the U.S. The diffusion pattern for the eastern seaboard counties is more complex, with numerous high prevalence foci and limited evidence of simple expansion diffusion.

Of interest to geographers, epidemiologists, and public health officials.

157. GAZZARD, B. "AIDS." *Balliere's Clinical Gastroenterology* 1 (1987): 567-587.

A discussion of the etiology, transmission, and high risk groups, diseases caused by HIV, and immunological abnormalities of AIDS.

Review

A review and discussion of various aspects of AIDS, from the perspective and experience in Great Britain.

Of general interest to health professionals and specifically immunologists.

158. GERSTOFT, Jan. "AIDS in Denmark 1980-1984." *Danish Medical Bulletin* 34 (1987): 217-234.

The identification and epidemiological, clinical, and immunological characterization of Danish patients with AIDS.

Research

A comprehensive discussion of the epidemiology, clinical manifestations, immunology, natural history of the AIDS virus, and risk group studies in Denmark.

Of interest to epidemiologists and international health experts.

159. GOULD, Peter. "Geographic dimensions of the AIDS epidemic." *Professional Geographer* 4 (1989): 71-78.

A summary of the major trends and implications of AIDS on a global basis.

Commentary

Modeling efforts at the national and regional scales in this country have much to offer the international community. Global models have already shown their worth in predicting transmittable diseases. More geographically specific data may be released at the Center for Disease Control. Some states are willing to supply diagnosed cases at county and zipcode scales. There are gaps. Some states refuse to release data. Regional models may provide valuable expertise until national data sets become available.

Of interest to epidemiologists and public health officials.

160. HARDY, Ann M., E. Thomas Starcher II, W. Meade Morgan, Julie Druker, Alan Kristal, Jeanne M. Day, Chet Kelly, Earl Ewing, James W. Curran. "Review of death certificates to assess completeness of AIDS case reporting." *Public Health Reports* 102 (1987): 386-391.

An investigation of the completeness of reporting of AIDS cases.

Research

The comparison of death certificates with AIDS surveillance registries in Washington, DC, New York City, Boston, and Chicago during a three month period in 1985 revealed a high percentage (83 to 100%) of AIDS case reporting in all four cities. A review of death certificates provides an easy and rapid means of evaluating surveillance efforts and a useful adjunct to other methods of surveillance for AIDS.

Of particular interest to epidemiologists.

161. HAVERKOS, Harry, and Robert Edelman. "The epidemiology of acquired immunodeficiency syndrome among heterosexuals." *Journal of the American Medical Association* 260 (1988): 1922-1929.

Provides information for health care professionals about the extent to which HIV and AIDS are spreading to the heterosexual population in the U.S.

Discussion

Several recommendations are offered. Persons with negative HIV antibody tests should be counseled to reduce their risk of becoming infected. Infected persons should be counseled to prevent the further transmission of HIV. If a potential sexual partner is known to be at risk for HIV infection, it is prudent to assume that that sexual partner could be infectious. If both sexual partners are known to be infected with HIV, both should take precautions with each other as if only one were infected.

Of interest to health professionals, public health officials, and epidemiologists.

162. HOOPER, Ed. "AIDS in Uganda." *African Affairs* 86 (1987): 469-477.

Discusses the epidemiology and etiology of AIDS in Uganda.

Descriptive

AIDS is rampant in Uganda, where the principal mode of transmission appears to be heterosexual activity, followed by blood transfusions, and transmission by HIV seropositive mothers to their unborn or nursing babies. In one community, 76% of the prostitutes tested were seropositive. Most of the people seem to lean towards fatalism or religiosity in their attitudes, and local communities appear to be accepting and supportive of the ill. Misinformation is common, and the use of condoms, two million of which, in various colors, were donated by the United States Agency for International Development (USAID), has been met with local resistance. There is some evidence of behavior change, particularly among the educated elite, but in the smaller towns and rural communities, 'slim disease,' as AIDS is called by Ugandans, remains a mystery and the people behave as they always have, unaware that there are HIV carriers in their midst.

Of general interest.

163. HORSBURGH, C. Robert, Jr., and Scott D. Holmberg. "The global distribution of human immunodeficiency virus type 2 (HIV-2) infection." *Transfusion* 28 (1988): 192-195.

Published reports of infection with HIV-2 were reviewed to provide a picture of its geographic distribution, pathogenicity, modes of transmission, and risk to the blood supply.

Literature Review

Since the first reports of HIV-2 in 1986, 627 HIV-2-seropositive persons have been reported, 604 of whom are natives of West Africa. AIDS developed in 42 patients, while 8 had ARC. The usual reported mode of transmission was through sexual intercourse. Although HIV-1 and HIV-2 are thought to have the same modes of transmission, neither perinatal transmission of HIV-2 nor transmission by sharing of needles among IV drug abusers has, as yet, been reported. The virus has not been identified in blood donors in the U.S. or West Germany, but two HIV-2-infected blood donors were reported in France. Further epidemiologic studies are needed to define the spectrum of HIV-2 disease, its modes of transmission, and risk to the blood supply.

Of particular interest to epidemiologists, virologists, and public health officials.

164. HUNT, Charles W. "Africa and AIDS: Dependent development, sexism, and racism." *Monthly Review* 39, no. 9 (1988): 10-22.

Examines the demographic and clinical differences that are evident when AIDS in Africa is compared with AIDS in the U.S., and discusses the possible reasons for infection with the identical virus to manifest itself in such different ways.

Theoretical

AIDS in Africa is epidemiologically and clinically quite distinct from AIDS in Europe or North America. The author suggests that the answer to its differences lies in the social/historical environment in which the HIV acts. Since an epidemic is a social as well as a biological event, it must be addressed socially for its damage to be controlled and its spread halted. While the relationship of dependency continues in Africa, the simple introduction of Western medicine, which ignores social causation, will not attack the root cause of the epidemic. To address social causation and social cure, it is necessary to use an approach that stresses the social structures which shape the epidemic and give it direction.

Of particular interest to social scientists.

165. ITALIAN Multicentre Study. "Epidemiology, clinical features, and prognostic factors of pediatric HIV infection." *Lancet 2*, no. 8619 (1988): 1043-1046.

Examines the similarities and dissimilarities in HIV epidemiology and clinical disease in two groups of children: those infected perinatally and those infected later in childhood.

Research

In a study of 486 children born to HIV-positive mothers and 58 children infected later in childhood, it was found that children with perinatal infection had a more varied clinical history and a poorer prognosis than those whose infection was acquired later. HIV infection occurred in 33% of the infants born to seropositive mothers, with girls having a higher rate of infection than boys. Early onset of symptoms correlated with the poorest prognoses, and secondary infections, neurological disorders, and hepatitis were linked to a high mortality rate in perinatally infected children.

Of interest to pediatricians and epidemiologists.

166. KLOVDAHL, Alden S. "Social networks and the spread of infectious diseases: The AIDS example." *Social Science and Medicine* 11 (1985): 1203-1216.

Data related to AIDS were used to illustrate a network approach to evaluating the infectious agent hypothesis when studying a disease or disease outbreak of unknown etiology and to developing strategies to limit the spread of an infectious agent transmitted through personal relationships.

Research

Illustrates one use of network data and network analysis in epidemiology. Demonstrates how a network perspective could help to stimulate insights about some infectious diseases and assist in designing rational control strategies.

Of interest to social and behavioral scientists, public health professionals, and specialists in infectious diseases.

167. McCORMICK, Anna. "Trends in mortality statistics in England and Wales with particular reference to AIDS from 1984 to April 1987." *British Medical Journal* 1296 (1988): 1289-1292.

Estimates trends in mortality related to HIV and investigates the proportion of such deaths attributed to AIDS or HIV infection on death certificates or supplementary information.

Research

The precise monitoring of trends in mortality from AIDS and possible identification of unrecognized conditions associated with HIV infection, as a basis for predicting future deaths from the syndrome, requires accurate notification of the underlying cause of death and associated diseases. However, when mortality statistics with reference to AIDS in England and Wales were completed from death certificates, increases in deaths from selected causes likely to be associated with AIDS or HIV infection suggested that AIDS was not stated on the death certificates of some patients with HIV infection or subsequently notified by the doctors who signed the certificates. It was estimated, from calculations of excess deaths between the beginning of 1985 and the end of April 1987, that at least 495 deaths possibly associated with HIV infection occurred among men, aged 15–54, during that period. AIDS or HIV infection was stated on the original or amended death entry as the cause of death in 261.

Of particular interest to epidemiologists.

168. ———, Hilary Tillett, Barbara Bannister, John Emslie. "Surveillance of AIDS in the United Kingdom." *British Medical Journal* 295 (1987): 1466-1469.

The surveillance of cases of AIDS in the United Kingdom is described, and a preliminary analysis is made of 1,012 cases reported to the end of August 1987.

Research

Homosexuals constituted the largest risk group. The rate of increase of new cases shows no sign of slowing down. One third of the patients with AIDS lived in a different regional health authority from that in which their disease had been diagnosed. The geographical distribution varied with the risk group. The commonest presenting feature at diagnosis was *Pneumocystis carinii* pneumonia. Kaposi's sarcoma was considerably more common among homosexuals than among people in other groups at risk.

Of interest to health professionals in general.

169. McEVOY, Marian. "The epidemiology of the acquired immune deficiency syndrome (A.I.D.S.)." *Journal of the Royal Society of Health* 3 (1985): 88-91.

Describes the epidemiology of AIDS in terms of time, place, and personal characteristics of those affected.

Descriptive

Epidemiologists are attempting to define, precisely, the combination of risk factors that determines whether a person who becomes infected with HIV will develop opportunistic diseases. Much work remains to be done in this field, and it is extremely important that data continue to be collected and analyzed on a national basis in order that correct information may be provided for all concerned.

Of interest to epidemiologists, public health officials, and other health professionals.

170. MANN, Jonathan M. (Ed.).   "AIDS--a global perspective."
      Western Journal of Medicine 147 (1987): 691-745.

This review considers the methods and limitations of AIDS case reporting and HIV serologic studies, summarizes modes of HIV transmission, defines three geographic patterns of spread, and then examines, by continent, the epidemiology of HIV infection.

Special Journal Issue

A total of 62,811 cases of AIDS have been reported to the World Health Organization from throughout the world. Extensive epidemiologic studies have shown that HIV infections are transmitted by three routes: sexual, parenteral, and perinatal. Three geographic patterns of transmission have been defined. In pattern I, transmission occurs predominantly among homosexual and bisexual men and urban intravenous drug abusers; in pattern II, transmission is predominantly heterosexual and perinatal; in pattern III, AIDS cases are just being documented and are generally due to sexual exposure abroad or to imported blood products.

Of interest to health professionals, public health officials, and laymen.

171. MAY, Robert M., and Roy M. Anderson.   "Transmission
      dynamics of HIV infection."   *Nature* 326 (1987): 137-142.

A mathematical model of the transmission dynamics of HIV helps to clarify some of the essential relations between epidemiological factors, such as distributed incubation periods and heterogeneity in sexual activity, and the overall pattern of the AIDS epidemic.

Theoretical

The ideas presented here are based on relatively simple mathematical models with the aim of making clear some of the essential relations between epidemiological parameters and the overall course of HIV infection within various populations. Such models help to clarify what kinds of epidemiological data are needed to make predictions.

Of interest to epidemiologists and public health officials.

172. MORGAN, W. Meade, and James W. Curran.   "Acquired
      immunodeficiency syndrome: Current and future trends."
      Public Health Reports 101 (1986): 459-465.

Provides a detailed description of the demographic projections that serve as the basis for the "Public Health Service Plan" for the prevention and control of AIDS and the AIDS virus.

Research and Analysis

Epidemiologic models for projecting the future incidence of AIDS will require additional information on the incidence, prevalence, and natural history of HIV infection and on the effectiveness of efforts to prevent virus transmission. Our current understanding of the severity of AIDS and projections for the future underscore the need for continued commitment to research for a vaccine and therapy. Primary prevention and education activities must be widely implemented throughout the U.S. to curtail the future spread of infection and future AIDS cases.

Of interest to health professionals and the general public.

173. MOSS, Andrew R., Peter Bacchetti, Dennis Osmond, Walter Krampf, Richard E. Chaisson, Daniel Stites, Judith Wilber, Jean-Pierre Allain, James Carlson. "Seropositivity for HIV and the development of AIDS or AIDS related condition: Three year follow up of the San Francisco General Hospital cohort. *British Medical Journal* 296 (1988): 745-750.

Reports on progression to AIDS in a cohort of HIV positive homosexual men in San Francisco.

Research

The three year actuarial progression rate to AIDS in a cohort of seropositive men was 22%. An additional 19% developed ARC. Of the men who were abnormal by two or more predictive variables at the start of the study (24%), two thirds (57%) progressed to AIDS, while only 7% of those who tested normal by all predictors (40%) progressed to AIDS. The authors conclude from the observed rates and distribution of predictive variables that half of the men who were seropositive for HIV will develop AIDS by six years after the start of the study, and three quarters will develop AIDS or an AIDS related condition.

Of interest to epidemiologists, virologists, and public health officials.

174. NORMAN, Colin. "Africa and the origin of AIDS." *Science* 230 (1985): 1141.

A commentary on the origin of the AIDS virus.

Commentary

Researchers have long believed that the retrovirus that has been implicated as the primary cause of AIDS originated in Africa. This suggestion rests in part on the fact that antibodies to the virus have been detected in frozen serum samples collected in Africa many years ago, and the disease appears to have spread more widely in some parts of the continent than it has in the West.

Of interest to scientists and the general public.

175. ———. "Politics and science clash on African AIDS." *Science*
230 (1985): 1140-1142.

A commentary on the fact that not a single case of AIDS has been
reported from Central Africa.

Commentary

Political sensitivity is hampering efforts to understand the spread of
AIDS in Africa. In spite of the lack of official reporting of AIDS in
Africa, it is clear that the disease is appearing in many countries.
The extent to which the virus is spreading is a topic of intense
debate. Although the epidemiological evidence is hazy, spread of the
virus is through heterosexual contact.

Of interest to the general public.

176. NOVICK, Lloyd F., Donald Berns, Rachel Stricof, Roy Stevens,
Kenneth Pass, Judith Wethers. "HIV seroprevalence in
newborns in New York State." *Journal of the American
Medical Association* 261 (1989): 1745-1750.

Reports on HIV seroprevalence in infants born in New York State
between November 30, 1987 and November 30, 1988.

Research

Of 276,609 infants born in New York State, 1816 tested positive for
HIV, a seroprevalence rate of 0.66. The rate in Upstate New York was
0.16% and in New York City, 1.25%. Seropositivity was significantly
higher in infants born to mothers aged 20 to 39 than in those born to
mothers under 20; higher in black and Hispanic newborns than in white
newborns; and three times higher in zip code areas with higher rates
of drug use than in other New York City areas. It is estimated that
40% (726) of the HIV-infected newborns were true seropositives.

Of interest to obstetricians, pediatricians, hospital personnel,
epidemiologists, and public health officials.

177. NZILAMBI, Nzila, Kevin M. De Cock, Donald N. Forthal, et al.
"The prevalence of infection with human immunodeficiency
virus over a 10-year period in rural Zaire." *New England
Journal of Medicine* 318 (1988): 276-279.

The current seroprevalence in different groups and risk factors in
patients hospitalized with HIV-related diseases in rural Zaire was
studied, and a 10 year follow-up of a selected cohort living in this
region was carried out to assess the rate of seroconversion to HIV.

Research

The authors believe that the long-term stability of HIV infection in
residents of rural Zaire suggests that social change may have promoted
the spread of AIDS in Africa.

Of interest to epidemiologists and public health officials.

178. PARKER, Richard. "Acquired immunodeficiency syndrome in
      urban Brazil." *Medical Anthropology Quarterly* 1 (1987):
      155-175.

Discusses the Brazilian sexual culture and its relevance for understanding the transmission of AIDS in Brazil.

Descriptive

Sexuality in Brazil traditionally has been defined by sexual roles,
not by sexual identities. The penetrator's role symbolizes domination
and that of the penetrated, submission, and the dominant partner is
considered heterosexual and culturally normative, regardless of the
gender of his partner; the submissive male, called a viado or bicha,
is stigmatized. Only in Brazil's larger cities is the North American
subculture of gay identity and community emerging. Anal intercourse
is widespread in Brazil between both homosexual and heterosexual
partners; adolescents often practice it to avoid pregnancy and rupture
of the hymen, which is still regarded an important sign of sexual
purity. Men frequently visit prostitutes to participate in a range of
sexual acts shunned by "proper" women. The author concludes that
prejudice, short-sighted planning, and economic instability have left
the Brazilian society unprepared to confront the AIDS epidemic. AIDS
education and treatment must be considered within the sociocultural
context of Brazil.

Of interest to epidemiologists, anthropologists, public health
professionals, and health educators.

179. PINCHING, A.J., R.A. Weiss, D. Miller (Eds.). "AIDS and
      HIV infection--the wider perspective." *British Medical
      Bulletin* 44, no. 1 (1988): 1-234.

Examines the emerging pandemic of AIDS and HIV infection from a broad
perspective, in particular, its epidemiological and clinical features
and its wider impact, highlighting important contrasts between these
in developed and developing countries.

Special Journal Issue

Topics in this compilation of 14 articles include clinical aspects of
AIDS and HIV infection, the impact of AIDS in the developed world and
in the developing world, health care planning and special policy
issues, epidemiological and sociological issues, HIV and social
psychiatry, HIV testing, and the virology of HIV.

Of interest to all health professionals.

180. QUINN, Thomas C., Jonathan M. Mann, James W. Curran, Peter
      Piot. "AIDS in Africa: An epidemiologic paradigm." *Science*
      234 (1986): 955-963.

An overview of the epidemiological aspects of AIDS in Africa.

Review

Initial surveillance studies in Central Africa suggest an annual incidence of AIDS of 550 to 1000 cases per million adults, and the present annual incidence of HIV infection in Central and East Africa is approximately 0.75% among the general population. From one to 18% of healthy blood donors and pregnant women, and as many as 27 to 88% of female prostitutes, have antibodies to HIV. The male to female ratio of AIDS cases is one to one, with greater incidence in females less than 30 years of age and in males over 40. Transmission is predominantly by heterosexual activity, parenteral exposure through blood transfusions and unsterilized needles, and perinatally from infected mothers to their newborns, and rapid spread of the infection is likely to continue where economic and cultural factors favor these modes of transmission. The immediate public health priority for all African countries should be the prevention and control of HIV infection through educational programs and blood bank screening.

Of interest to epidemiologists, public health officials, and laymen.

181. RADEMAKER, M., R.H. Meyrick Thomas, G. Provost, M. McEvoy, P.C. Grint, R. Heath, J.D.T. Kirby. "Acquired immune deficiency syndrome without the recognized risk factors." *Postgraduate Medical Journal* 63 (1987): 877-879.

Reports on two cases of AIDS in which the usual exposure factors were not apparent.

Case Report

A 45 year old housewife was found to be HIV antibody positive and diagnosed as having AIDS after suffering from a series of infections, which included *Pneumocystis carinii* pneumonia. She had none of the usual risk factors, but recalled having provided home-nursing care several years earlier for a family friend, a 33 year old Ghanian man who subsequently died of an undiagnosed encephalitis. At the time, she had several small cuts as well as irritant dermatitis on her hands, which were exposed to the patient's body fluids. About eight weeks later she developed "glandular fever." A review of the man's post-mortem histology allowed a retrospective diagnosis of cerebral toxoplasmosis to be made, and analysis of stored serum and cerebrospinal fluid samples showed them both to contain HIV antibodies. He also had no apparent risk factors and had not returned to Africa for the ten years prior to his death. Investigation disclosed that he had worked in the entertainment industry several years before his death, at which time he may have had contact with drug users.

Of interest to physicians, health care workers, and epidemiologists.

182. REEVES, William C., Marina Cuevas, Juan Ramon Arosemena, et al. "Human immunodeficiency virus infection in the Republic of Panama." *American Journal of Tropical Medicine and Hygiene* 39 (1988): 398-405.

Reports on studies to identify risk factors for HIV infection in homosexuals and to estimate seroprevalence in high risk populations.

Research

Thirty-one documented cases of AIDS occurred in Panama during 1984-1987. Twenty-three (74%) patients were homosexual males. All but two patients recognized prior to June 1987 have died. To identify HIV risk factors, 287 male homosexual residents of Panama City were enrolled in a cross-sectional study. Nine were seropositive. Travel to the U.S., homosexual relations with U.S. nationals in Panama, and sexual contacts in Panamanian clubs were associated with HIV infection. Number of male sex partners per year was not. No seropositivity was found among 183 Panama City prostitutes or 55 rural homosexual males. Two of 182 sickle cell anemia patients, 15 of 7,720 blood donors, and 84% of Panamanian hemophiliacs were found to be seropositive.

Of interest to epidemiologists and public health officials.

183. ROTHENBERG, Richard, Mary Woelfel, Rand Stoneburner, John Milberg, Robert Parker, Benedict Truman. "Survival with the acquired immunodeficiency syndrome: Experience with 5833 cases in New York City." *New England Journal of Medicine* 317 (1987): 1297-1302.

Reports an analysis of the pattern of survival among 5833 persons in New York City who were diagnosed with AIDS before January 1986, assessing the relative influence of sex, race or ethnic background, age, risk group, and manifestations of illness on survival.

Research

White homosexual men, 30 to 34 years old, who presented with Kaposi's sarcoma only, had the most favorable survival rate, while black women who contracted the disease through intravenous drug abuse had a particularly poor prognosis. The manifestations of disease at diagnosis had the most influence on survival, followed by age, race or ethnicity, risk group, and sex in that order. Four and one-half percent of the risk was attributed to interaction between variables. A significant improvement in the one-year cumulative probability of survival was found among subjects with *Pneumocystis carinii* pneumonia, but not among subjects without.

Of interest to physicians, public health professionals, and medical researchers.

184. RUBINSTEIN, Arye, and Larry Bernstein. "The epidemiology of pediatric acquired immunodeficiency syndrome." *Clinical Immunology and Immunopathology* 40 (1986): 115-121.

Analyzes the rates and routes of transmission of AIDS to children.

Research/Analysis

In most cases of pediatric AIDS, the disease is transmitted in utero; 35-65% of HTLV-III-positive women give birth to an infected child. In fewer cases, the disease is acquired through blood transfusions, and in exceptional cases, transmission may occur in young children by way of sexual abuse or use of needles. There is no evidence of intra-familial horizontal transmission from child to child. The number of cases of pediatric AIDS, which constitute approximately one percent of the total cases at the time of this report, is expected to increase as the disease spreads to more women of child-bearing age.

Of interest to epidemiologists, public health officials, and pediatricians.

185. SELIK, Richard M., Kenneth G. Castro, Marguerite Pappaioanou. "Racial/ethnic differences in the risk of AIDS in the United States." *American Journal of Public Health* 78 (1988): 1539-1545.

Presents the results of a study to determine more precisely the magnitude of the association between AIDS and racial/ethnic groups for different means of acquiring HIV infection and the variation in this association by geographic area and over time.

Research

Relative risks in blacks and Hispanics were highest in the northeast region, and higher in suburbs than in central cities or metropolitan areas. Relative risks in blacks and Hispanics were greatest for AIDS directly or indirectly associated with intravenous drug abuse by heterosexuals and were also high for AIDS associated with male bisexuality, suggesting that these behaviors may be more prevalent in blacks and Hispanics than in whites. Prevention strategies should take into account these racial/ethnic differences.

Of interest to health professionals, epidemiologists, and policymakers.

186. SHANNON, Gary W., and Gerald F. Pyle. "The origin and diffusion of AIDS: A view from medical geography." *Annals of the Association of American Geographers* 79 (1989): 1-24.

An overview of AIDS from a medical geographical point of view.

Descriptive

Using available hypotheses, theories, and data, the authors explore questions pertaining to the origin, etiology, and spatial diffusion of the disease. The specific geography of HIV-1 origin and diffusion remains incomplete, involving the interaction of a plethora of factors and forces of particular geographic interest. Mapping the spread of AIDS is a useful geographical exercise, but an entire complex of factors and relationships must be recognized as contributing to the problem. The social-ecological disease model, stressing the impor-tance of personal behavioral factors is essential to understanding the disease experience. As such, personal behavior represents an important factor mediating the ecological relationships expressed between the host, disease agent, and environment.

Of interest to epidemiologists, public health officials, and physicians.

187. SONNET, Jean, Jean-Louis Michaux, Francis Zich, Jean-Marie Brucher, Marc De Bruyere, Guy Burtonboy. "Early AIDS cases originating from Zaire and Burundi (1962-1976). *Scandinavian Journal of Infectious Diseases.* 19 (1987): 511-518.

Reports and discusses several cases of AIDS and HIV infection contracted in Central Africa prior to the present outbreak.

Case Histories

Although the current outbreak of AIDS occurred almost simultaneously in the United States, Western Europe, and Central Africa in the early 1980's, earlier case reports with a retrospective diagnosis of AIDS have suggested that AIDS had already occurred in Zaire prior to its emergence elsewhere. The case histories of three additional fatal cases that were retrospectively diagnosed are discussed together with those of four HIV seropositive patients who contracted the virus during the seventies or earlier in Central Africa without any risk factor other than heterosexual exposure. These data and simultaneous information from other sources contribute to the assumption that AIDS is an old disease in Central Africa that presented itself as a sporadic, ill-defined entity and remained unrecognized until the present outbreak.

Of interest to medical and scientific researchers, particularly epidemiologists and virologists.

188. STEHR-GREEN, Jeanette K., Janine M. Jason, Bruce L. Evatt, and the Hemophilia-Associated AIDS Multicenter Study Group. "Potential effect of revising the CDC surveillance case definition for AIDS." *Lancet* 1, no. 8584 (1988): 520-521.

Reports a study to determine the impact of the Centers for Disease Control's August 1987 revision of the surveillance case definition for AIDS.

Research

Information was extracted from the medical charts of 630 patients receiving comprehensive medical care at six hemophilia treatment centers as of 1980 who were, therefore, likely to have been infected with HIV. Thirty-eight (6%) met the 1985 case definition and 47 (7%) the 1987 case definition, an increase of 22%. These data suggest the revision of the AIDS case definition will have a substantial impact on AIDS surveillance trends in persons with hemophilia and, possibly, in other risk groups.

Of particular interest to epidemiologists.

189. TENNISON, B.R., and S. Hagard. "AIDS: Predicting cases nationally and locally." *British Medical Journal* 297 (1988): 711-713.

A two stage approach, using trend extrapolation, was chosen to predict the numbers of AIDS cases in the United Kingdom, in East Anglia, and in Cambridge, for the national case reports.

Analytical

The method predicted that about 2,700 cases would be reported nationally during 1990 and about 6,000 during 1992. The number of people with AIDS expected to present for treatment in East Anglia was 48 during 1990 and 105 during 1992; the corresponding figures for Cambridge were 20 and 43.

Of interest to epidemiologists and public health officials.

190. WEISS, Arthur, Harry Hollander, John Stobo. "Acquired immunodeficiency syndrome: Epidemiology, virology, and immunology." *Annual Review of Medicine* 36 (1985): 545-562.

Examines epidemiology, virology, and immunology associated with AIDS.

Review

AIDS is indicated by opportunistic infection or unusual malignancy associated with a marked deficiency of cell mediated immunity in the absense of any other cause of the immune defect. It appears to be caused by infection of at-risk individuals by a retrovirus that has tropism for a specific population of T lymphocytes.

Of interest to epidemiologists, virologists, immunologists, physicians, and public health professionals.

191. WOOD, William B. "AIDS North and South: Diffusion patterns of a global epidemic and a research agenda for geographers." *Professional Geographer* 40 (1988): 266-279.

Contributes three general regionally based models of AIDS diffusion and suggests programs for geographic research towards that goal.

Descriptive

Reviews the disease and its transmission; then, proposes three models of AIDS diffusion to assess the implications of the epidemic on various regions. AIDS North, of North America and Western Europe, is urban based and primarily confined to homosexuals and IV drug users. AIDS South, in Central Africa and the Caribbean, is spreading from cities to rural regions and affects, primarily, heterosexuals. An AIDS North/South hybrid is postulated as a model of diffusion of the disease in other Third World regions. Addresses the potential contribution of geographic research to policymakers in their attempts to cope with the diffusion of AIDS and to curb the epidemic's advance.

Of interest to public health professionals, health educators, and international health specialists.

c. Chapters

192. BRUNET, Jean-Baptiste, Elizabeth Bouvet, Veronica Massari. "Epidemiological aspects of acquired immune deficiency syndrome in France." *In* Irving J. Selikoff, Alvin S. Teirstein, Shalom Z. Hirschman (Eds.). *Acquired Immune Deficiency Syndrome.* New York: New York Academy of Sciences, 1984.

An epidemiological study of AIDS in France.

Research

This epidemiological study of AIDS in France reveals several differences with respect to the situation in the U.S. The first difference concerns cases with cutaneous nonextensive Kaposi's sarcoma. The second difference is, AIDS has not spread to the IV drug abuser group in France. The third, most interesting difference is the existence of AIDS cases in Africans, particularly in Belgium.

Of interest to epidemiologists and virologists.

193. CLUMECK, Nathan, Jean Sonnet, Henri Taelman, Sophie Cran, Philippe Henrivaux, and reported by Jan Desmyter. "Acquired immune deficiency syndrome in Belgium and its relation to Central Africa." *In* Irving J. Selikoff, Alvin S. Teirstein, Shalom Z. Hirschman (Eds.). *Acquired Immune Deficiency Syndrome.* New York: The New York Academy of Sciences, 1984.

Reports the epidemiological data regarding AIDS in Belgium during 1979 to 1983.

Research

The vast majority of AIDS cases diagnosed in Belgium were in African patients who lived in Belgium or traveled to Belgium for medical care.

Of interest to epidemiologists and virologists.

194. FISCHL, Margaret A., and Gordon M. Dickinson. "An acquired immunodeficiency syndrome among Haitians: An update." *In* Irving J. Selikoff, Alvin S. Teirstein, Shalom Z. Hirschman (Eds.). *Acquired Immune Deficiency Syndrome.* New York: New York Academy of Sciences, 1984.

Reports the authors' experience with 60 Haitian patients with the diagnosis of AIDS, seen between 1980 and 1983.

Research

The immunologic abnormalities and clinical manifestations of AIDS in Haitians reported here are similar to those described in other risk groups. The incidence of Kaposi's sarcoma among Haitians with AIDS in Miami was relatively low (10%). One striking difference is the high frequency of tuberculosis in Haitian patients with AIDS. Toxoplasma encephalitis was seen in 25% of the patients. The most common infections associated with death were *Pneumocystis carinii*, disseminated cytomegalovirus, and toxoplasma encephalitis.

Of interest to epidemiologists and virologists.

195.   SPIRA, Thomas J., and Kenneth G. Castro. "The epidemiology of the acquired immunodeficiency syndrome." *In* Eva Klein (Ed.). *Acquired Immunodeficiency Syndrome.* Basel: Karger, 1986.

Reviews the epidemiology of AIDS.

Review

Discusses the nature and cause of AIDS, groups at risk, modes of transmission, distribution, and epidemiological linkages. Concludes that lacking an effective treatment for AIDS, a better understanding of its epidemiology will aid in designing better strategies for its prevention.

Of particular interest to public health professionals.

2. ETIOLOGY AND TRANSMISSION

a. Books

196.   MASTERS, William H., Virginia E. Johnson, Robert C. Kolodny. *Crisis: Heterosexual Behavior in the Age of AIDS.* New York: Grove Press, 1988.

Documents how extensively infection with HIV has spread beyond the original high risk groups, explains the necessity for a personal and public commitment to prevention as a primary issue, and presents information regarding risks of infection.

Text

This controversial book contains some background information plus information on the virus and its transmission, clinical facts regarding AIDS, evidence regarding heterosexual infection, the safety of the nation's blood supply, modes of transmission, aspects of sexual behavior relating to the risk of transmission, the impact of the epidemic on sexual behavior, and AIDS prevention as an issue for society.   Three appendices cover clinical features of the AIDS epidemic, the research questionnaires used by the authors, and a technical reanalysis of the Harvard Study Group's analysis of the predicted effectiveness of a mandatory premarital HIV screening program.

Of general interest.

197. MATSUMARA, Kenneth N.   *Heterosexual AIDS: Myth or Fact?*
      Berkeley, CA: Alin Foundation Press, 1988.

Summarizes current research on heterosexual transmission of AIDS, describes, in detail, the most significant research reports, and analyzes the validity of their conclusions.

Text

Brief sections are presented on: what AIDS is; what causes AIDS; where AIDS came from; newer treatments for AIDS; a review of articles dealing with heterosexual AIDS; comments and recommendations.

Of interest to health professionals and the general public.

198. PETRAKIS, Peter L. (Ed.).   *Acquired Immune Deficiency
      Syndrome and Chemical Dependency.*   Rockville, MD: U.S.
      Department of Health and Human Services, Public Health
      Service, Alcohol, Drug Abuse, and Mental Health
      Administration, National Institute on Alcohol Abuse and
      Alcoholism, DHHS Publication No. (ADM) 87-1513, 1987.

Summarizes a symposium to examine the potential for modulating the AIDS epidemic by understanding how addictive substances contribute to it, sponsored in April 1986 in San Francisco by the American Medical Society on Alcoholism and Other Drug Dependencies, Inc. and the National Council on Alcoholism.

Symposium Report

Focuses on the following subject areas: the nature of AIDS; chemical dependency and AIDS; barriers to the recognition of links between drug and alcohol abuse and AIDS; alcohol and the immune system; parallels between AIDS and alcoholism; counseling gay men about substance abuse and AIDS; a clinical perspective on co-dependency in AIDS; alcohol abuse, suicidal behavior, and AIDS. Concludes that AIDS can be a major stressor in people who are recovering from substance abuse, and AIDS-focused Alcoholics Anonymous groups might help them develop the strength to cope with their ordeal and provide them with some quality of life.

Useful to health professionals, mental health professionals, and social workers involved with substance abuse programs or substance abusers.

199. RAPPOPORT, Jon. *AIDS, Inc.: Scandal of the Century.* San Bruno, CA: Human Energy Press, 1988.

Presents an alternative etiology to viral causation of AIDS.

Theoretical

Basing his arguments primarily on anecdotal reports, the author posits that the HIV virus has not been proven to cause disease and that there is no disease entity called AIDS, nor a contagious epidemic. He contends that the use of legal and illegal drugs is responsible for most symptoms of AIDS and pre-AIDS. Inflated reports of AIDS cases promote widespread marketing of pharmaceutical drugs, costly research, and scientific ambitions. The author recommends that a "Scopes" test case of HIV be tried in the courts to gain media coverage and exposure of errors.

Of interest to virologists, epidemiologists, and public health officials.

200. ROSS, Michael W. *Psychovenereology: Personality and Lifestyle Factors in Sexually Transmitted Diseases in Homosexual Men.* New York: Praeger, 1986.

An investigation of the social, psychological, and political contributors to sexually transmitted diseases in homosexual men.

Monograph

Provides basic data and discussion on the psychological and social concomitants of STDs in homosexual men. Points out the fact that some forms of sexual behavior carry a greater risk of STD transmission than others; in the case of AIDS, the risks are major. When the risks of infection, in terms of morbidity and mortality, outweigh the pleasures of particular behaviors, those behaviors need to be modified. Since some forms of homosexual behavior are less risky than others, a shift to alternative homosexual practices may be appropriate.

Of interest to medical and scientific researchers and public health professionals.

b. Articles

201. "AIDS and sex." *Lancet* 1, no. 8575/6 (1988): 31.

A meeting was held to further a better understanding of the relationship between HIV infection and human sexuality.

Conference Findings

To assess the potential for the spread of AIDS among the heterosexuals of industrialized nations, much more quantitative and qualitative information is needed on human sexual behavior. Clinicians and epidemiologists should realize that conventional labels of human sexual behavior can be very misleading.

Of interest to epidemiologists, physicians, and public health officials.

202. BACKINGER, Cathy. "Personal service workers: A critical link in the AIDS education chain?" *AIDS Education and Prevention* 1, no. 1 (1989): 31-38.

Discusses the potential for HIV transmission by personal service workers (PSW) in acupuncture, ear piercing, tattooing, and cosmetology and their need for AIDS education.

Review

Since hepatitis B has been reported to be transmitted by acupuncture, ear piercing, and tattooing, it is possible that these procedures can also transmit HIV. Infection control mandated by licensing boards and/or law varies according to state and personal service group. The author recommends that all PSW groups follow CDC guidelines for infection control and provide HIV educational programs for their members. Differences in the level of HIV knowledge, attitudes, and behaviors should be considered in planning educational programs.

Of interest to personal service workers, professional organizations, and public policymakers.

203. BOVE, Joseph R. "Transfusion-associated hepatitis and AIDS: What is the risk?" *New England Journal of Medicine* 317 (1987): 242-245.

Discusses the risk associated with transfusions and the benefits of screening donors and testing blood.

Discussion

The risk of transfusion-transmitted infectious disease will always exist, and each transfusion will have to be considered in terms of benefit versus risk. However, current approaches, which include steps to exclude high-risk donors and testing for antibody to HIV, antibody to hepatitis B core antigen, and alanine aminotransferase, have a beneficial effect on the blood supply and are highly effective in minimizing the risk of transfusion-transmitted infection.

Of interest to all health professionals.

204. BOWIE, Cameron, and Nicholas Ford. "Sexual behaviour of young people and the risk of HIV infection." *Journal of Epidemiology and Community Health* 43 (1989): 61-65.

A representative sample of 400 young people, 16 to 21 years of age, were surveyed, using quota sampling, in 40 randomly selected electoral wards in Somerset, England, prior to the mounting of a local education campaign on AIDS.

Research

Ninety-two percent of those surveyed considered themselves to be heterosexual. Nearly half had engaged in sexual intercourse by age 16, with the number increasing to 89% by age 21. Mean frequency of sexual intercourse among the sexually active was 62 per year. The frequency of change in partners decreased with increasing age from 2.1 per year for 16-year-olds to 1.5 for 21-year-olds. This level of sexual activity could eventually give rise to prevalence rates of HIV infection similar to those found in Africa (15-100 HIV antibody positives per 1000).

Of interest to epidemiologists, educators, counselors, and public health officials.

205. BRETTLER, Doreen B., Ann D. Forsberg, Peter H. Levine, Charla A. Andrews, Sharon Baker, John L. Sullivan. "Human immunodeficiency virus isolation studies and antibody testing: Household contacts and sexual partners of persons with hemophilia." *Archives of Internal Medicine* 148 (1988): 1299-1301.

Virus isolation studies and HIV antibody testing were performed on household contacts of HIV antibody-positive hemophiliac patients to determine the extent that HIV could be transmitted through heterosexual or intimate contact.

Research

Results demonstrated the lack of transmission of HIV in intimate but nonsexual settings, and suggested that heterosexual transmission may be relatively uncommon in hemophiliac couples when the male and female partner have no other risk factors.

Of interest to physicians, especially hematologists.

206. CASTRO, Kenneth G., Alan R. Lifson, Carol R. White, Timothy J. Bush, Mary E. Chamberland, Anastasia M. Lekatsas, Harold W. Jaffe. "Investigations of AIDS patients with no previously identified risk factors." *Journal of the American Medical Association* 259 (1988): 1338-1342.

Two thousand and fifty-nine patients with AIDS and no recognized risk factors were reported to the Centers for Disease Control and followed to determine changes in risk status.

Research

This follow-up of AIDS patients with no apparent risk factors suggests that modes of transmission for AIDS have remained stable.

Of interest to all health professionals and public health officials.

207. CLAVEL, Francois, Kamal Mansinho, Sophie Chamaret, Denise
      Guetard, Veronique Favier, Jaime Nina, Marie-Odette
      Santos-Ferreira, Jose-Luis Champalimaud, Luc Montagnier.
      "Human immunodeficiency virus type 2 associated with AIDS in
      West Africa." *New England Journal of Medicine* 316 (1987):
      1180-1185.

Reports evidence of infection with HIV-2 in 30 patients, almost all
from West Africa, 17 of whom presented with a clinical syndrome
indistinguishable from AIDS, while the others had either ARC or no
HIV-related symptoms.

Research

All of these patients were found to be infected with HIV-2, which is
related to, but distinct from HIV-1. Cross-reactivity of serum
antibodies with HIV-1 was found in a minority of patients, but varied
according to the assay used. The findings indicate that some cases of
AIDS in West Africa may be caused by HIV-2. Careful epidemiological
investigation will be required to determine the extent of the spread
of this virus and its clinical correlates.

Of particular interest to epidemiologists and virologists.

208. COOPER, David A., Julian Gold, Warwick May, Lawrence S.
      Kaminsky, Ronald Penny, Jay A. Levy. "Contact tracing in
      the acquired immune deficiency syndrome (AIDS): Evidence
      for transmission of virus and disease by an asymptomatic
      carrier." *Medical Journal of Australia* 141 (1984): 579-582.

The sexual contacts of a patient diagnosed with AIDS in 1983 were
traced, and clinical, immunological, and serological evidence was
obtained and evaluated.

Research

It was determined that the patient had been in contact with a
homosexual man who had no symptoms, but in whom laboratory evidence of
exposure to the AIDS-associated retrovirus was found. The findings
suggest that AIDS can be acquired from a carrier who has no symptoms,
but whose antibodies do not protect against infectivity.

Of interest to epidemiologists, virologists, and medical historians.

209. DARROW, William W., Dean F. Echenberg, Harold W. Jaffe, Paul
      M. O'Malley, Robert H. Byers, Jane P. Getchell, James W.
      Curran. "Risk factors for human immunodeficiency virus
      (HIV) infections in homosexual men." *American Journal of
      Public Health* 77 (1987): 479-483.

A sample of 492 randomly selected homosexual men who had participated
in studies of Hepatitis B in San Francisco in 1978-80 were enrolled in
a follow-up study of AIDS to clarify risk factors for infection with
HIV.

Research

The 240 subjects (67%) who were found to have developed antibodies to HIV were compared to the 119 who remained seronegative. Receptive anal intercourse with ejaculation by non-steady partners, many sexual partners per month, and other indications of high levels of sexual activity were highly associated with HIV seroconversion. No sexual activities involving exposure to the semen, blood, or excretions of infected persons were shown to be safe.

Of interest to physicians and counselors, health educators, and homosexual men.

210. EUROPEAN Collaborative Study. "Mother-to-child transmission of HIV infection." *Lancet* 2, no. 8619 (1988): 1039-1043.

Reports on a study to determine rates of transmission, factors that influence transmission, and the natural history of perinatal HIV infection.

Research

Two hundred and seventy-one infants born to HIV-infected women in eight European centers were studied. HIV-infected infants were defined as those who had antibodies at 15 months. A transmission rate of 24% was determined, but this was considered an underestimate because of the insensitivity of virus and antigen tests to the presence of the virus in infants. Mothers' clinical status at delivery, mode of delivery, and breastfeeding did not appear to influence transmission rates. A dysmorphic syndrome in children with AIDS was not confirmed.

Of interest to pediatricians and epidemiologists.

211. FRIEDLAND, Gerald H., and Robert S. Klein. "Transmission of the human immunodeficiency virus." *New England Journal of Medicine* 317 (1987): 1125-1135.

Reviews current information related to the routes of transmission of HIV infection.

Review

The likely routes of transmission of AIDS and the likelihood of its having an infectious cause were suggested by its appearance in disparate populations connected only by the probable routes of transmission before an etiologic agent was discovered. The discovery, in 1983, of HIV, the recovery of the virus from substantial numbers of patients, and the presence of antibodies to HIV in populations at increased risk of AIDS served to confirm the earlier hypotheses of specific routes of transmission of an infectious agent. Despite the worldwide spread of the disease, the three initially described routes of transmission--inoculation of blood, sexual, and perinatal--still remain the only ones demonstrated to be important.

Of interest to epidemiologists, public health professionals, health educators and counselors, and persons at risk for AIDS.

212. FRIEDLAND, Gerald H., Brian R. Saltzman, Martha F. Rogers, Patricia A. Kahl, Martin L. Lesser, Marguerite M. Mayers, Robert S. Klein. "Lack of transmission of HTLV-III/LAV infection to household contacts of patients with AIDS or AIDS-related complex with oral candidiasis." *New England Journal of Medicine* 314 (1988): 344-349.

Nonsexual household contacts of patients with AIDS or ARC with oral candidiasis were studied to determine the risk of transmission of human T-cell lymphotropic virus type III/lymphadenopathy associated virus (HTLV-III/LAV).

Research

This study indicates that household contacts who are not sexual partners of, or born to, patients with AIDS are at minimal or no risk of infection with HTLV-III/LAV.

Of interest to public health officials and all health professionals.

213. GLASER, Jordan B., Theodore J. Strange, Diane Rosati. "Heterosexual human immunodeficiency virus transmission among the middle class." *Archives of Internal Medicine* 149 (1989): 645-649.

The clinical experience of a private infectious disease practitioner on Staten Island.

Research

Thirty-nine heterosexual contacts of HIV infected individuals were evaluated by a private infectious diseases practice located in a predominantly white middle class borough of New York City. Thirty-five of the 39 patients were white. The mean household income was $41,200. Source cases were predominantly IV drug abusers. Heterosexual HIV spread is occurring among the middle class with the predominant source being IV drug abusers who do not fit the stereotype of being minorities and lower class. Condoms were not regularly utilized in these relationships, even though 23 of 32 contacts became aware of their partner's risk behaviors before the diagnosis of HIV infection and 23 of 32 IV drug abusers had attended a methadone program.

Of interest to health educators and physicians.

214. GREENBERG, Alan E., Phuc Nguyen-Dinh, Jonathan M. Mann, et al. "The association between malaria, blood transfusions, and HIV seropositivity in a pediatric population in Kinshasha, Zaire." *Journal of the American Medical Association* 259 (1988): 545-549.

The relationships between malaria, blood transfusions, and HIV seropositivity were investigated in a pediatric population in Kinshasha, Zaire.

Research

Malaria and AIDS are both major public health problems in tropical Africa, and concerns have been raised about potential mechanisms of interaction between the two diseases. In a cross-sectional survey of 167 hospitalized children in Kinshasha, 112 (67%) had malaria, 78 (47%) had received transfusions during the current hospitalization, and 21 (13%) were seropositive. Ten of the 11 seropositive malaria patients had received transfusions during the current hospitalization, and pretransfusion specimens, available for four of these children, proved to be seronegative. Of all blood transfusions, 87% were administered to malaria patients, and there was a strong dose-response association between transfusions and HIV seropositivity. A review of 1000 emergency ward records showed 69% of transfusions were administered to malaria patients. Treatment of malaria with blood transfusions appears to be an important factor in the exposure of Kinshasha children to HIV infection.

Of interest to epidemiologists and public health officials.

215.   HAUCK, Walter W., George Fein, John M. Neuhaus.   "A comment on the CDC study of nonsexual household transmission of AIDS and on Cameron's correction to that study." *Psychological Reports* 64 (1989): 468.

A comment on the CDC study of nonsexual household transmission of AIDS and on a published correction to that study.

Commentary

The authors challenge Cameron's paper, "Corrected statistical analysis suggests casual transmission of AIDS in the African study of the Centers for Disease Control," which reports a reanalysis of the CDC's statistical analysis on the risks due to household, nonsexual contact with persons with AIDS. Although they agree that the original study was inadequate and improperly analyzed, they argue that Cameron's alternate analysis was also incorrect because he failed to take family size into consideration.

Of interest to epidemiologists, statisticians, and public health officials.

216.   HEBERT, James R., and Jeanine Barone.   "On the possible relationship between AIDS and nutrition." *Medical Hypotheses* 27 (1988): 51-54.

Because of its effect on cellular immunity, nutritional stress is proposed as a plausible determinant of increased risk for AIDS.

Discussion

It is noted that host resistance or susceptibility factors are important in determining the probability of contracting many diseases. Though AIDS has been studied primarily in terms of exposure to disease agents, it is proposed that factors affecting susceptibility or resistance be considered. Specific mechanisms are discussed and a connection between diverse risk groups is proposed.

Of interest to health professionals and nutritionists.

217. JOHNSON, Anne M. "Heterosexual transmission of human immunodeficiency virus." *British Medical Journal* 296 (1988): 1017-1020.

Reviews the epidemiology of heterosexually acquired HIV and discusses the potential for a heterosexual epidemic in the United States and Europe.

Review

Although heterosexual transmission is probably the commonest way that HIV is spread, and parts of Africa already have a heterosexual epidemic, the potential for a major heterosexual epidemic in the U.S. or Europe remains a subject for speculation. Two key factors are likely to determine future heterosexual spread: patterns of sexual and needle sharing behavior, and the probability of transmission of HIV from men to women and from women to men. The future of the heterosexual epidemic in Europe and the United States will depend on rates of partner change in the heterosexual population. Since heterosexuals far outnumber male homosexuals, heterosexually acquired HIV may eventually account for a higher proportion of the population, but a heterosexual epidemic is also likely to develop more slowly.

Of interest to epidemiologists and public health officials.

218. KAPLAN, Edward H. "What are the risks of risky sex? Modeling the AIDS epidemic." *Operations Research* 37 (1989): 198-209.

Uses mathematical models to examine the risks of risky sex among gay men.

Analytical

The use of models allows for the consideration of arbitrary probability distributions for risky sex rates, the duration of sex lives, and the incubation of AIDS following HIV infection. The analysis suggests what must happen for the epidemic to subside (barring a cure) by generalizing known formulas for the reproductive rate of HIV infection. Several scenarios illustrating the time frame necessary for changes in the AIDS case rate and the prevalence of HIV infection to occur are presented. Even under optimistic scenarios, the model predicts that it will take over 15 years to eradicate AIDS in gay communities, where HIV prevalence is currently close to 50%.

Of special interest to public health officials and policymakers.

219. KIECOLT-GLASER,   Janice   K.,   and   Ronald   Glaser.
      "Psychosocial moderators of immune function." *Annals of
      Behavioral Medicine* 9 (1987): 16-20.

Reviews evidence linking major and minor stressful events to changes
in immune function in humans.

Review

Declines in immune function are a very frequent concomitant of the
heightened distress associated with even commonplace stressful events
like academic examinations. Moreover, chronic stress does not appear
to lead to adaptation to the level of well-matched comparison
subjects. These data are consistent with epidemiological studies that
have found greater morbidity and mortality in certain distressed
populations.

Of interest to social and behavioral scientists.

220. LEDERER, Robert.   "Origin and cause of AIDS: Is the West
      responsible?" *Covert Action Information Bulletin* 28 (1987):
      43-54.

The first article in a two-part series poses the question of whether
AIDS is a natural or a human-made disease.

Analytical

In response to questions that have arisen regarding whether AIDS is a
natural development, the author discusses and analyzes four
alternative theories of its origin and spread: HIV derived from
monkeys (the "official" theory); HIV genetically engineered by the
U.S. government in chemical-biological warfare research; dioxin, the
contaminant in Agent Orange; and maguari and dengue, two insect borne
tropical viruses.

Of interest to epidemiologists, virologists, and political theorists.

221. ————.   "Origin and cause of AIDS: Is the West responsible?
      (Conclusion.)" *Covert Action Information Bulletin* 29 (1988):
      52-65.

The second article in a two-part series analyzing theories regarding
the origin and spread of AIDS.

Analytical

Begins with the conclusion of part I of this two-part article, in
which two more alternative theories of the cause of AIDS are reviewed:
African swine fever virus, and multiple factors (no single microbe).
Part II analyzes various proposed co-factors, which spread the
causative microbe or make individuals more vulnerable to developing
AIDS, once exposed. It is argued that clarification of co-factors

among those vulnerable to AIDS and those who already have it could point up holistic therapies to reverse some of the immune damage which triggers and results from AIDS. The author concludes that Western institutions, probably through their "normal" functioning rather than any specific conspiracy, played a major role in the origin and spread of AIDS.

Of interest to epidemiologists, virologists, and political theorists.

222. LEHRMAN, Nathaniel S. "Is AIDS non-infectious? The possibility and its CBW implications." *Covert Action Information Bulletin* 28 (1987): 55-62.

Discusses possible non-viral causes of AIDS.

Theoretical

The author argues that the commonly accepted explanations of the origins of AIDS are wrong, and suggests that AIDS may really be an accidental byproduct or even a deliberate result of chemical-biological warfare research. He concludes that the epidemiological and public health measures to investigate whether AIDS may be a deliberately created disease, and its possible toxic causes, are not being implemented. Unless all of the causes of this disease are understood, it cannot be prevented or treated properly.

Of interest to epidemiologists, public health officials, and political theorists.

223. LIFSON, Alan R. "Do alternate modes for transmission of human immunodeficiency virus exist? A review." *Journal of the American Medical Association* 259 (1988): 1353-1356.

Discusses the ways in which HIV is and is not transmitted.

Review

All individuals need to be aware of how HIV is and is not transmitted so that high risk behaviors may be reduced and unnecessary fears and actions avoided. Transmission of HIV is known to occur perinatally, through sexual contact, and after exposure to infected blood and blood products. The possibility that breast milk may transmit HIV is being evaluated. Because HIV has, in rare cases, been isolated from saliva, tears, and urine, guidelines have been developed to reduce extensive exposure to these fluids; however, no epidemiological evidence of HIV infection resulting from contact with any of these body fluids exists. Data strongly indicate that HIV is not transmitted through gamma globulin preparations, the hepatitis B vaccine, contact with insects, or casual contact.

Of interest to the general public.

224. MOLGAARD, Craig A., Chester Nakamura, Melbourne Hovell, John P. Elder. "Assessing alcoholism as a risk factor for acquired immunodeficiency syndrome (AIDS)." *Social Science and Medicine* 27 (1988): 1147-1152.

Reviews alcohol abuse as a prominent feature of the homosexual experience, and suggests that it may merit consideration as a risk factor in relation to AIDS.

Review

The presumably high prevalence of alcohol abuse among homosexuals and the damaging effects of alcohol on the immune system are discussed as a basis for linking alcoholism, homosexuality, and AIDS. The implications of the potentiating effects of alcohol misuse as HIV infiltrates the heterosexual population are presented in terms of high risk populations and the need for additional preventive measures.

Of interest to health professionals, especially epidemiologists, virologists, and preventive medicine specialists.

225. PADIAN, Nancy S. "Heterosexual transmission of acquired immunodeficiency syndrome: International perspectives and national projections. *Reviews of Infectious Diseases* 9 (1987): 947-960.

Examines epidemiologic data on heterosexual transmission of AIDS obtained from the surveillance program of the Center for Disease Control (CDC), from prostitutes around the world, and from studies conducted in Africa and Haiti.

Review

The efficacy of heterosexual transmission and related risk factors remain unclear. Viral transmission from males to their female sexual partners is well documented, although, in the U.S., instances of female-to-male transmission have been observed less frequently. On the other hand, in parts of Africa and Haiti, AIDS appears to be a bidirectional, heterosexually transmitted disease that often occurs concurrently with other sexually transmitted diseases.

Of interest to virologists, infectious disease specialists, and public health officials.

226. PERKINS, Herbert A., Susan Samson, Jane Garner, Dean Echenberg, James R. Allen, Morton Cowan, Jay A. Levy. "Risk of AIDS for recipients of blood components from donors who subsequently developed AIDS." *Blood* 70 (1987): 1604-1610.

Reported cases of AIDS in San Francisco, as of March 31, 1986, include 92 individuals who had donated blood subsequent to 1978. The status of 336 of the 406 recipients, through transfusion, of their blood components, as of April 1, 1986, is reported.

Follow-up

Of 336 recipients whose current status is known, 2% have developed AIDS. Of the 46 living recipients who do not have AIDS, 24 (25%) have antibody to HIV and seven meet the criteria for ARC. The blood components transfused from the donors who developed AIDS included all routine components. This fact confirms the previous CDC report that AIDS can be transmitted by whole blood, RBC and platelet concentrates, and fresh frozen plasma.

Of interest to blood bank specialists, public health officials, and virologists.

227. PETERMAN, Thomas A. "Sexual transmission of human immunodeficiency virus." *Journal of the American Medical Association* 256 (1986): 2222-2226.

Examines the sexual transmission of HIV, the precautions that individuals can take to avoid transmission, potential public health interventions, and the present evidence for the effectiveness of prevention efforts.

Commentary

The most effective way to prevent HIV transmission is to develop a cure or vaccine, but we cannot afford to wait for these developments. Confidential counseling and HIV antibody testing should be available for anyone who is concerned about possible infection. Studies are needed to refine estimates of risk of infection, to evaluate the efficacy of safe sex practices, and to evaluate methods of encouraging people to use them consistently. Studies of effectiveness should consider costs and benefits, both financial and psychological.

Of interest to public health officials, health educators, and virologists.

228. PETERSON, Edwin P., Nancy J. Alexander, Kamran S. Moghissi. "A.I.D. and AIDS--too close for comfort." *Fertility and Sterility* 49 (1988): 209-210.

Discusses the American Fertility Society's precautionary changes in its guidelines for artificial insemination.

Editorial

Semen donors in the U.S. have seroconverted while actively participating in an artificial insemination by donor program, and four of eight women in Australia became seropositive after donor insemination with a seropositive donor. Since it is possible for HIV to be transmitted by fresh donor semen before the donor has become seropositive, the potential for HIV infection with fresh semen cannot be eliminated entirely. The American Fertility Society, therefore, has revised its

New Guidelines for the Use of Semen Donor Insemination: 1986, and now recommends that all donor semen be frozen and quarantined for 180 days and the donor retested and found to be seronegative before release of any specimen.

Of particular interest to health professionals working in fertility programs.

229. QUINN, Thomas C. "Perspectives on the future of AIDS."
      Journal of the American Medical Association 253 (1985):
      247-249.

Discusses what has been learned about HTLV-III/LAV and its implications for the future of AIDS.

Editorial

Discovery of the biological agent responsible for a disease represents only the beginning of our understanding of that disease. The availability of a diagnostic test makes us capable of limiting transmission in some groups, but sexual transmission of AIDS will probably not be affected until an effective vaccine or treatment becomes available. It is not known whether heterosexual transmission will ever become important in the epidemiology of AIDS in the United States. Certain factors, such as genetic susceptibility, differences in virologic strains, cultural differences in sexual practices, coinfection with other pathogens, and immunologic status at the time of exposure, may limit the spread of AIDS via heterosexual activity. However, until effective treatment and control programs are developed, the incidence of HTLV-III/LAV infection and AIDS will continue to increase and its consequences to be felt throughout the world.

Of general interest.

230. REES, Malcolm. "HIV infectiousness and the AIDS epidemic."
      Scandinavian Journal of Social Medicine 17 (1989): 33-38.

Outlines a theory of the AIDS epidemic based on assumptions regarding the changes in infectiousness over the life cycle of the disease.

Descriptive

The author suggests a short initial period of infectiousness followed by a long dormant period, which in turn is succeeded by another period of infectiousness, longer than the first period. Each of the periods of infectiousness can generate an associated epidemic. It is suggested that the Western homosexual epidemic is based on initial stage infectiousness, while the African heterosexual epidemic is mainly the result of end stage infectiousness.

Of interest to epidemiologists and public health officials.

231. SANDE, Merle A. "Transmission of AIDS: The case against casual contagion." *New England Journal of Medicine* 314 (1986): 380-382.

Discusses the belief that the AIDS virus can be transmitted by casual contact.

Commentary

The AIDS virus is spread sexually, by the injection of contaminated blood, and vertically from mother to fetus. Other modes of transmission are extremely rare.

Of interest to health professionals and laymen.

232. SCHMIDT, Casper G. "The group fantasy origins of AIDS." *Journal of Psychohistory* 12 (1984): 37-78.

Proposes an alternative hypothesis for the etiology of AIDS, namely a psychosocial origin of the AIDS epidemic.

Descriptive

The author hypothesizes that AIDS is a typical example of epidemic hysteria; that the epidemic has, at its core, an unconscious group delusion, which can be called the group-fantasy of scapegoating; that the fantasy complex underlies this scapegoating ritual as was found for leprosy; that the causes of the tensions giving rise to the epidemic can be found in the group psychology of the U.S.; and that among the more distal causes are the effects of drastic changes in cultural ethos, such as the development of nuclear arsenals, the introduction of birth control, and the invention of recreational sex. The author suggests that the only attempts at cure from the lay public have been reducing sexual activity or the numbers of sexual partners. He states that until the public awakens from their "group trance," it will not be possible to deal with other aspects of the epidemic.

Of interest to historians, psychologists, and social scientists.

233. SEALE, John. "Origins of the AIDS viruses, HIV-1 and HIV-2: Fact or fiction?" *Journal of Biosocial Science* 20 (1988): 445-451.

Presents the idea that the AIDS virus could have been introduced by accident or design.

Discussion

The various theories of the origin of the AIDS viruses, HIV-1 and HIV-2, are discussed--natural selection, artificial selection, and accident or design. The author proposes that the AIDS epidemic in the U.S. may be the result of a deliberate act of biological warfare that may not be as fictitious as it might seem.

Of interest to health professionals and laymen.

234. SHIRLEY, L. Reed, and Steven A. Ross. "Risk of transmission
      of human immunodeficiency virus by bite of an infected
      toddler." *Journal of Pediatrics* 114 (1989): 425-427.

Reports on the long-term follow-up of exposure to the saliva of an
HIV-infected child.

Case Study

An HIV-infected three-year-old, on several occasions, bit four cousins
on the face and the extremities. Although the skin remained intact
and, in some cases, was protected by clothing, a moist impression was
visible after each biting episode. The cousins were tested for seropositivity just after the bites and at 3, 6, 12, and 20 months. No
antibody was detected, and all the exposed children have remained
clinically healthy. Other cases of biting by HIV-infected persons are
reviewed.

Of particular interest to school and day care personnel and to members
of the general public.

235. SOLOMON, George F. "The emerging field of psychoneuroimmu-
      nology with a special note on AIDS." *Advances* 2 (1985):
      6-19.

The author seeks to identify the links between the central nervous and
immune systems and the mechanisms through which they might influence
each other.

Descriptive

The author sees 14 connections between immunology and the central
nervous system, which he lists and discusses as hypotheses. For each,
he adduces illustrative supporting data.

Of interest to social and behavioral scientists.

236. VERRUSIO, A. Carl. "Risk of transmission of the human
      immunodeficiency virus to health care workers exposed to
      HIV-infected patients: A review." *Journal of the American
      Dental Association* 118 (1989): 339-342.

Summarizes national surveillance data and prospective studies on the
risk of HIV transmission to health care workers.

Review

Data indicate that HIV infection in health care workers in the United
States results primarily from exposure outside the health care
setting, although a small number of health care workers have been

infected by occupational exposure. The risk of seroconversion after needlestick exposure to HIV-infected blood is about 0.5%. Risk from exposure of mucous membranes or nonintact skin is lower.

Of interest to health care workers, laboratory personnel, and administrators of patient care facilities.

237. "VERTICAL transmission of HIV." *Lancet* 2, no. 8619 (1988): 1057-1058.

Reports on pediatric AIDS and comments on the limitations of pediatric studies and the implications for counseling pregnant women.

Commentary

Studies of pediatric AIDS have been limited by the following conditions: small sample sizes, lack of measurement standardization, clinical symptoms in antibody-negative children, and a lack of long-term studies. Blanket recommendations of termination of pregnancy or sterilization of seropositive women are inappropriate until more is known about vertical transmission.

Of interest to obstetricians/gynecologists and epidemiologists.

238. WARD, John W., Scott D. Holmberg, James R. Allen, et al. "Transmission of human immunodeficiency virus (HIV) by blood transfusions screened as negative for HIV antibody." *New England Journal of Medicine* 318 (1988): 473-478.

Thirteen persons who seroconverted after receiving blood from donors screened, at the time of donation, as antibody-negative were investigated to identify instances of HIV transmission by antibody-negative donations.

Research

Twelve of the recipients had no identifiable risk factors for HIV other than the transfusions they received. Eight to 20 months after transfusion, three developed HIV-related illnesses and one developed AIDS. All seven donors were found to be HIV infected. Six reported a risk factor for HIV infection and five had engaged in high-risk behavior or had an illness suggestive of acute retroviral syndrome within the four months preceding their seronegative donation. They apparently had been infected only recently, and were negative, according to available antibody tests, at the time of donation. The authors conclude that a small but identifiable risk of HIV infection exists for recipients of screened blood. Donors at high risk need to be informed more effectively of the reasons for deferral of donation, and new assays that detect HIV infection earlier need to be evaluated for effectiveness in screening donated blood.

Of interest to blood bank personnel and public health officials.

239. WORLD Health Organization. "WHO consensus statement: Sexually transmitted diseases as a risk factor for HIV transmission." *Journal of Sex Research* 26 (1989): 272-275.

A consultation on sexually transmitted diseases (STD) as a potential risk factor for HIV transmission was convened by the WHO's Global Programme on AIDS (GPA) and Sexually Transmitted Disease Programme (VDT) in Geneva on January 4-6, 1989.

Descriptive

Recent studies have suggested that STD may facilitate the transmission of the HIV, Type 1. A total of 32 participants from 21 countries, including experts in public health, epidemiology, biomedical and social science aspects of STD and AIDS, participated in the consultation convened by WHO to develop a consensus based on the critical analysis of available evidence regarding the potential role and importance of STD as a risk factor for HIV-1 transmission. Included in this article are the consultation objectives and the consultation consensus statement.

Of interest to health professionals, epidemiologists, and public health officials.

c. Chapters

240. GOEDERT, James J. "Recreational drugs: Relationship to AIDS." *In* Irving J. Selikoff, Alvin S. Teirtein, Shalom Z. Hirschman (Eds.). *Acquired Immune Deficiency Syndrome.* New York: The New York Academy of Sciences, 1984.

Review data concerning the relationship between recreational drugs, immune alterations, and AIDS.

Review

The current evidence concerning use of nitrate inhalants and the risk of AIDS is inconclusive, as is true for two other recreational drugs, heroin and cocaine.

Of interest to epidemiologists and virologists.

241. SONNABEND, Joseph A. "A multifactorial model for the development of AIDS in homosexual men." *In* Irving J. Selikoff, Alvin S. Teirtein, Shalom Z. Hirschman (Eds.). *Acquired Immune Deficiency Syndrome.* New York: The New York Academy of Sciences, 1984.

The author proposes that there is no specific AIDS agent.

Theoretical

A model is presented illustrating how AIDS could have developed in homosexual men as a result of an interaction of the known or likely effects of repeated exposures to specific environmental factors. Rather than invoke a single common infectious etiology, it is suggested that different pathways may lead to similar disorders of immune regulation.

Of interest to virologists, public health officials, and epidemiologists.

d. Dissertation

242. PADIAN, Nancy Schwartz. "The heterosexual transmission of human immunodeficiency virus." Ph.D. dissertation, University of California, Berkeley, 1987.

The frequency of heterosexual transmission of HIV and the factors that influence this transmission were investigated.

Literature Review/Research

A critical review of the literature and scientific evidence bearing upon the issues led to the conclusion that a widespread heterosexual epidemic is unlikely in the U.S., although "pockets" of epidemic may spread in communities mimicking demographic and sociological factors found in African communities. A heterosexual partner study was conducted. About 20% of the long-term sexual partners of infected men were found to have developed antibodies to HIV. Transmission was associated with repeated exposures to the infected male partner and with the practice of anal intercourse. Some infection may have been through vaginal intercourse. Female-to-male transmission was much less common. Eight men who began sexual contact with a woman after she was infected were followed and, despite sustained high risk contacts, none became infected. However, larger samples need to be recruited before generalizations can be made about these results. Suggestions are made for further studies.

Of interest to epidemiologists and virologists.

3. GROUPS AT RISK

a. Books

243. HAMMETT, Theodore M. *AIDS in Correctional Facilities: Issues and Options.* Washington, DC: National Institute of Justice, U.S. Department of Justice by Abt Associates, 1986.

Presents the basic facts about AIDS, sets out a range of possible correctional system responses to the disease, and discusses the advantages and disadvantages of each.

Report/Manual

Divided into two sections: the problem of AIDS, and policy options
for correctional administrators.   Appendices include a resource list;
training, education, and counseling materials; and guidelines for
preventing the transmission of infection.

Intended for prison administrators and medical staff as well as
legislators and other policymakers for correctional institutions, but
may be of interest to other institutional administrators and staff.

244.   KASSLER, Jeanne.   *Gay Men's Health: A Guide to the AIDS
       Syndrome and Other Sexually Transmitted Diseases.*   New
       York: Harper & Row, 1983.

Describes the sexually transmitted diseases that affect gay men.

Text

Discusses the sexually transmitted diseases that affect gay men, their
symptoms, which sexual practices are likely to transmit them, how they
are diagnosed and treated, and what can be done to prevent them.
Contains a chapter describing the medical examination, a discussion of
the male anatomy, and a list of clinics, hotlines, and referral
centers.

Intended for members of the gay community, but should also interest
health educators.

b. Articles

245.   CHAISSON, Richard E., Peter Bacchetti, Dennis Osmond,
       Barbara Brodie, Merle A. Sande, Andrew R. Moss.   "Cocaine
       use and HIV infection in intravenous drug users in San
       Francisco."   *Journal of the American Medical Association* 261
       (1989): 561-565.

Risk factors for HIV infection were assessed in 633 heterosexual drug
users.

Research

HIV seroprevalence was 26% in blacks, 10% in Hispanics, and 6% in
whites.   Intravenous cocaine use significantly increased the risk of
HIV infection, with a seroprevalence of 35% in daily cocaine users.
Black subjects were more likely to use cocaine regularly.   Drug use in
shooting galleries and sharing of drug injection equipment were also
associated with HIV infection and were more common in cocaine users.

Of interest to public health professionals.

246. CHAISSON, Richard E., Andrew R. Moss, Robin Onishi, Dennis Osmond, James R. Carlson. "Human immunodeficiency virus infection in heterosexual intravenous drug users in San Francisco." *American Journal of Public Health* 77 (1987): 169-172.

The prevalence of antibodies to HIV was determined in 281 heterosexual drug users from community-based settings in San Francisco who had been recruited for an investigation of their risk of infection with the human immunodeficiency virus.

Research

Addicts who reported regularly sharing needles when injecting, particularly those sharing with two or more persons, showed an increased risk of seropositivity. Blacks and Latins had a greater prevalence of seropositivity than whites, even after adjustment for needle sharing. Seropositivity was not associated with age, sex, duration of drug use, or history of prostitution. The data indicate that an epidemic of AIDS in intravenous drug users, similar to that which occurred among homosexuals in San Francisco, is possible.

Of interest to public health professionals, epidemiologists, physicians, counselors, and health educators.

247. CLEARY, Paul D., Eleanor Singer, Theresa F. Rogers, Jerome Avorn, Nancy Van Devanter, Steven Soumerai, Samuel Perry, Johanna Pindyck. "Sociodemographic and behavioral characteristics of HIV antibody-positive blood donors." *American Journal of Public Health* 78 (1988): 953-957.

Describes the sociodemographic and behavioral characteristics of 173 blood donors who were confirmed by Western blot tests to have antibodies to HIV.

Research

Seropositive donors were predominantly young, unmarried, and male, and major risk factors could be identified for almost all. However, more than 20 percent of the study participants were women, and many participants were not aware that they were at risk of infection.

Of interest to physicians, blood bank professionals, and public health officials.

248. COATES, Randall A., Liviana M. Calzavara, Colin L. Soskolne, Stanley E. Read, Mary M. Fanning, Frances A. Shepherd, Michel H. Klein, J. Kenneth Johnson. "Validity of sexual histories in a prospective study of male sexual contacts of men with AIDS or AIDS-related conditions." *American Journal of Epidemiology* 128 (1988): 719-728.

Seventy-five AIDS or ARC patients and their corresponding sexual contacts were asked details concerning the sexual activities involved in their sexual encounters.

Research

There was a tendency for primary cases to report greater numbers of various activities than their sexual contacts. The agreement between the primary respondents and their sexual contacts appeared to be affected by the time lapsed from the last sexual encounter with the contact and the date of the primary case interview. Such data can be compared with sufficient reliability and validity for use in epidemiological investigations to assess risk of HIV infection for the more common forms of sexual activities.

Of interest to epidemiologists, health educators, and physicians.

249. COLEMAN, Rosie M., and David Curtis. "Distribution of risk behavior for HIV infection amongst intravenous drug users." *British Journal of Addiction* 83 (1988): 1331-1334.

One hundred and sixty-two intravenous drug users attending two London clinics were questioned about their sexual and equipment sharing behavior.

Research

Four individuals accounted for 90% of all sexual contacts and 39 individuals accounted for 90% of all equipment sharing contacts. Individuals with multiple sexual contacts were more likely to have multiple equipment sharing contacts. It is suggested that the concentration of high risk behavior in only a few subjects may contribute to the overall levels of HIV infection among drug users in London.

Of interest to drug counselors and mental health professionals.

250. DOLAN, Michael P., John L. Black, Horace A. Deford, John R. Skinner, Ralph Robinowitz. "Characteristics of drug abusers that discriminate needle-sharers." *Public Health Reports* 102 (1987): 395-398.

To identify variables that discriminate needle-sharing among drug abusers, 224 male drug abusers were studied.

Research

Three variables were identified that discriminated needle-sharers from other drug abusers. Compared with other drug abusers, needle-sharers used more multiple drugs, were more likely to use a "shooting gallery," and had more problems related to drug use. No demographic or personality variables discriminated needle-sharers from non-sharers.

Of interest to drug abuse counselors and mental health professionals.

251. FLAVIN, Daniel K., and Richard J. Frances. "Risk-taking behavior, substance abuse disorders and the acquired immune deficiency syndrome." *Advances in Alcohol and Substance Abuse* 6, no. 3 (1987): 23-32.

The authors address the relationship between the addictions and disinhibition, suicidal behavior, and the clinical and therapeutic needs of patients, their families and staff.

Descriptive

While basic science and clinical research continues into the biological aspects of AIDS, emphasis and priority should be given to co-factors in disease such as the disinhibiting effects of alcohol and drugs. More study is needed of the evolution, progression, and spread of AIDS in relation to substance use vs. abuse and addiction with associated psychiatric illness in a variety of high risk populations. Development and use of standardized research interviews will help in comparing different studies.

Of interest to health educators and substance abuse counselors.

252. FRANCHESCHI, S., U. Tirelli, E. Vaccher, et al. "Risk factors for HIV infection in drug addicts from the northeast of Italy." *International Journal of Epidemiology* 17 (1988): 162-167.

Prevalence and determinants of HIV infection were assessed in 313 parenteral drug addicts admitted to five Centers for Drug-Addict Assistance and two prisons located in northeast Italy.

Research

The overall prevalence of HIV positivity was high (30%). The most important risk factors beside syringe sharing were of a geographical nature, i.e. living in Pordenone Province (where a U.S. military base is located) or coming from other endemic areas and having travelled long distances in the past three years. Prostitution also increased the risk of infection, but duration of drug addiction had little effect.

Of interest to epidemiologists.

253. GERBERDING, J. Louise, Cheryl E. Bryant-LeBlanc, Kathleen Nelson, et al. "Risk of transmitting the human immunodeficiency virus, cytomegalovirus, and hepatitis B virus to health care workers exposed to patients with AIDS and AIDS-related conditions." *Journal of Infectious Diseases* 156 (1987): 861-864.

This prospective cohort study was designed to evaluate the risk of occupational transmission of HIV, hepatitis B virus, and cytomegalovirus to health care workers with intensive exposure to HIV-infected patients.

Research

Results indicate that health care workers are at minimal risk for HIV, CMV, and HBV transmission from occupational exposure to patients with AIDS or ARC, even when intensively exposed for long periods of time.

Of interest to all health care workers and health professions students.

254. GINZBURG, Harold M. "Intravenous drug users and the acquired immune deficiency syndrome." *Public Health Reports* 99 (1984): 206-212.

Discusses the occurrence and transmission of AIDS in IV drug abusers.

Descriptive

AIDS occurs most commonly among homosexual and bisexual males with multiple sex partners and among users of IV drugs. It appears to be spread by contact with blood products and body fluids. Not only heroin users, but also occasional users of recreational drugs who share needles and syringes when self-administering cocaine or amphetamines at a weekend party, are at risk of contracting AIDS. Data from surveys indicate that drug users entering treatment are aware of the increased risks associated with AIDS. Treatment staff have expressed concerns about their own susceptibility to the disease. Special education programs, which have been instituted in New York City to provide health workers with information and reassurance, have met with success. To date, no health worker providing direct assistance to substance abusers with a history of IV drug use has contracted AIDS.

Of interest to epidemiologists, mental health professionals, and health care workers in substance abuse treatment centers.

255. GRABAU, John C., Benedict I. Truman, Dale L. Morse. "A seroepidemiologic profile of persons seeking anonymous HIV testing at alternate sites in upstate New York." *New York State Journal of Medicine* 88 (1988): 59-62.

Questionnaire data were obtained from 1,635 persons for development of an epidemiologic profile of persons attending alternate sites for HIV counseling and testing in New York State in 1985.

Research

Most attendees were white males, born in the U.S., who were well and sought testing because they had risk factors or had sex with persons at risk. Higher rates of HIV seropositivity were found among blacks, Hispanics, males, and those with symptoms than among those without these characteristics.

Of interest to epidemiologists, public health officials, and virologists.

256. GREEN, John, Lydia Temoshok, Jane Zich. "Editorial: Drug abuse and AIDS." *Psychology and Health* 1 (1987): 147-148.

Discusses the spread of HIV infection among intravenous drug users.

Editorial

The HIV virus is spread by needle sharing, probably assisted by drawing blood into the syringe and reinjecting it. Infected drug users spread it to their sexual partners, a risk magnified by the common practice of prostitution to support the drug habit. Pregnant mothers can infect their unborn children and both are at increased risk for developing AIDS. Since individuals in this population may be suspicious of authority figures and difficult to reach by public health campaigns, there is a need for appropriately targeted, culturally sensitive public health education efforts, developed in collaboration with community leaders, and new models of health education and behavior change that take into account the needs and circumstances of this group.

Of interest to health educators and public health professionals.

257. GUINAN, Mary E., and Ann Hardy. "Epidemiology of AIDS in women in the United States: 1981 through 1986." *Journal of the American Medical Association* 257 (1987): 2039-2042.

An analysis of 1819 cases of AIDS in women, reported between 1981 and 1986.

Descriptive

The majority of women with AIDS were intravenous drug users. The second most common risk factor was heterosexual contact with a person at risk for AIDS. The proportion of women with AIDS in this risk group increased significantly between 1982 and 1986, from 12% to 26%. This trend may prove to be a good marker for following trends in heterosexual transmission. Since the majority of childhood AIDS cases are a result of perinatal transmission from the mother, trends in AIDS cases for women may also predict future trends for AIDS in children.

Of interest to public health officials and epidemiologists.

258. HARDY, Ann M., James R. Allen, W. Meade Morgan, James W. Curran. "The incidence rate of acquired immune deficiency syndrome in selected populations." *Journal of the American Medical Association* 253 (1985): 215-220.

Describes efforts to estimate denominator figures and presents approximate incidence rates of AIDS in single (never married) men, IV drug users, Haitians living in the United States, persons with hemophilia A and B, female sexual contacts of male IV drug users, and blood transfusion recipients.

Descriptive

The highest rates of disease (82 to 268.9 per 100,000) were found among single men in San Francisco and Manhattan, IV drug users in New York City and New Jersey, hemophilia A patients, and recent Haitian entrants to the U.S. Male IV drug users and male Haitians were two to four times as likely to develop AIDS as were females in each group. Persons with hemophilia A had six times the incidence rate of AIDS as those with hemophilia B, and those with severe hemophilia A had three times the rate as those with moderate and seven times the rate of those with mild clotting factor deficiency. Blood transfusion recipients and female sexual contacts of male IV drug users had much lower average yearly rates than did persons in the other four groups (0.4 to 9.4 per 100,000), but still had a higher incidence rate than did persons not belonging to any of these groups (0.1 per 100,000).

Of interest to epidemiologists and public health officials.

259. HOFMANN, Bo, Peter Kryger, Nils Strandberg Pedersen, et al. "Sexually transmitted diseases, antibodies to immunodeficiency virus, and subsequent development of acquired immuno-deficiency syndrome: Visitors of homosexual sauna clubs in Copenhagen: 1982-1983. *Sexually Transmitted Diseases* 15 (1988): 1-4.

Sera from 260 men from Denmark and elsewhere attending two Copenhagen sauna clubs for homosexual men during nine months of 1982-1983 were investigated for markers for syphilis, hepatitis A and B, and HIV.

Research

Markers for sexually transmitted diseases were found with very high frequencies among the high risk group studied. Among individuals tested twice, seroconversion for antibodies to hepatitis A, hepatitis B, and HIV was observed and indicates a continuous spread of hepatitis viruses and HIV among men who visited the saunas. When one considers that only seven cases of AIDS were registered in Denmark at the time of this study, the prevalence of antibodies to HIV was very high.

Of interest to virologists and epidemiologists.

260. JASON, Janine, Kung-Jong Lui, Margaret V. Ragni, Nancy A. Hessol, William W. Darrow. "Risk of developing AIDS in HIV-infected cohorts of hemophilic and homosexual men." *Journal of the American Medical Association* 261 (1989): 725-727.

To examine whether the latency period and/or incidence of AIDS differs in persons infected with HIV by different routes or having different "cofactors," 79 hemophilic men in Pennsylvania and 117 homosexual men in California, all having known dates of infection and long post-infection observation periods, were compared.

Research

By 1987, 21% of the hemophilic and 27% of the homosexual men had developed AIDS. Seroconversion patterns differed for the two groups, and when this was taken into account, the conditional odds ratio for AIDS was 1:20. No significant difference in the cumulative proportion with AIDS from time of infection was shown by Kaplan-Meier survival analysis. Although limited by the small size and geographically localized nature of the study population, the results suggest that, currently, the relative length of HIV infection is of primary importance in comparing disease outcome for different populations.

Of interest to epidemiologists, virologists, and public health officials.

261. KAPLAN, Mark H.   "The AIDS epidemic and the drug substance
     abuse patient."   *Journal of Substance Abuse Treatment* 4
     (1987): 127-136.

An overview of AIDS for drug abuse counselors.

Review

A discussion of the epidemiological and immunological aspects of AIDS, transmission, signs and symptoms, and the role of the drug treatment counselor in the AIDS epidemic.

Of particular interest to drug and alcohol abuse counselors and mental health professionals treating drug abusers.

262. KOPLAN, Jeffrey P., Ann M. Hardy, James R. Allen.
     "Epidemiology of the acquired immunodeficiency syndrome in
     intravenous drug abusers."   *Advances in Alcohol and
     Substance Abuse* 5 (1986): 13-23.

Describes the epidemiology of AIDS in IV drug users and discusses unanswered questions arising from the limited data that are available.

Descriptive

AIDS in IV drug users seems relatively geographically confined to the metropolitan New York area. The epidemic curve of all AIDS cases, and that of heterosexual IV drug users as well, appears to have decreased its rate of ascent. Drug user cases have a different disease pattern than non-users with more *Pneumocystis carinii* pneumonia, less Kaposi's sarcoma, and a higher case-fatality rate.

Of interest to drug abuse counselors, epidemiologists, and infectious disease specialists.

263. LANDESMAN, Sheldon H.   "Human immunodeficiency virus
     infection in women: An overview."   *Seminars in Perinatology*
     13 (1989): 2-6.

Reviews the magnitude and consequences of HIV infection in women in the inner city.

Review

HIV infection in women is marked by geographic, ethnic, and economic clustering and is closely associated with drug abuse. Most infected women are black or Hispanic. The infection rate among women giving birth in municipal hospitals along the eastern seaboard ranges from 1.0% to 3.6%. Steady female partners of infected hemophiliacs have an infection rate of seven to 21%, and 40% or more of women who are steady sexual partners of men with AIDS or ARC are infected. About 20% to 50% of the babies born to HIV-infected women will be infected. Although pregnancy appears to accelerate the progress of HIV infection, this has not been documented, and it is not known whether the infection retards intrauterine growth or promotes embryopathy. Delivery by Caesarean section does not appear to reduce the risk of perinatal infection. Breast milk is a potential means of HIV transmission. Social support systems for infected women and foster care systems for infants are generally inadequate.

Of interest to health professionals, social service professionals, public health professionals, and public policymakers.

264. LAWRENCE, Dale N., Janine M. Jason, Robert C. Holman, Peggy Heine, Bruce L. Evatt, and the Hemophilia Study Group. "Sex practice correlates of human immunodeficiency virus transmission and acquired immunodeficiency syndrome in heterosexual partners and offspring of U.S. hemophilic men." *American Journal of Hematology* 30 (1989): 68-76.

Reports on an assessment of the risk of HIV transmission from seropositive hemophilic men to their female sex partners, which was conducted during 1984 to 1987.

Research

Five percent of 21 female partners of asymptomatic men and 11% of 35 partners of HIV-symptomatic hemophilic men had been infected when first tested. One of 19 seronegative women seroconverted during the following year. Only 18% of the women said their partners used condoms "nearly always." Over 60% engaged in oral-genital sex in addition to vaginal intercourse. Only 12% of the seronegative women reported avoidance of oral-genital sex and consistent condom use by their male partner. Further evidence of women who acquired HIV infection through heterosexual contact with U.S. hemophilic men and of children whose infection was acquired through exposure of their mothers to hemophilic partners, which was taken from the CDC national AIDS surveillance reports, is discussed.

Of interest to epidemiologists, virologists, and public health officials.

265. McCUSKER, Jane, Anne M. Stoddard, Kenneth H. Mayer, David N. Cowan, Jerome E. Groopman. "Behavioral risk factors for HIV infection among homosexual men at a Boston community health center." *American Journal of Public Health* 78 (1988): 68-71.

Cross-sectional data from homosexual and bisexual male clients of a Boston community health center were used to analyze social and behavioral factors associated with HIV infection.

Research

Partners from California, a previous period of greater sexual activity (high period), and the frequency of receptive anogenital intercourse, both during the high period and during the last six months, were independently associated with positive HIV antibody status.

Useful to epidemiologists and public health professionals.

266. MESSIAH, A., J.Y. Mary, J.B. Brunet, W. Rozenbaum, M. Gentilini, A.J. Valleron. "Risk factors for A.I.D.S. among homosexual men in France." *European Journal of Epidemiology* 4 (1988): 68-74.

To identify risk factors for AIDS among homosexual men in France, the authors undertook a case-control study in Paris and its suburbs.

Research

Cases were more likely than controls to belong to upper socioeconomic classes, to have used local corticosteroids, to have regularly inhaled nitrites, to report a history of syphilis and of herpes infections, to have a higher level of promiscuity with occasional partners, and to have had sexual encounters in the U.S.A. History of syphilis, promiscuity with occasional partners, and the use of local corticosteroids appeared to be the main risk factors.

Of interest to epidemiologists and public health officials.

267. MOSS, Andrew R., Dennis Osmond, Peter Bacchetti, Jean-Claude Chermann, Francoise Barre-Sinoussi, James Carlson. "Risk factors for AIDS and HIV seropositivity in homosexual men." *American Journal of Epidemiology* 125 (1987): 1035-1047.

Reports a case-control study of risk factors for AIDS and HIV seropositivity in which homosexual AIDS cases in San Francisco were compared with two groups of controls.

Research

AIDS risk was strongly associated with number of sexual partners, doubling with every 20-30 partners, when cases were compared with antibody-negative neighborhood controls. Rectal receptivity was clearly the primary sexual behavior leading to the transmission of HIV. There was no consistent evidence in the study for oral-genital, oral-anal, or other sexual transmission of HIV. No drugs, except possibly nitrites, consistently were associated with risk.

Of interest to virologists and epidemiologists.

268. MULLEADY, Geraldine. "A review of drug abuse and HIV infection." *Psychology and Health* 1 (1987): 149-163.

A comprehensive overview of the issues and problems associated with HIV infection in drug abusers.

Review

The rising prevalence of HIV infection and AIDS among IV drug users necessitates increased contact with drug abusers in the community and an increase in the availability of treatment alternatives if effective health education and preventive measures are to take place. Heterosexual transmission, pregnancy, and syringe availability are issues of particular importance for this group. Possible options for service provision are considered.

Of interest to mental health professionals, public health professionals, public policymakers, and anyone involved in drug abuse programs.

269. O'FARRELL, N., and I. Windsor. "Prevalence of HIV antibody in recurrent attenders at a sexually transmitted disease clinic." *South African Medical Journal* 74 (1988): 104-105.

The prevalence of antibodies to the human immunodeficiency virus among recurrent attenders at a sexually transmitted disease clinic was investigated.

Research

Four of 140 recurrent attenders at a sexually transmitted disease clinic for blacks were seropositive to HIV, a prevalence rate of 2.9%. All denied engaging in any risk behaviors for AIDS other than heterosexual activity. The authors recommend that existing STD clinics be used for HIV testing, counseling, assessment, and follow-up, rather than the proposed development of new HIV diagnostic centers.

Of interest to personnel working in STD clinics and alternative HIV testing sites, public health officials, and South African policy makers.

270. OSMOND, Dennis, Peter Bacchetti, Richard E. Chaisson, Thomas Kelly, Robert Stempel, James Cohen, Andrew R. Moss. "Time of exposure and risk of HIV infection in homosexual partners of men with AIDS. *American Journal of Public Health* 78 (1988): 944-948.

Reports on an analysis of risk factors for seropositivity to HIV antibody in a group of homosexual men who were regular sexual partners of men who developed AIDS.

Research

Receptive anal intercourse with the index AIDS cases and number of different sexual partners with whom subjects were anally receptive were both risk factors. Risk was not associated with the duration or frequency of contact. The data suggest that the potential for sexual transmission from an HIV-infected person may be greater close to or after the onset of the disease.

Of interest to virologists, epidemiologists, and public health officials.

271. PETERMAN, T.A., K.-J. Lui, D.N. Lawrence, J.R. Allen. "Estimating the risks of transfusion-associated acquired immune deficiency syndrome and human immunodeficiency virus infection." *Transfusion* 27 (1987): 371-374.

Presents a mathematical model to estimate the number of transfusion associated AIDS cases that will develop in persons who received blood transfusions from 1978 to 1984. Then uses that estimate plus the prevalence of HIV in blood donors in 1985 to estimate the number of recipients who have acquired a transfusion associated infection.

Theoretical

Mathematical modeling suggests there may eventually be 2100 cases of AIDS among persons, aged 13 to 65, who received transfusions between 1978 and 1984. An estimated 12,000 living recipients of all ages from those years are infected with HIV. However, the likelihood of infection in any single recipient is small. Secondary transmissions may be prevented by testing and counseling recipients.

Of interest to epidemiologists, virologists, and public health professionals.

272. PETERMAN, Thomas A., Rand L. Stoneburner, James R. Allen, Harold W. Jaffe, James W. Curran. "Risk of human immuno-deficiency virus transmission from heterosexual adults with transfusion-associated infections." *Journal of the American Medical Association* 259 (1988): 55-58.

The families of patients with transfusion-associated HIV infections were studied to determine the risk of HIV transmission by female-to-male and male-to-female heterosexual contact and by casual family contact.

Research

Two (8%) of 25 husbands and ten (18%) of 55 wives who had had sexual contact with infected spouses were seropositive for HIV. Seropositive wives were older and actually reported somewhat fewer sexual contacts with their infected husbands than seronegative wives. There was no difference in the types of sexual contacts or methods of contraception of the seropositive and seronegative spouses. Most husbands and wives remained uninfected despite repeated sexual contacts without protection, but some acquired infection after only a few contacts, which is consistent with an as yet unexplained biologic variation in transmissibility or susceptibility. There was no evidence of HIV transmission to the 63 other family members who had no sexual contact with the index patient.

Of interest to clinicians, counselors, and public health officials.

273. PIOT, Peter, and Marie Laga. "Prostitutes: A high risk group for HIV infection?" *Social and Preventive Medicine* 33, no. 7 (1988): 336-339.

Reviews the occurrence of HIV infections in prostitutes, the current evidence for prostitutes as a reservoir of STD's, and policy implications.

Review

The HIV prevalence rate among prostitutes varies geographically, with the highest rates occurring in Africa and in areas with large numbers of IV drug users. In Europe, the most important risk factors for HIV infection in prostitutes are IV drug use and unprotected intercourse with non-paying partners. There is, as yet, no evidence that female prostitutes are a source of HIV infection for the heterosexual population in Europe; however, they are playing a major role in the spread of HIV in Africa. Education about safe sex practices should be included in prevention programs aimed at IV drug users. HIV infection should be monitored in prostitutes, and health education on AIDS prevention should be offered to prostitutes and their clients.

Of interest to public health professionals and health educators.

274. QUINN, Thomas C., David Glasser, Robert O. Cannon et al. "Human immunodeficiency virus infection among patients attending clinics for sexually transmitted diseases." *New England Journal of Medicine* 318 (1988): 197-203.

To assess the prevalence and associated risk factors for HIV infection in patients attending inner-city clinics for sexually transmitted diseases in Baltimore, the authors screened 4,028 patients anonymously.

Research

These data suggest that patients at clinics for sexually transmitted diseases represent a group at high risk for HIV infection, and that screening, counseling, and intensive education should be offered to all patients attending such clinics.

Of interest to virologists, infectious disease specialists, and public health officials.

275. RAGNI, Margaret V., Phalguni Gupta, Charles R. Rinaldo, Lawrence A. Kingsley, Joel A. Spero, Jessica H. Lewis. "HIV transmission to female sexual partners of HIV antibody-positive hemophiliacs." *Public Health Reports* 103 (1988): 54-58.

Twenty-one HIV antibody-positive hemophiliacs and their 21 spouses/ sexual partners were evaluated in a study of heterosexual transmission of HIV.

Research

HIV antibody was detected in four of the female partners. None of the couples engaged in anal intercourse. These data confirm the low frequency of heterosexual transmission of HIV from HIV antibody-positive hemophiliacs to their female partners and suggest that this may be due to a low rate of HIV infectivity in HIV seropositive hemophiliacs.

Of interest to health professionals, health educators, and public health officials.

276. ROSS, Michael W. "Prevalence of classes of risk behaviors for HIV infection in a randomly selected Australian population." *Journal of Sex Research* 25 (1988): 441-450.

Describes a randomized, geographically stratified survey to determine prevalence of high risk behaviors in 2600 Australians, 16 years of age and older.

Research

Prevalence of male and female homosexual behavior and contact with prostitutes was substantially lower than the estimates by Kinsey *et al.* Prevalence of HIV risk behaviors appears to be lower in Australia than in the U.S., but higher than previously has been assumed. Implications for HIV preventive education are discussed.

Of interest to public health officials, epidemiologists, and health educators.

277. ROSSER, B.R. "Auckland homosexual males and AIDS prevention: A behavioural and demographic description." *Community Health Studies* 12 (1988): 328-338.

A report of the first major study of male homosexual behavior in New Zealand.

Research

This study found that men who have sex with other men form a heterogeneous sub-group of Auckland society.   The wide diversity of
responses on demographic factors of age, ethnicity, sexual orientation, and sexual identity, as well as the source of information
about the study and differences in socializing, suggest that the
term "gay community," as a global description of this sample, is
somewhat inappropriate. Rather, there would appear to be a variety of
lifestyles, identities, and subgroups operating in Auckland.   The
pattern of sexual activity also reflects this diversity.

Of interest to health educators and public health officials.

278.   SAMUEL, Michael C., and Robert R. Engel.   "Selected aspects
       of AIDS among homosexual men."   *Social and Preventive
       Medicine* 33, no. 7 (1988): 331-335.

A brief summary of important points concerning AIDS and homosexual
men.

Review

Presents the current overall figures of the cumulative AIDS incidence
for Switzerland, the U.S., and the world and similar figures for
homosexual men in Switzerland, the U.S., and the world.   A brief
history of the epidemic is included, with a focus on the role of
homosexual men.   The main risk factors for acquiring HIV infection
among homosexual men, including large numbers of sexual partners,
receptive anal intercourse, and rectal douching, are mentioned, with
emphasis on results from the San Francisco Men's Health Study.   The
development of education and prevention programs is outlined, as is
the role, in these areas, of the Swiss AIDS Foundation and Swiss
Federal Office of Public Health.

Of interest to public health professionals, epidemiologists,   and
health educators.

279.   SCHNEIDER, Beth E.   "Women and AIDS: An international
       perspective." *Futures* 21 (1989): 72-90.

Examines the status of women with AIDS and the prevention campaigns
directed at them.

Descriptive

The author speculates on what the future may hold for women with AIDS,
looking at prospects for health care and social support systems, and
at how AIDS may affect the social and economic status of women.
Several geographic areas are focused upon, and three epidemiological
patterns of HIV infection are presented.

Of interest to women and to social and behavioral scientists.

280. STIMSON, Gerry V., Martin Donoghoe, Lindsey Alldritt, Kate
      Dolan. "HIV transmission risk behaviour of clients attending
      syringe exchange schemes in England and Scotland." *British
      Journal of Addiction* 83 (1988): 1449-1455.

Reports on the HIV risk behavior of British clients interviewed during
the first year of a syringe exchange program.

Research

Most clients had accurate knowledge of the risk of infection from
shared syringes, but few considered themselves to be at risk for HIV
infection. About one-third reported sharing needles and syringes at
or shortly after acceptance into the program. Most clients were
sexually active, many with partners who did not inject drugs. The two
main reasons for participation in the program were scarcity of
injection equipment and worry about AIDS. A majority of clients
reported changes in their injecting practices because of AIDS, and
some reported changes in sexual behaviors.

Of interest to drug abuse counselors, health educators, and public
health professionals.

281. VALDISERRI, Edwin V. "Fear of AIDS: Implications for mental
      health practice with reference to ego-dystonic homosex-
      uality." *American Journal of Orthopsychiatry* 56 (1986):
      634-638.

Examines psychological symptoms caused by fear of AIDS, particularly
in males displaying ego-dystonic homosexuality.

Descriptive

Discusses three cases in which physically healthy homosexual men
suffer from fear of AIDS complicated by major depressive disorder and
premorbid personality dysfunction with reference to psychotherapeutic
intervention.

Of interest to mental health professionals.

282. Van GRIENSVEN, Godfried J.P., Robert A.P. Tielman, Jaap
      Goudsmit, Jan Van der Noordaa, Frank De Wolf, Ernest M.M.
      De Vroome, Roel A. Coutinho. "Risk prevalence of HIV
      antibodies in homosexual men in the Netherlands." *American
      Journal of Epidemiology* 125 (1987): 1048-1057.

Concerned with the relation between lifestyle characteristics and the
prevalence of HIV antibodies.

Research

When the number of sexual partners is considered a risk factor for
HIV, a clear distinction should be made between the sexual techniques
practiced by these partners. A positive relation was found between

the number of partners with whom anal receptive techniques were performed and the presence of anti-HIV. The riskiness of anal receptive sexual techniques confirms the results of other studies. The use of cannabis and nitrite were found to be related to anti-HIV.

Of interest to virologists and epidemiologists.

283. WINKELSTEIN, Warren, Jr., David M. Lyman, Nancy Padian, et al. "Sexual practices and risk of infection by the human immunodeficiency virus: The San Francisco Men's Health Study." *Journal of the American Medical Association* 257 (1987): 321-325.

Reports on a prospective study of the epidemiology and natural history of AIDS in a cohort of 1,034 single men, 25 to 54 years of age, recruited by probability sampling.

Research

The seropositivity rate for HIV infection among homosexual/bisexual study participants was 48.5% at entry (June 1984 through January 1985). No heterosexual participants were HIV seropositive. Homosexual/bisexual men reporting no male sexual partners in the two years prior to entry had a seropositivity rate of 17.6%. The seropositivity rate for those reporting more than 50 partners was 70.8%. Only receptive anal/genital contact had a significantly elevated risk of infection. Douching was the only ancillary sexual practice that contributed significantly to risk of infection.

Of interest to health educators, epidemiologists, and public health officials.

284. WINKELSTEIN, Warren, Jr., Michael Samuel, Nancy S. Padian, James A. Wiley, William Lang, Robert E. Anderson, Jay A. Levy. "The San Francisco Men's Health Study: III. Reduction in human immunodeficiency virus transmission among homosexual/bisexual men, 1982-86." *American Journal of Public Health* 77 (1987): 685-693.

Describes a study of 1,034 single men living in the area of San Francisco where the AIDS epidemic has been most intense to determine the prevalence and incidence of HIV infection.

Research

Prevalence of infection among homosexual/bisexual subjects increased from about 22.8% during the first half of 1982 to 48.6% during the second half of 1984. During the next 18 months, it remained stable at approximately 50%. Annual infection rates, estimated at 18.4% per year from 1982 to 1984, decreased to 5.4 and 3.1% during the first and second halves of 1985 and to 4.2% during the first six months of 1986. The declines were associated with reductions of 60% or more in the prevalence of high risk sexual behavior associated with acquiring and disseminating infection by HIV.

Of interest to epidemiologists, public health officials, physicians, and social and behavioral scientists.

Chapter 3

AIDS AND SOCIETY

1. Social and Cultural Issues, 113-150
2. Ethical Issues, 150-174
3. Public Health and Public Policy Issues, 174-205
4. Economic Issues, 205-217
5. Legal Issues, 217-234
6. Workplace Issues, 234-248

1. SOCIAL AND CULTURAL ISSUES

a. Books

285. AGGLETON, Peter, and Hilary Homans (Eds.). *Social Aspects of AIDS*. London: The Falmer Press, 1988.

Papers written for the first UK Conference on Social Aspects of AIDS, held in 1986, plus additional contributions, which help map out areas of research interest in Britain.

Book of Readings

Central among the themes that recur throughout the book's ten chapters is the extent to which popular and professional understandings of AIDS have been influenced by racism, homophobia, and heterosexism. The processes by which AIDS has been progressively individualized as a disease of lifestyle or choice are examined, and the authors point out the need for research into the political economy of AIDS and the nature and consequences of health education in relation to AIDS.

Of interest to social and behavioral scientists, political scientists, and policymakers.

286. ALTMAN, Dennis. *AIDS in the Mind of America*. Garden City, NY: Anchor Press/Doubleday, 1986.

A discussion of the impact of the AIDS epidemic on the various factions of American society.

Monograph

Deals with living through an epidemic; the politicization of the disease; the conceptualization of AIDS; fear and stigma; the gay community's response; politics and money; sex and disease; and the perception of AIDS as a gay American disease. Concludes that AIDS is a major social and cultural catastrophe that requires political will, public education, and rational thought to find ways to cure and prevent the illness and overcome the panic associated with it.

Excellent reading for concerned laypersons as well as social and behavioral scientists.

287. BAYER, Ronald, Daniel M. Fox, David P. Willis (Eds.). *AIDS: The Public Context of an Epidemic*. New York: Milbank Memorial Fund, 1986.

This supplement to the *Milbank Memorial Quarterly* explores the social environment--the public context--of the AIDS epidemic.

Book of Readings

Eight essays address three broad themes: the influence of social and economic arrangements on the spread and control of the disease; the adequacy of public health measures for controlling the spread of the disease, and how these measures have been shaped by the political and legal systems; and how Americans have collectively met the burden of AIDS, including the costs of care and the tasks of control and caring.

Of particular interest to public health professionals and public policymakers.

288. BERK, Richard A. (Ed.). *The Social Impact of AIDS in the U.S.* Cambridge, MA: Abt Books, 1988.

A collection of essays that are meant to highlight various aspects of social life that may be affected by AIDS.

Book of Readings

The nine essays cover a range of topics including: gender, sexuality, and AIDS; the social consequences of AIDS; AIDS and pornography; hospital responses to epidemics and AIDS; AIDS-related competencies of primary care physicians; AIDS and the Catholic church; an attributional analysis of changing reactions to persons with AIDS; how to cover a plague, a journalist's view; and implications of AIDS for East Africa and the Eastern United States.

Of interest to social and behavioral scientists, health educators, clergy, and the lay public.

289. BRANDT, Allan M.   *No Magic Bullet: A Social History of Venereal Disease in the United States Since 1880*.   Expanded Edition. New York: Oxford University Press, 1987.

Traces the historical record of sexually transmitted diseases from the late nineteenth century to the current epidemics of herpes and AIDS.

Originally published in 1985, *No Magic Bullet* has been expanded to include additional material on the AIDS epidemic.

Text

Attempts to evaluate how shifting attitudes and perceptions concerning sexually transmitted diseases among laypeople and physicians during the last century impacted upon medical practice, public health and military programs, and social behavior. Analyzes the meaning and impact of the AIDS epidemic, examining attitudes and responses to the disease. Contends that venereal disease has engendered a number of social fears about class, race, ethnicity, and sexuality and the family, and that the social and cultural uses of venereal disease as a means of controlling sexuality have greatly complicated attempts to deal effectively with the diseases from a therapeutic standpoint.

Has appeal for a wide audience, including social and behavioral scientists, medical historians, and interested laypersons.

290. CRIMP, Douglas (Ed.). *AIDS: Cultural Analysis/Cultural Activism.* Cambridge, MA: The MIT Press, 1988.

A compilation of essays by a variety of contributors, some activists, some analysts, on the topic of AIDS.

Book of Readings

This exploration of the representational issues is an important intervention by people who combine their lived experience of the AIDS crisis with their analytic insights. The essays challenge the assumptions of AIDS education and policy and expose the images produced by both scientific discourse and the mass media.

Of interest to members of the gay community and to social and behavioral scientists.

291. HALL, Lynn, and Thomas Modl (Eds.). *AIDS: Opposing Viewpoints.* St. Paul, MN: Greenhave Press, 1988.

Presents opposing points of view on the topic of AIDS.

Book of Readings

Each of the five chapters in this volume contains a series of opposing views by various authors on the following questions: How serious is AIDS? How can AIDS be controlled? Will controlling AIDS undermine civil rights? Is the government's response to AIDS adequate? How will AIDS affect society?

Of interest to the general public.

292. IDE, Arthur Frederick. *AIDS Hysteria.* Dallas: Monument Press, 1986.

Chronicles the history and development of the fear of AIDS, and offers information to minimize and deal with the hysteria.

Monograph

The five chapters cover the background to the hysteria, the growing fear, the reality of AIDS, the immunological aberration of AIDS, and guidelines for safe sex.

Of interest to members of high risk groups as well as concerned laypersons.

293. JUENGST, Eric T., and Barbara A. Koenig (Eds.). *The Meaning of AIDS: Implications for Medical Science, Clinical Practice, and Public Health Policy.* New York: Praeger, 1989.

Identifies and analyzes the cultural values and assumptions that color our interpretations of AIDS and determine our response to the disease, and discusses the implications for medical science, clinical practice, and public policy.

Book of Readings

AIDS can be discussed as a disease entity, an illness experience, a contagious infection, a fatal affliction, an epidemic disease, or a challenge to individual liberty. Each interpretation has its own implications for our responses to the disease, and each can be loosely aligned with different professional, personal, and social points of view on the crisis. The relations among the different interpretations are the key to their individual explication and assessment. Effective and appropriate responses to AIDS will require a critical awareness of all those visions of AIDS, the links between them, and the implications we draw from them. The chapters in this volume analyze the various interpretations from a wide range of disciplinary perspectives, including the humanities and the medical and social sciences.

Of interest to health professionals, social and behavioral scientists, and concerned laypersons.

294. LEE, Robert E. *AIDS in America: Our Chances, Our Choices.* Troy, NY: Whitston, 1987.

The future of AIDS in America is discussed. Information about the scientific struggle, the potential magnitude of the disease, the social impact, and individual protection is presented.

Text

The author presents the AIDS epidemic in America as it may develop. The potential impact on the government's ability to continue the provision of social welfare programming, and the impact on medical costs, health insurance, and civil liberties are discussed.

Of interest to health professionals and laymen.

295. McCUEN, Gary E. *The AIDS Crisis: Conflicting Social Values.*
      Hudson, WI: GEM, 1987.

Focuses on the political, moral, and social issues of AIDS. Written
for students.

Textbook

Each chapter presents an overview of a different aspect of AIDS
followed by an exercise for discussion. The four major sections of
the book contain a series of articles that present different
viewpoints on an issue--for example, religious and moral conflicts or
the politics of AIDS. A bibliography, a list of national AIDS-related
organizations, and AIDS research and experimental therapies are
included.

For junior and senior high school students.

296. PATTON, Cindy. *Sex and Germs: The Politics of AIDS.*
      Boston: South End Press, 1985.

Deals with the political implications for the gay and lesbian communities of the AIDS epidemic.

Monograph

AIDS presents a wide social problem as well as a serious public health
concern. It threatens the progress towards sexual freedom and civil
rights made by the gay/lesbian liberation movement and liberal social
activist groups and places a weapon in the hands of right-wingers who
see it as "God's punishment for unnatural behavior" or an opportunity
to squash the homosexual movement in the United States. People with
AIDS and related illnesses and those in high risk groups need to
recognize their common interests and work together to organize a broad
agenda for influencing medical and social policies regarding AIDS.

Of particular interest to members of groups at risk for AIDS.

297. RICHARDSON, Diane. *Women and AIDS.* New York: Methuen,
      1988.

Provides an informative account of the issues that AIDS raises for
women, and challenges the racism, sexism, and homophobia surrounding
the disease.

Text

The eight chapters include such topics as: what AIDS is, AIDS in
women, safer sex, lesbians and AIDS, living with AIDS, caring for
people with AIDS, policies and prevention, and the challenge of AIDS.
A resource list and glossary are provided.

Aimed at women who are concerned about AIDS as well as women who
already have AIDS.

298. SABATIER, Renée. *Blaming Others: Prejudice, Race and
      Worldwide AIDS*. London: The Panos Institute, 1988.

The stated purpose of this book is to reduce the burden of people
likely to suffer double oppression from AIDS.

Monograph

The ten chapters cover topics such as: AIDS and race; origins of
AIDS; sex and race; blame and counterblame; who pays the price of
blame; and different peoples, different messages. In the short term,
AIDS control necessarily concerns itself with emergency measures, but
bringing the pandemic under control will require as long as it takes
to develop a vaccine.

Of interest to the general public.

299. SHILTS, Randy. *And the Band Played On: Politics, People,
      and the AIDS Epidemic*. New York: St. Martin's Press, 1987.

Tells the story of the first five years of the AIDS epidemic in the
United States.

Social History

The story of the AIDS epidemic in America, between the years of 1980
and 1985, is a story of failure--the failure of government to allocate
adequate funding for AIDS research, the failure of scientists to
devote proper attention to a "homosexual affliction," the failure of
political leaders and public health authorities to take the necessary
measures to curb the epidemic's spread, the failure of gay community
leaders to put the preservation of life ahead of political dogma, and
the failure of the mass media to adequately cover a situation that
involved homosexuals and gay sexuality--and it is a story of courage,
the courage of a handful of individuals who fought against the tide of
institutional indifference to bring about an appropriate response to a
profoundly threatening medical crisis.

Of interest to general audiences.

300. SONTAG, Susan. *AIDS and its Metaphors*. New York: Farrar,
      Straus and Giroux, 1989.

Discusses the history of metaphoric thinking about the body. Military
metaphors contribute to stigmatizing certain diseases and those who
are ill. Cancer, syphilis, and AIDS are examples.

Text

Proposes to retire the "military metaphor" of AIDS, which overmobilizes, overdescribes, and contributes to excommunicating and stigmatizing the ill.

Of general interest.

301. UNITED States Department of Health and Human Services, Centers for Disease Control. *AIDS Knowledge and Attitudes of Black Americans*. DHHS Publication No. 165, March 30, 1989.

One of two special reports examining knowledge and attitudes about AIDS and HIV among minority subgroups in the U.S. population.

Report

Based on data collected in the National Health Interview Survey (NHIS), the report describes various aspects of AIDS-related knowledge, attitudes, and behavior for black adults, 18 years of age and over. It presents differentials by age, sex, and education for the black population and compares selected measures for black and white individuals.

Of use to epidemiologists and researchers of AIDS.

302. ———. *AIDS Knowledge and Attitudes of Hispanic Americans*. DHHS Publication No. 166, April 11, 1989.

One of two special reports examining knowledge and attitudes about AIDS and HIV among minority subgroups in the U.S. population.

Report

Based on data collected in the National Health Interview Survey (NHIS), this report describes various aspects of AIDS-related knowledge, attitudes, and behavior for Hispanic adults, 18 years of age and over. It presents differentials by age, sex, education, and specific Hispanic ancestry and compares selected measures for Hispanic and non-Hispanic individuals.

Of use to epidemiologists and researchers of AIDS.

303. VASS, Antony A. *AIDS: A Plague in Us: A Social Perspective: The Condition and its Social Consequences*. St. Ives, Combs: Venus Academica, 1986.

A sociological perspective of AIDS.

Text

An attempt to consider the social aspects of AIDS and its social effect on individuals. The five chapters include: consideration of public opinion and consequences, medical aspects of AIDS, AIDS as a social problem. The book also includes a bibliography.

Of interest to the general public.

304. WATNEY, Simon. *Policing Desire: Pornography, AIDS and the Media.* Minneapolis: University of Minnesota Press, 1987.

A book about the media's representation of homosexuality and AIDS.

Text

Chapter topics include: sex, diversity and disease; infectious desires; moral panics; AIDS, pornography and law; AIDS and the press; AIDS on television; safer representations; and epilogue.

Of interest to the general public.

305. WELLS, Nicholas. *The AIDS Virus: Forecasting its Impact.* London: Office of Health Economics, 1986.

Assesses the validity of predictions regarding the magnitude of the future burden of HIV on the community and on health services, and explores the potential for containing the spread of the virus.

Monograph

Presents information on the nature and origin of human immunodeficiency virus; the consequences of HIV infection; who is at risk; and containing the spread of HIV infection. Concludes that we lack sufficient data to make accurate forecasts about the future impact of HIV, and that since there is, as yet, no specific antiviral therapy or vaccine, health education and public awareness constitute the most effective preventive measures.

Useful to public health professionals, policymakers, and health care workers.

306. WITT, Michael D. (Ed.). *AIDS and Patient Management: Legal, Ethical, and Social Issues.* Owings Mills, MD: National Health Publishing, 1986.

Based on lectures presented at a conference entitled "AIDS: The Ethical, Legal and Social Considerations," which was held on April 24-25, 1985 and jointly sponsored by Tufts New England Medical Center and Public Responsibility in Medicine and Research, plus supplementary material.

Book of Readings

This book begins with a review of the scientific, health policy, and legal aspects of the AIDS epidemic. The articles which follow were written by people from a wide variety of backgrounds and have been divided into eight categories: the public health response to the AIDS crisis; the complications of AIDS research; legal problems of AIDS patients and health care providers; the impact of AIDS on the patient, family, friends, and community; HTLV-III screening and the blood supply; cultural and historical perspectives; issues in social science research; and guidelines for the management of AIDS patients.

Appropriate for a diverse audience including social and behavioral scientists, researchers, health professionals, members of the helping professions, lawyers and legislators, policymakers, and concerned laypersons.

b. Articles

307. ALLARD, Robert. "Beliefs about AIDS as determinants of preventive practices and of support for coercive measures." *American Journal of Public Health* 79 (1989): 448-452.

A telephone survey of 1,072 persons, aged 18 to 65, in the Montreal health region was conducted to explore relationships between knowledge, beliefs, and AIDS-preventive practices.

Research

AIDS-preventive practices were more frequent among young or single people and those with one of four health beliefs: perceiving oneself as particularly susceptible to AIDS, perceiving the disease as particularly severe, perceiving AIDS as particularly amenable to prevention, or having a strong health motivation. Support for coercive measures to control the epidemic was widespread, but was particularly strong among the less educated, married people, and those with a high level of one of the following beliefs about AIDS: perceived severity, susceptibility, curability, or barriers to treatment. AIDS preventive practices and support for coercion share two modifiable determinants: perceived severity of AIDS, and perceived susceptibility to it. This finding suggests that emphasizing them may promote preventive practices, but may also increase support for coercive measures toward people with or at high risk of AIDS.

Of interest to health educators and public health officials.

308. "ANTHROPOLOGY and AIDS." *Medical Anthropology Review* 17 (1986): Entire Issue.

Describes the role of anthropologists in the AIDS epidemic.

Special Journal Issue

A series of articles describe how anthropologists can document aspects of AIDS, their role in the development of community-based prevention efforts, and their role in formulating public policy.

Of interest to social and behavioral scientists.

309. BENNETT, F.J.   "AIDS as a social phenomenon."   *Social
      Science and Medicine* 25 (1987): 529-539.

Views AIDS as a social phenomenon and explores its social repercussions.

Review

Describes political, behavioral, economic, and legal reactions to
AIDS, as well as such social responses as stigmatization, changes in
the sick role, the growth of voluntary organizations, and international collaboration. Considers the communication, education, and
information aspects of AIDS, and concludes that a massive educational
approach to modify behavior must be the basis for any program for its
control.

Of interest to social and behavioral scientists, public health
professionals, health educators, and health planners and policymakers.

310. BERK, Richard A.   "Anticipating the social consequences of
      AIDS: A position paper."   *The American Sociologist* 18
      (1987): 211-227.

A discussion of the social consequences of AIDS, focusing on the role
available to sociologists in anticipating and evaluating the long-term
social impact of the disease.

Discussion

Intelligent planning is seen as impossible without a reduction in the
uncertainty regarding the future. Efforts should be expended to fill
this void in information.

Of particular interest to social and behavioral scientists.

311. BLENDON, Robert J., and Karen Donelan.   "Discrimination
      against people with AIDS: The public's perspective."   *New
      England Journal of Medicine* 319 (1988): 1022-1026.

Reports on data from 53 national and international opinion surveys
conducted between 1983 and 1988.

Research

Findings suggest that persons being tested for AIDS cannot be
reassured regarding the potential discriminatory consequences of a
positive finding, and that public health education, alone, is
inadequate to prevent discrimination. Some rational action beyond the
provision of more public education may be required, especially if

widespread voluntary HIV testing is to be encouraged. New legislation is one way of creating a safe climate for persons who are infected with HIV and might allow public health officials to better carry out their responsibilities to control the epidemic.

Of interest to social scientists, public health officials, health educators, and public policymakers.

312. BLUMENFIELD, Michael, Peggy Jordano Smith, Jane Milazzo, Stuart Seropian, Gary P. Wormser. "Survey of attitudes of nurses working with AIDS patients."

Reports the results of a survey about caring for AIDS patients that was given to nurses at Westchester County Medical Center in July 1983 and January 1984.

Research

Two-thirds of the responding nurses reported that their friends or family had expressed concern about associating with hospital personnel who have contact with AIDS patients. Between one fourth and one half of the nurses had a fear of caring for homosexual men and male prisoners because of their awareness of AIDS. Half the nurses believed that AIDS could be transmitted to hospital personnel because of contact with patients despite precautions. The fear of caring for AIDS patients, as opposed to caring for hepatitis patients, was highest in the staff of the intensive care unit. Eight-five percent of the respondents believed that pregnant nurses should not care for AIDS patients, and half of the respondents indicated they would ask for a transfer if they had to care for an AIDS patient on a regular basis. The implications of these findings for future treatment programs, medical and nursing education, and psychologic support for staff are discussed.

Of interest to health professionals, hospital administrators, and health professions educators.

313. BOUTON, Richard A., Peggy E. Gallaher, Paul Arthur Garlinghouse, Terri Leal, Leslie D. Rosenstein, Robert K. Young. "Scales for measuring fear of AIDS and homophobia." *Journal of Personality Assessment* 51 (1987): 606-614.

Discusses two scales, one for measuring attitudes toward the fear of AIDS and one for measuring attitudes towards homosexuality, which were constructed using Thurstone's method of equal-appearing intervals.

Research

The scales were given to 528 students to determine their respective reliabilities, and factor analyses were done to determine what factors underlie the attitudes measured by the scales and to determine if fear of AIDS and homophobia are both facets of fear of homosexuals. The results indicated high reliability of both scales and a low correlation between the two scales, suggesting that they do measure different attitudes.

Of interest to social and behavioral scientists.

314. BOYTON, Rosemary, and Graham Scambler. "Survey of general
     practitioners' attitudes to AIDS in the North West Thames and
     East Anglian regions." *British Medical Journal* 296 (1988):
     538-540.

A survey was carried out among general practitioners to determine
their attitudes to AIDS and to the issues AIDS raises for them.

Research

One hundred and thirty-seven questionnaires were returned, and four
factors underlying the doctors' attitudes identified: concern with
disease control, general practitioner care, patient support, and
perception of seriousness. There were wide divergencies of attitude
among the general practitioners, younger doctors being more in line
with specialists' thinking on AIDS than older colleagues, and evidence
of important gaps between policies advocated by AIDS specialists and
bodies of opinion in general practice.

Of interest to general practitioners and family physicians.

315. BRANDT, Allan M. "AIDS and metaphor: Toward the social
     meaning of epidemic disease." *Social Research* 55 (1988):
     413-432.

Compares the process by which venereal diseases and AIDS acquired
social meaning and affected interventions.

Theoretical

Venereal disease became a metaphor for the concerns of the early
1900s, reflected by social values about sexuality, contagion, and
social organization. Interventions in the epidemic included antisex
education in the public schools, case reporting, testing, closing of
red light districts, and the incarceration of alleged carriers.
Responses to the AIDS epidemic reflect social concerns and
interventions similar to those related to venereal disease, and
demonstrate that individual behavior is subject to complex social
forces.

Of interest to social and behavioral scientists, public health
officials, and public policymakers.

316. BUISMAN, Noelyn, Andrew Chan Mow, Thomas Currie, Fenella
     Devereux, Bernard Fanning, Dorothy Hawkins, Helen Holden.
     "AIDS: Knowledge and attitudes in Otago." *New Zealand
     Medical Journal* 101 (1988): 241-243.

A questionnaire, sent to 307 randomly selected people in small towns
and rural areas of Southern New Zealand, examined public knowledge and
attitudes about AIDS, methods of obtaining information, and demographic data.

Research

Two hundred and three questionnaires were returned, a response rate of 66%. The mean score for knowledge was 80% with respondents in the 45-59 year age group scoring highest, closely followed by those in the 18-29 and 30-44 year groups; elderly people had the lowest scores. More than 10% of the respondents answered the most basic questions incorrectly, many were unaware that all blood donations in New Zealand are screened for HIV, and confusion regarding modes of transmission was widespread. However, many people were unconcerned about working with an AIDS virus carrier. Attitudes reflected the current controversy regarding availability of free needles and condoms. Compulsory blood testing was favored by 55% of the respondents. A majority of the respondents wanted more information about AIDS. Only 13% felt they were personally at risk, and 59% believed AIDS was not a major health problem in Otago and Southland.

Of interest to health educators and public health officials.

317. BURDA, David, and Suzanne Powills. "AIDS: A time bomb at
      hospitals' door." *Hospitals* 60, no. 1 (1986): 54-61.

Reviews the impact of AIDS on hospitals.

Descriptive

Discusses the cost for caring for AIDS patients, the issues surrounding the isolation of AIDS patients in hospitals, the impact of AIDS on hospital staff, and the issue of testing.

Of interest to hospital administrators and health professionals.

318. CHODOFF, Paul. "Fear of AIDS." *Psychiatry* 50 (1987):
      184-191.

The author offers a series of vignettes illustrating reactions to the threat of AIDS that range from the distinctly maladaptive to the appropriately adaptive.

Descriptive

Discusses some of the psychodynamic mechanisms operative in four cases, and makes general observations about the fear of AIDS in target populations.

Of interest to health professionals, health educators, and mental health professionals.

319. COLEMAN, Rosie M., David Curtis, Charlotte Feinmann.
      "Perception of risk of infection by injecting drug users and
      effects on medical clinic attendance." *British Journal of
      Addiction* 83 (1988): 1325-1329.

One hundred and sixty-two injection drug users attending two London clinics were asked if they thought they were at risk for HIV infection.

Research

There was no evidence that perception of risk influenced subjects in their intention to attend a medical clinic, and subjects who attended the medical clinic did not differ significantly from others attending the drug depending unit.

Of interest to drug abuse counselors and mental health professionals.

320.   COTTON, Deborah J.   "The impact of AIDS on the medical care
        system." *Journal of the American Medical Association* 260
        (1988): 519-523.

Discusses the impact of AIDS on health care manpower, risks to health care workers, and the impact on hospitals.

Commentary

The medical care system will be changed by AIDS. The effect of having so many young people dying of the same disease will be exceedingly depressing to health care workers. Prejudices and barriers in the health care system to treating gay and bisexual men and IV drug users as well as their sexual partners and children will have to be acknowledged and overcome. The ethical issues of allocation of scarce medical resources to the treatment of AIDS instead of to prenatal care, cancer, heart disease, and geriatrics will have to be addressed head on.

Of interest to all health professionals, ethicists, and laymen.

321.   COVELL, R.G.   "HIV infection and adoption in Scotland."
        Scottish Medical Journal 32 (1987): 117-119.

Discusses AIDS and adopted children.

Review

Discusses the effect of fear, attitudes, health effects, and family impact of adoption of HIV infected children and children suffering from AIDS.

Will interest a general audience.

322.   CUNNINGHAM, Ineke.   "The public controversies of AIDS in
        Puerto Rico." *Social Science and Medicine* 29 (1989): 545-553.

All articles using the word "AIDS" that appeared in the five major daily newspapers in Puerto Rico were studied to analyze the way in which AIDS has been presented in the daily press.

Descriptive

Virtually all newspaper articles regarding AIDS that pertained to Puerto Rico presented controversies; those about prevalence, incidence, and sources of funding were presented as controversies between the two main political parties, while those regarding risk factors, prevention, and treatment were presented as controversies between elected and appointed representatives of the people. Homosexuals, drug users, and hemophiliacs generally were not included as participants in the controversies. The controversies were generally nonmedical and nonscientific, suggesting that the public perceives insufficient interest on the part of medical and scientific leaders and is expropriating the problem. The proposed solutions were directed more toward the victims than the virus, a situation which is characteristic of past epidemics. The author concludes that unless an apolitical, socially organized assault is made on AIDS by the people, Puerto Rican society will have difficulty surviving the epidemic.

Of interest to social scientists, politicians, and public health officials.

323. DARROW, William W., Harold W. Jaffe, Pauline A. Thomas, *et al.* "Sex of interviewer, place of interview, and responses of homosexual men to sensitive questions." *Archives of Sexual Behavior* 15 (1986): 79-88.

Effects of sex of interviewer and place of interview on the responses of 57 AIDS patients and 145 other homosexual men were studied.

Research

Patients with AIDS tended to be interviewed in hospitals and doctors' offices, other men tended to be interviewed in hotel rooms, and patients tended to be different from other men. After adjustments were made for confounding, sex of interviewer and place of interview seemed to have little influence on the answers obtained.

Of interest to social and behavioral scientists.

324. DHOOPER, Surjit Singh, David T. Royse, Than V. Tran. "Social work practitioners' attitudes toward AIDS victims." *Journal of Applied Social Sciences* 12 (1987-88): 108-123.

Reports on a study of social work practitioners' fear of AIDS, their knowledge about it, and their attitudes towards its victims.

Research

Social workers, aged 35 or younger, were found to be more empathetic than older social workers; a greater proportion of single social workers and of recent graduates were less homophobic than were their married counterparts and those who graduated more than five years before. Fear of AIDS and empathy for AIDS victims were found to be inversely correlated. Knowledge of AIDS was associated with lower levels of fear and social distance concerns and greater empathy.

Of special interest to social workers and other mental health professionals.

325. DOUGLAS, Carolyn J., Concetta M. Kalman, Thomas P. Kalman. "Homophobia among physicians and nurses: An empirical study." *Hospital and Community Psychiatry* 36 (1985): 1309-1311.

Thirty-seven medical house officers and 91 registered nurses in a large teaching hospital treating many patients with AIDS completed a questionnaire designed to measure attitudes about homosexuality.

Research

Mean scores for both physicians and nurses fell in the low-grade homophobic range. There were no significant differences between the scores of doctors and nurses, but women were significantly more homophobic than men. Respondents who had a homosexual friend or relative were less homophobic than those who did not. Nearly 10% of the respondents agreed with the statement that homosexuals who contract AIDS are getting what they deserve. The authors consider this to be an alarming statistic and conclude that homophobia is higher than desirable among this group of health professionals.

Of interest to physicians, nurses, hospital administrators, and health professions educators.

326. DUPRAS, André, Joseph Levy, Jean-Marc Samson, Dominique Tessier. "Homophobia and attitudes about AIDS." *Psychological Reports* 64 (1989): 236-238.

A random sample of 407 French Canadian adults responded to a questionnaire about the perception of AIDS.

Research

This study shows that homophobia is a key indicator of sexual conservatism associated with negative attitudes about AIDS. That homosexuals have been the first AIDS victims may explain this situation. To modify attitudes about AIDS, the survey suggests that information campaigns should clearly indicate that homosexuality and AIDS are different phenomena. Indeed, mass media increasingly convey this information, since more cases of heterosexually contracted AIDS have been reported.

Of interest to health educators and social and behavioral scientists.

327. ENGEL, Wayne. "AIDS: Dealing with the hysteria." *Virginia Medical* 113 (April 1986): 222-224.

Discusses appropriate responses to what has become a psychological as well as a medical emergency.

Essay

Education and the dissemination of knowledge are the key tools that must be used to allay irrational fears about AIDS. Prevention requires understanding of how infection occurs and what actions or precautions will avoid it. Health professionals must take a personal responsibility for learning the facts about AIDS, its transmission, and its prevention and be prepared, at all times, to offer reliable information about contributing factors and the disease's transmissibility in a secure, nonjudgmental fashion.

Useful for physicians, nurses, and other health professionals.

328. EPSTEIN, Steven. "Moral contagion and the medicalizing of gay identity: AIDS in historical perspective." *Research in Law, Deviance and Social Control* 9 (1988): 3-36.

Examples of past epidemics that were interpreted as a punishment and led to the stigmatization of a particular group are given, and commonalities in these cases are isolated to develop a model that applies to AIDS.

Essay

AIDS is but the most recent example of a dangerous epidemic, linked to sex, that has been endowed with moral significance and presumed to be constitutive of the social identity of some stigmatized group. The author argues that in such a situation, medicine, by its very nature, becomes an institution that helps to displace social anxieties onto a scapegoat. In the case of AIDS, the focus on the "gay lifestyle" and gay "promiscuity" detoured society's ability to meet the threat of AIDS, and set in motion the forces of control and stigmatization. In asserting their identity, homosexuals have made themselves vulnerable to forms of social control that repress identifiable groups as being different in a biological sense. Gays and lesbians need to consider carefully the strategies they employ for social and political legitimization. Legitimization may be dangerous if it erodes conceptions of a shared humanity.

Of interest to social and behavioral scientists and to members of the gay community.

329. ERGAS, Yasmine. "The social consequences of the AIDS epidemic: A challenge for the social sciences." *Social Science Research Council* 41, nos. 3/4 (1987): 33-39.

Highlights the kinds of problems on which research and theoretical work must focus in order to set a framework for studying the social consequences of the AIDS epidemic.

Review

The AIDS epidemic has exerted, or may soon exert, a powerful influence on a wide variety of social organizations and processes. AIDS has led to the formation of new organizational structures and new solidarities; it may eventually lead to new definitions of rights and obligations, to new understandings of death and dying, and to new rituals for coping with disease. It has and will probably continue to lead to new scientific research and discoveries. Ultimately, the effects of the epidemic will reflect society's ability to use the knowledge at its disposal and to generate new knowledge to limit the spread and damage of the disease.   Social scientists have a complex task in determining the social consequences of the epidemic.   It requires understanding to what extent and how this epidemic will affect the structures of everyday life, reorder social groupings, harden boundaries, redefine gender and sex roles, affect life cycles and family cycles, and exert an impact on basic social structures.

Of interest to social scientists.

330. FAN, David P., and Gregory McAvoy. "Predictions of public opinion on the spread of AIDS: Introduction of new computer methodologies." *Journal of Sex Research* 26 (1989): 159-187.

Describes a computer methodology, which has several important advantages for studies of the impact of the media on public opinion.

Descriptive

The authors show the usefulness of a new methodology whereby opinion, e.g., of the spread of AIDS, can be estimated using the mathematical model of idiodynamics. As input, the model uses information in the mass media scored by computer, using the technique of successive filtrations. Such opinion computations can be made over any period of time, however long or short, so long as the mass media provide the major information about the issue.

Of interest to public opinion analysts.

331. FINK, Raymond. "Changes in public reaction to a new epidemic: The case of AIDS." *Bulletin of the New York Academy of Medicine* 63 (1987): 940-949.

This report describes the results of public opinion and attitude surveys in the United States which included questions about AIDS.

Research

The results suggest that one possible approach to educating the public in what it should know about AIDS might be conveying different messages to different target populations. This would require that the messages be appropriate to the specific target groups to which they are directed.

Of interest to health professionals and the public.

332. FRIEDLAND, Gerald. "AIDS and compassion." *Journal of the American Medical Association* 259 (1988): 2898-2899.

Cites three reasons for lack of compassion towards AIDS patients—fear of transmission, negative views of the social worth of individuals at risk, and the nature of plagues in our mind and human history—and shows why each is inappropriate.

Commentary

Normal daily interactions do not transmit HIV; treating at-risk or infected individuals as if they were highly infectious is unwarranted and uncompassionate. Behavior, not group identity, results in HIV transmission. Many individuals became infected before anything was known about HIV, and a substantial reduction in high risk behavior has been reported in recent years. "Blaming the victim" is inappropriate; rather, we should be openly talking about risky behaviors, advocating broader, targeted education about risky behaviors, and working to eliminate social conditions that promote unhealthy behaviors. Failure to comprehend the magnitude of the plague has resulted in the lack of a national plan to contain the epidemic and an inadequate marshalling of resources for health care, prevention, and research. As the AIDS epidemic progresses, the strength of our culture will be measured by the level of compassion evidenced by society, health professionals, and individuals.

Of general interest.

333. FRIEDMAN, Samuel R., Jo L. Sotheran, Abu Abdul-Quader, *et al.* "The AIDS epidemic among blacks and Hispanics." *The Milbank Quarterly* 65, Supplement 2 (1987): 455-499.

This article has three themes: AIDS has disproportionately affected minorities; there is a great need for minority community mobilization to deal with the epidemic; and blacks and Hispanics have developed resources and relationships that offer many benefits in fighting AIDS.

Descriptive

Blacks and Hispanics are more likely than whites to get AIDS. This is true among gays, among IV drug users and their heterosexual partners, and among children. There is considerable evidence that blacks have been at least as likely as whites to attempt to reduce their risk. Many IV drug users have cut back on behaviors that put them and others at risk. Several recommendations are offered.

Of interest to social and behavioral scientists, public health officials, and health policymakers.

334. GAINES, Josephine, Albert F. Iglar, Mary L. Michal, and Robert D. Patton. "Attitudes towards AIDS." *Health Values* 12, no. 4 (1988): 53-60.

Reports on the attitudes of a select group of college students in rural Appalachia towards AIDS and people with AIDS.

Research

The attitudes found in this study would stigmatize persons with AIDS, as well as lead to physical and social isolation. The feelings that were reported would exclude persons, generally, from the job market. The findings reflected moralistic and judgmental attitudes towards persons with AIDS. However, there was recognition by the majority of the students that AIDS was a social problem. The preponderance of negative attitudes and misconceptions indicates the need for expanded AIDS educational programs.

Of interest to health educators and social and behavioral scientists.

335. GINZBURG, Harold M. (Ed.). "The psychosocial aspects of AIDS." *Psychiatric Annals* 16 (1986): 135-185.

A collection of five articles, designed to explore the psychosocial implications of HTLV-III diseases.

Special Journal Issue

Begins with a brief epidemiologic overview of HTLV-III diseases; addresses the neurological complications associated with HTLV-III diseases; discusses the social dimensions of AIDS; presents a therapeutic model for addressing the clinical and social problems of infected patients; and explores the legal and ethical issues that have evolved in dealing with patients with HTLV-III diseases.

Of interest to health care, mental health, and social service professionals.

336. GRIEGER, Ingrid, and Joseph G. Ponterotto. "Students' knowledge of AIDS and their attitudes toward gay men and lesbian women." *Journal of College Student Development* 29 (1988): 415-422.

A convenience sample of 198 predominantly white university students was surveyed to determine the students' level of knowledge of AIDS and their attitudes toward people with AIDS and toward homosexuals.

Research

Data indicated that a majority of the students were accurately informed on AIDS. Overall, the students did not have negative views regarding homosexuality or punitive attitudes toward persons with AIDS. They did not advocate exclusionary policies, nor did they view AIDS as a punishment. Closeness with a gay person was found to be the most discriminatory variable among attitudes toward homosexuals.

Should interest health service personnel and educators in universities and colleges.

337. GRÖNFERS, Martti, and Olli Stålström. "Power, prestige, profit: AIDS and the oppression of homosexual people." *Acta Sociologica* 30 (1987): 53-66.

Discusses the negative social and psychological impact of AIDS on homosexual people.

Descriptive

The appearance of the AIDS virus has resulted in a renewal of overt and covert hostility to gays, who are frequently considered a threat to "decent" values in society and to the "decent" members of society. Careers and monetary gain can be made out of AIDS. The news media has been exploiting public curiosity and fear, satisfying the need for villains and heroes, entering and feeding the general rush for emotion, using and being used, all for profit. The medical profession's attempt to define the AIDS issue as a medical problem largely has to do with power, prestige, and profit. In the midst of all of these secondary issues, those suffering from AIDS or fearing it tend to be forgotten.

Of interest to social and behavioral scientists.

338. HARDING, T.W. "AIDS in prison." *Lancet* 2, no. 8570 (1987): 1260-1263.

A survey, carried out in 17 countries, shows how prison doctors and administrators have reacted to the AIDS epidemic.

Research

The pressing need to control HIV infection in prison, to counsel and support seropositive prisoners, to care for prisoners who get AIDS, and to cope with the psychosocial pressures within a closed, authoritarian environment poses a serious challenge to prison medical services. It is far from certain that they have sufficient resources and professional independence to cope.

Of special interest to prison administrators and health professionals working in prisons, as well as judicial and law enforcement personnel.

339. HARRINGTON, Eugene. "A fatal bias: AIDS and minorities." *Human Rights* 14, no. 3 (1987): 34-37, 52.

Discusses differences in the response to AIDS and the care given its sufferers depending upon the risk group to which the patient belongs.

Commentary

Blacks and Hispanics in the United States make up a disproportionate number of persons with AIDS, but leaders in the minority communities have been slow to respond to the problem. Because members of the black and Hispanic communities frequently have less access to adequate health care, more unbalanced nutrition, less effective, or nonexistent, health insurance, and are less apt to perceive themselves and their partners as being at risk than their white counterparts, medical intervention is later in coming, and, due in part to the high

cost of treatment, probably of a poorer quality. In addition to
sensitizing the gay/lesbian support groups to minority issues, there
is a need to educate some special interest groups, such as advocates
for the handicapped, advocates for prison reform, and drug program
workers, regarding the legal and ethical issues involved in the AIDS
epidemic.

Of interest to health educators, public health officials, social
welfare workers, and concerned laypersons.

340.   HEAVEN, Patrick C.L.   "Beliefs about the spread of the
       acquired immunodeficiency syndrome."   *Medical Journal of
       Australia* 147 (September 21, 1987): 272-274.

Beliefs about the spread of AIDS were determined among a community
sample of Australians.

Research

No sex differences were found, although age and educational level
appeared to have some influence on beliefs.   The findings are
discussed in light of a recent television advertising campaign about
AIDS.

Of interest to health professionals, health educators, and public
health officials.

341.   HEIN, Karen, and Marsha Hurst.   "Human immunodeficiency
       virus infection in adolescence: A rationale for action."
       Adolescent and Pediatric Gynecology 1 (1988): 73-82.

Aspects of adolescent physiology, sexual and drug-related behavior,
and development are examined in the context of AIDS risk.   Legal,
ethical, and sociopolitical ramifications are explored.

Review

A model is proposed that provides a conceptual framework for analysis
of relative risk of HIV infection in various adolescent subgroups.
This model can be used as a basis for recommendations related to HIV
infection in adolescents.

Of interest to pediatricians, health educators, teachers, and school
administrators.

342.   HILL, Ronald Paul.   "An exploration of the relationship between
       AIDS-related anxiety and the evaluation of condom advertise-
       ments.   *Journal of Advertising* 17, no. 34 (1988): 35-42.

The relationship between AIDS-related anxiety and the evaluation of
condom advertisements was investigated.

Research

Data suggest that subjects' attitudes toward condom ads and brands may
have been the product of different causes of anxiety. Attitudes
toward the condom ads may have been based on a subject's level of
anxiety concerning the spread of AIDS in society. However, attitudes
toward the condom brands may have been based on the extent of personal
threat from infection through sexual contact. Data show that subjects
held more positive attitudes for the moderate fear appeal than the
high fear and non-fear appeals.

Of interest to health educators and public health officials.

343. HOGAN, Tom. "Psychophysical relation between perceived
     threat of AIDS and willingness to impose social restrictions."
     Health Psychology 8, No. 2 (1989): 255-266.

Psychophysical methods were applied to measure and analyze attitudes
toward the threat and control of AIDS.

Research

Participants rated and gave magnitude estimations for the amount of
social restriction in 12 possibilities for controlling AIDS. The
relation between ratings and magnitude estimations were curvilinear.
Perceived threat to society increased as the estimated number of
people with the virus increased. The amount of social restriction
imposed was a negatively accelerated growth function of increasing
levels of threat. The negative acceleration was probably due to
ethical considerations associated with more stringent methods of
control.

Of interest to social and behavioral scientists.

344. HOPKINS, Donald R. "AIDS in minority populations in the
     United States." *Public Health Reports* 102 (1987): 677-681.

Discusses the implications for public health policy of the disproportionate number of cases of AIDS among blacks and Hispanics in the
United States.

Review/Commentary

Blacks and Hispanics in the United States, who compose 12% and seven
percent of the population, respectively, constitute 24% and 14% of the
AIDS cases. Seventy-eight percent of all children with AIDS are black
or Hispanic, as are 71% of all women with AIDS. IV drug abuse is
associated with much of the transmission of AIDS in these populations, and parenterally acquired infections are spread secondarily by
sexual and perinatal transmission. Intervention programs are needed,
which are intended especially for the black and Hispanic communities,
take into account important differences in the understanding of AIDS
and HIV infection, and emphasize greatly intensified prevention and
treatment of IV drug abuse, to supplement programs aimed at the
general public. In combatting AIDS, the black and Hispanic communities have the opportunity to greatly reduce some serious social
problems, including IV drug abuse, other sexually transmitted
diseases, and teenage pregnancy.

Of particular interest to public health officials and social scientists.

345. HUNT, Charles W. "AIDS and capitalist medicine." *Monthly Review* 39, no. 8 (1988): 11-25.

The author proposes that the AIDS crisis is likely to accent the threefold crisis in North American medicine by drastically increasing costs and per capita medical expenses, by decreasing confidence in the medical care system, and by increasing the maldistribution of health care.

Essay

Concludes that the AIDS crisis will make the crisis in North American medicine more extreme. By exerting pressure for increases in the cost of medicine and decreasing confidence in North American medicine, the AIDS epidemic is likely to bring about an even greater maldistribution of medical care than that which presently exists. AIDS will increase the existing contradictions of the health care system, and these contradictions will, in turn, make the health care system's responses to AIDS less effective and successful.

Particularly interesting to social and behavioral scientists.

346. JOHNSON, Stephen D. "Factors related to intolerance of AIDS victims." *Journal for the Scientific Study of Religion* 26 (1987): 105-110.

Randomly selected residents of Muncie, Indiana were administered a questionnaire that included two items measuring the rejection of AIDS victims.

Research

The only variable found to relate independently to rejection of AIDS victims was the perception that the U.S. had not recognized the contributions of Christian fundamentalists.

Of interest to students of religion and social scientists.

347. KORCOK, Milan. "AIDS hysteria: A contagious side effect." *Canadian Medical Association Journal* 133 (1985): 1241-1248.

A discussion of the problems caused by unreasonable fears regarding AIDS.

Descriptive

Together with the reliable information being propagated in public health education is a lot of misinformation about AIDS, often resulting in unreasonable fear. AIDS hysteria is disruptive and costly and has become a major problem for the public health service.

348. LESTER, David. "Attitudes toward AIDS." *Personality and Individual Differences* 10 (1989): 693-694.

A scale to measure attitudes toward AIDS patients and to explore correlates of these attitudes was developed in an effort to further understanding of the prejudice against patients suffering from AIDS.

Research

The scale was administered to 78 male and 45 female undergraduate college students, aged 18-22. Results showed an independence between negative and positive attitudes toward AIDS patients. Males had stronger negative attitudes toward AIDS patients than females and, for males only, scores on a hysteroid-obsessoid questionnaire were positively associated with positive attitudes towards AIDS patients.

Of interest to social and behavioral scientists.

349. "LIVING with AIDS." *Daedalus* 118, no. 2 (1989): Entire Issue.

The first of two issues dedicated to the dissemination of useful knowledge for living and coping with AIDS and the political, moral, and social dilemmas it creates.

Special Journal Issue

AIDS is not likely to depart from the scene. Therefore, it is important to determine how the disease can be lived with; how the ill and the soon to be ill can be cared for; how the uninfected can remain so; what specific social conditions can be changed to contain the spread of AIDS; what hopes there are for behavior change that will make new infection unlikely; what institutional changes will curb the spread of the disease; and what new knowledge is needed to cope with the social and economic problems created by AIDS. The nine articles in this issue deal with: AIDS in historical perspective; the challenge AIDS presents to biomedical research; AIDS in the U.S.: patient care and politics; clinical care in the AIDS epidemic; living with AIDS; AIDS policies in Britain, Sweden, and the U.S.; international interests in AIDS control; AIDS as human suffering; and the epidemiology and transmission dynamics of HIV-AIDS.

Of interest to social and behavioral scientists, health professionals, mental health professionals, public health officials, public policymakers, legislators, and laypersons.

350. "LIVING with AIDS." *Daedalus* 118, no. 3 (1989): Entire Issue.

The second of two issues dedicated to the dissemination of useful knowledge for living and coping with AIDS and the political, moral, and social dilemmas it creates.

Special Journal Issue

The issues discussed in the ten articles that make up this issue
include: prospects for the medical control of the AIDS epidemic;
social policy concerning AIDS and IV drug use; disease and desire;
AIDS, privacy, and responsibility; AIDS and the law; public health and
the politics of AIDS prevention; AIDS, blood banking, and the bonds of
community; AIDS in Africa: diversity in the global pandemic; and AIDS
prevention through effective education.

Of interest to social and behavioral scientists, health professionals,
mental health professionals, public health officials, public
policymakers, legislators, and laypersons.

351. McCOMBIE, S.C.   "The cultural impact of the AIDS' test: The
       American experience." *Social Science and Medicine* 23 (1986):
       455-459.

Discusses the cultural impact of the HIV test in the U.S.

Discussion

All of the emotions and attitudes associated with AIDS have been
projected on to those who test positive. A review of the circumstances surrounding the release of this test illustrates the extent to
which cultural beliefs and attitudes affect public health and medical
practice. It suggests that contagion has a social definition, even in
the context of Western scientific medicine.

Of interest to health professionals and social and behavioral
scientists.

352. MACK, Arien (Ed.).   "In time of plague: The history and social
       consequences of lethal epidemic disease." *Social Research* 55
       (1988): 323-528.

Papers presented at a conference held at the New School for Social
Research in January 1988 in an attempt to put the AIDS epidemic into
perspective by considering it in the context of the social history of
past lethal epidemics.

Special Journal Issue

The editor states, in his introduction, that this conference was
organized with the hope that focusing attention on the many ways in
which diseases, particularly catastrophic infectious diseases, are and
have been both biologically and socially defined might help lead the
way to a calmer and more effective public response to the problem of
AIDS. The text that follows is divided into four sections: the
definition and control of disease; science and health--possibilities,
probabilities, and limitations; case histories; and moral dilemmas.
The sections parallel the four conference sessions, and each is
introduced by the moderator of the session in which the papers were
presented.

Of general interest.

353. MARKOVA, Ivana, and Patricia Wilkie. "Representations, con-
      cepts and social change: The phenomenon of AIDS." *Journal
      for the Theory of Social Behavior* 17 (1987): 389-409.

Discusses the AIDS epidemic as a social phenomenon.

Discussion

Discusses the social history of AIDS, its public impact, and the
cognitive and emotional responses of the public. Compares public
responses to syphilis in the past to public responses to AIDS today,
demonstrating how those responses are shaped by and contribute to
changes in the social climate of the times, and shows how two major
social factors, the gay community and the media, have influenced the
formation of public representations of AIDS.

Of particular interest to social scientists.

354. MARKS, Gary, Jean L. Richardson, L. Thomas Lochner,
      Kimberly A. McGuignan, Alexandra Levine. "Assumed
      similarity of attitudes about AIDS among gay and heterosexual
      physicians." *Journal of Applied Psychology* 18 (1988):
      774-786.

Samples of heterosexual and gay physicians were requested to indicate
their own attitudinal positions on several issues related to the AIDS
epidemic and to attribute a position on each issue to the target
group, "most people."

Research

The heterosexual physicians' attitudes were more negative than those
of the gay physicians. Both groups judged that "most people" hold
attitudes more negative than their own. The distance between own and
attributed position was much greater for the gay individuals.

Of interest to social psychologists and social and behavioral
scientists.

355. MAYS, Vickie M., and Susan D. Cochran. "Acquired
      immunodeficiency syndrome and black Americans: Special
      psychosocial issues." *Public Health Reports* 102 (1987):
      224-231.

Examines three areas of concern when focusing on AIDS in the black
population: differences from whites in patterns of transmission of the
infection, cultural factors that may affect health education efforts,
and ethnically relevant issues in the provision of medical care to
black persons with AIDS.

Discussion

The epidemiologic pattern of infection in the black population differs from that of whites. Blacks make up nearly 25% of reported AIDS cases. It is estimated that between one and 1.4% of the black population may be infected with HIV. Educational interventions designed to slow the rate of infection need to be sensitive to cultural and behavioral differences between blacks and whites who are at risk for acquiring or transmitting HIV. The psychological, sociocultural, and medical care issues are important to take into account when caring for black AIDS patients.

Of interest to public health officials, health educators, and social and behavioral scientists.

356. MEISENHELDER, Janice Bell, and Christopher L. LaCharite. "Fear of contagion: A stress response to acquired immunodeficiency syndrome." Advances in Nursing Science 11, no. 2 (1989): 29-38.

Suggests education on cross-cultural, sexual, and death-related issues, as well as factual information on AIDS to decrease fear.

Descriptive

Fear of contagion is an effective stress response to the neurocognitive activity that leads to a perceived threat of AIDS. This perception of danger is based largely on the symbolic meaning of this disease, its association with mystery, death, punishment, and sexuality. The stress response of fear results in avoidance, extreme caution, and fearful verbal behaviors. The research implications include verification of the model, its concepts and relationships, as well as exploration of the impact of fear of contagion on nursing care.

Of interest to nurses and other health care professionals.

357. MORTON, A.D., and I.C. McManus. "Attitudes to and knowledge about the acquired immune deficiency syndrome: Lack of a correlation." British Medical Journal 293 (1986): 1212.

The authors examined attitudes about AIDS among preclinical medical students.

Research

Attitudes to AIDS and its treatment among a group of preclinical medical students did not correlate with knowledge about the condition, but generally related to attitudes concerning homosexuality. The implication for health education is clear; if we are to reduce the prejudice about AIDS and to increase public awareness of the problems of patients with AIDS, there should be increased emphasis on general education about homosexuality rather than on the specific, factual details of the disease.

Of interest to health educators and public health officials.

358. NUTBEAM, Don, John C. Catford, Simon A. Smail, Colin Griffiths. "Public knowledge and attitudes to AIDS." *Public Health* 103 (1989): 205-211.

Three independent cross-sectional surveys of public knowledge and attitudes about AIDS were conducted on a representative sample of people, age 15-54, in Wales.

Research

The results show that most people knew that having sexual intercourse or sharing needles with people with AIDS represented a high risk of catching AIDS. However, there appeared to be considerable misunderstanding about the nature of HIV infection; one in three thought that a man and woman with a single heterosexual partner was at high or moderate risk for catching AIDS. The high level of concern, coupled with considerable confusion, appears to have contributed to both unnecessary anxiety and prejudice.

Of interest to health educators and public health officials.

359. ORTON, Simon, and John Samuels. "What we have learned from researching AIDS." *Journal of the Marketing Research Society* 30 (1988): 3-34.

A case history setting out what the authors have learned from a major program of research into public knowledge, attitudes, and behavior in relation to AIDS, with emphasis on research methodology.

Case History

Section I discusses the background, presenting data on the incidence and spread of AIDS in Britain and projections for the future. Section II describes the sample design for the general public and homo-sexuals. Section III is devoted to questionnaire design. Section IV covers the reactions of the interviewers to working on a project obtaining such sensitive information. Section V explains how the project was extended from the general public to include young people. Section VI gives some results to demonstrate changes in knowledge, attitudes, and behavior. Section VII presents four concluding observations.

Of particular interest to social and behavioral scientists, public opinion analysts, and public health officials.

360. PAXTON, Cynthia, and David Susky. "AIDS, homophobia, and sexual attitudes." *Health Values* 12, no. 4 (1988): 39-43.

A discussion about the association between AIDS and homosexuality, which has resulted in a dismissal of the realities of this sexually transmitted disease.

Essay

If it is possible that any good can come from the AIDS epidemic, it will be that this disease will have enabled us to correct many long-standing prejudices in our understanding of human sexuality.

Of interest to health educators.

361. PETERSON, Candida C., and James L. Peterson. "Australian students' ratings of the importance of AIDS relative to other community problems." *Australian Journal of Sex, Marriage & Family* 8, no. 4 (1987): 194-200.

The perceptions of 87 university students in western Australia regarding the seriousness of AIDS relative to the seriousness of other community problems were assessed.

Research

Thirty-seven percent of the students ranked AIDS as a greater threat to the community than any other problem, including unemployment, crime, drugs, and nuclear weapons. There was a significant gender difference in the results; women evaluated AIDS as a more serious threat than did men.

Of interest to social scientists and public health professionals.

362. POIRIER, Richard. "AIDS and traditions of homophobia." *Social Research* 55 (1988): 461-475.

Cites evidence of the historic stigmatization of homosexuality and decries efforts to use the AIDS crisis as a campaign against homosexuality.

Review/Commentary

Homosexuality has been characterized as unnatural in the writings of early church founders, St. Thomas, Dante, Freud, Pope John Paul II, and Patrick Buchanan. This characterization has contributed, throughout the AIDS epidemic, to the scapegoating of homosexuals, campaigns against anal intercourse, and withholding of funds for safe sex education.

Of interest to social and behavioral scientists and the lay public.

363. POLAKOFF, Phillip L. "Irrational fear: Another AIDS infection pervading and paralyzing the country." *Occupational Health and Safety* 55, no. 12 (1986): 50.

Proposes that AIDS is generating a secondary, societal infection: irrational fear and revulsion among people not otherwise affected.

Commentary

Advocates that physicians and health care providers create as calm and enlightened an atmosphere as possible for the victims and the fearful as the search for prevention and cure goes on.

Of interest to health professionals and laymen.

364. PRYOR, John B., Glen D. Reeder, Richard Vinacco, Jr., Teri L. Kott. "The instrumental and symbolic functions of attitudes toward persons with AIDS." *Journal of Applied Social Psychology* 19 (1989): 377-404.

Five studies explored the psychological bases of attitudes toward persons with AIDS, examining both the instrumental and symbolic bases of these attitudes.

Research

In Studies 1, 2, and 3, both instrumental (beliefs about the probability of one's own child contracting AIDS) and symbolic factors (general attitudes toward homosexuality) contributed to the prediction of attitudes toward having one's child attend classes with a non-homosexual person with AIDS. In Study 4, attitudes toward homosexuality, and not beliefs about contagiousness, related to students' expression of a desire to transfer from a class with an AIDS-infected professor. In Study 5, subjects role played the situation experienced by subjects in Study 4, and a wider array of instrumental concerns was assessed. Both instrumental and symbolic factors were related to attitudes, but the specific instrumental concerns of importance were related to beliefs about feeling comfortable with the professor, not to fear of contagion. The findings are discussed with regard to their relevance for understanding the varying functions of attitudes and for understanding the stigmatization of disease.

Of interest to social and behavioral scientists.

365. ROSS, Michael. "Components and structure of attitudes toward AIDS." *Hospital and Community Psychiatry* 39 (1988): 1306-1312.

A study was carried out to determine the structure of attitudes toward AIDS in the general public.

Research

A strong correlation was found between homonegative opinions and social conservatism. The most homonegative individuals also had the most unreasonable concerns about AIDS and the least recognition that AIDS can be transmitted nonsexually. People who knew homosexual individuals were less homophobic. No significant age or gender related differences were noted. Fear of death and of the unknown are also significant components of attitudes toward AIDS and are significantly correlated.

Of interest to health educators and public health professionals.

366. ROSS, Michael W. "AIDS phobia: Report of 4 cases." *Psycho-
      pathology* 21 (1988): 26-30.

Illustrates the course, psychodynamics, and treatment of AIDS phobia
through the use of case reports.

Case Reports

AIDS phobia may be triggered by life stresses and media publicity
about AIDS. It often presents a hypochondria and is associated with
guilt over sexual behavior. Symptoms can usually be resolved by brief
interpretive counseling that focuses on the underlying conflicts and
stresses.

Of interest to psychologists, psychotherapists, counselors, and social
workers.

367. ————. "Distribution of knowledge of AIDS: A national study."
      Social Science and Medicine 27 (1988): 1295-1298.

Knowledge of, and attitudes toward, AIDS were assessed in a random
sample of over 2600 individuals, aged 16 and over, in all states and
territories of Australia.

Research

There were no differences in knowledge of AIDS across states or
between sexes. Individuals with lower knowledge of AIDS were more
likely to be separated, divorced, widowed, older, more conservative,
and more personally concerned about AIDS; they had greater fear of
homosexuals, more unrealistic concerns about AIDS, and were more apt
to blame the infected and more afraid of the unknown aspects of AIDS
than those with higher knowledge. Individuals who had used IV drugs
ever and in the past year had significantly lower knowledge of AIDS.
Individuals who personally knew homosexual people had higher knowledge
of AIDS.

Of interest to health educators, social scientists, and public health
officials.

368. ROUNDS, Kathleen A. "AIDS in rural areas: Challenges to
      providing care." *Social Work* 33 (1988): 257-261.

Examines the development and provision of services to persons with
AIDS and their families in rural areas and barriers to the delivery of
care.

Research

Several barriers to providing care to persons with AIDS and their
families living in rural areas emerged during the analysis of
interviews of 15 persons involved in coordinating or delivering such
services in a Southeastern state in which 48% of the population is
rural. The distance to health care facilities that treat AIDS

patients and the difficulties associated with transportation constitute a major problem in the provision of health and social care to
AIDS patients in rural areas. Another serious problem, which isolates
people when they are most in need of support, is fear of disclosure
and maintenance of confidentiality in communities where "everyone
knows everyone and everyone knows your business." Fear of contagion
and homophobia also cause difficulty in arranging for services in
certain communities. Proposals are made for social work interventions, focusing on coordinating, strengthening, and expanding existing
community resources and networks, to provide the care and support
needed by AIDS patients and their families.

Of interest to social workers and health care providers.

369. ROYSE, David, Surjit Singh Dhooper, Laurie Russell Hatch.
"Undergraduate and graduate students' attitudes towards
AIDS." Psychological Reports 60 (1987): 1185-1186.

An exploration of the association of fear of AIDS with knowledge about
AIDS and empathy towards AIDS victims.

Research

An available sample of 219 students at the University of Kentucky
responded to a questionnaire about AIDS that had been constructed
from a review of salient issues appearing in the popular press.
Undergraduate or graduate status was not found to be a good predictor
of empathy towards AIDS victims, fear of AIDS, or knowledge of AIDS.
Knowledge about AIDS was a better predictor of fear than was age,
race, or sex. Greater knowledge was associated with greater empathy.

Of interest to social and behavioral scientists.

370. SELIK, Richard M., Kenneth G. Castro, Marguerite
Pappaioanou, James W. Buehler. "Birthplace and the risk of
AIDS among Hispanics in the United States." American
Jouranal of Public Health 79 (1989): 836-839.

The authors compared U.S. residents born in different Latin American
countries and computed the cumulative incidence of AIDS and the
distribution of cases by mode of exposure.

Research

The reference group was the non-Hispanic white population. In the
South and West, the rate in Mexican-born Hispanics was half the
reference rate. In each U.S. region, the cumulative incidence of AIDS
in heterosexual IV drug abusers in Puerto Rican-born persons was
several times greater than that for other Latin American-born persons;
most of these cases occurred in heterosexual IV drug abusers. The data
suggest that resources for preventing AIDS are needed most among those
of Puerto Rican ethnicity addicted to drug abuse.

Of interest to health educators and public health officials.

371. SINGER, Eleanor, Theresa F. Rogers, Mary Corcoran.
      "Report: AIDS." *Public Opinion Quarterly* 51 (1987):
      580-595.

A summary of several nationwide opinion polls about AIDS.

Research

The data indicate no trend of increasing concern about AIDS as a
problem for one's own health. The data on beliefs about transmission
indicate widespread accuracy at the extremes with some confusion about
intermediate modes. The evidence is mixed with regard to attitudes
about regulation. There is a slight increase in the number of people
reporting that they are changing their behavior as a result of AIDS.
The data also provide evidence that the public credits the media with
being an important source of information about AIDS.

Of interest to public opinion analysts, public health officials, and
health professionals.

372. STIPP, Horst, and Dennis Kerr. "Determinants of public opinion
      about AIDS." *Public Opinion Quarterly* 53 (1989): 98-106.

A study of determinants of public opinion about AIDS.

Research

Findings from analyses presented in this paper, using data from a
Roper survey, suggest that the role of attitudes toward homosexuals
should be at the center of future explorations of the relationship
between the media coverage of AIDS and public opinion. While the data
are limited, the authors' analyses raise the possibility that anti-gay
attitudes constrain the ability of the media to effectively
communicate information about risk factors and how the disease is
transmitted. Researchers need to explore the possibility that
anti-gay attitudes stand between media information and public
knowledge and public opinion.

Of interest to social and behavioral scientists and health educators.

373. TRIPLET, Rodney G., and David B. Sugarman. "Reactions to
      AIDS victims: Ambiguity breeds contempt." *Personality and
      Social Psychology* 13 (1987): 265-274.

The causes of negative reactions towards AIDS victims were
investigated.

Research

A questionnaire, administered to 58 subjects, required rating the
personal responsibility and interactional desirability of eight
hypothetical victims of disease who varied only on their sexual
preference and on their diagnosis (AIDS, serum hepatitis,
Legionnaire's disease, genital herpes). Homosexual victims were rated

more personally responsible for their disease, and AIDS victims were rated least desirable interactionally. However, no support was found for a victim derogation interpretation of the ratings. The results were interpreted as suggesting that the reaction against AIDS victims reflects a fear of the unknown causes of the disease and a general prejudice against homosexuals.

Of interest to social and behavioral scientists engaged in research on AIDS.

374. VALDISERRI, Ronald O. "Epidemics in perspective." *Journal of Medical Humanities and Bioethics* 8 (1987): 95-100.

Irrational responses to AIDS patients, particularly in regard to HIV transmissibility, are examined from a historical and psychosocial perspective.

Discussion

Although societal responses to AIDS are similar to those reported during past epidemics, they are in direct conflict with today's level of medical understanding. Their genesis may be related to the reaction to AIDS as a metaphor. In order to allay public concern about AIDS, it is essential to recognize the metaphor associated with venereal disease in general and AIDS in particular.

Of interest to health professionals, educators, social workers, ethicists, and public health officials.

375. VELIMIROVIC, B. "AIDS as a social phenomenon." *Social Science and Medicine* 25 (1987): 541-552.

Discusses AIDS as a social as well as an infectious disease, speculating about the effects that AIDS may have on complex social structures in general, on health structures in particular, and on the problems which may shape future attitudes, values, and morals.

Review/Theoretical

AIDS has created social, political, ethical, and legal problems that extend far beyond traditional medical interests and create polarization among the public, politicians, the press, and among physicians. The fear among major risk groups is more pronounced than is warranted by society's response, and conflicts between perceived individual versus collective rights are bound to grow. However, the position of major risk groups is changing in various ways, and society is no longer reluctant to address issues of sexual behavior openly. Information is accumulating rapidly about social influences in the spread of the disease, although little is known, as yet, about the influence of social factors on control efforts and the effectiveness of preventive behavioral strategies. The long term effects of AIDS upon societal structure, attitudes, and values cannot be delineated with any accuracy, but can only be guessed at.

Of general interest.

376. WITT, L. Alan.   "Authoritarianism, knowledge of AIDS, and
     affect toward persons with AIDS: Implications for health
     education." *Journal of Applied Social Psychology* 19 (1989):
     599-607.

A sample of 406 undergraduate university students were asked to
indicate their knowledge of AIDS and affect toward persons with AIDS
and to take the California F-scale.

Research

Results indicated a significant relationship between authoritarianism
and affect toward persons with AIDS.   Knowledge of AIDS was very
slightly related to affect toward persons with AIDS, but it did not
moderate the relationship between authoritarianism and affect toward
persons with AIDS.   The findings are interpreted as having possible
implications for health education.

Of interest to social and behavioral scientists and health educators.

c. Chapter

377. HIRSCH, Dan Alan, and Roger W. Enlow.   "The effects of the
     acquired immune deficiency syndrome on gay lifestyle and the
     gay individual."   *In* Irving J. Selikoff, Alvin S. Teirstein,
     Shalom Z. Hirschman (Eds.).   *Acquired Immune Deficiency
     Syndrome.*   New York: New York Academy of Sciences, 1984.

The authors discuss the multifaceted psychosocial reactions to AIDS
and illustrate the range of behaviors they have observed in healthy
gay men in the New York gay community.

Discussion

The shifting rates of sexually transmitted diseases denote a more
conservative pattern of sexual activity in the gay community.   The
presence of AIDS may bring about a change in public attitude towards
homosexuality.   Further research on this population is indicated to
investigate these changes.

Of interest to psychiatrists and other mental health professionals
treating AIDS patients.

d. Dissertations

378. ELWELL, Patricia A.   "Psychological correlates of attitudes
     towards and knowledge of AIDS in a college population."
     Ph.D. dissertation, Boston College, 1988.

A survey of a 320-subject random sample of students at Bentley
College, MA, stratified by class, seeking information about student
attitudes towards and knowledge of AIDS.

Research

A 66-item attitudinal scale and a 22-item knowledge scale were used to determine whether the subject's anger level, anxiety level, personal causality orientation, and dogmatism level affect his or her response to AIDS; in what ways these personality characteristics are interdependent, and what developmental changes occur in these attitudes and personality characteristics. Sex differences were found for all AIDS factors, with females being less rejecting and hostile towards AIDS victims, more interested in behavioral response and change, less opposed to mandatory testing, less into denial, more sympathetic towards AIDS victims, and more worried about AIDS. Females perceived themselves as more autonomous and were more anxious than males. No sex differences were found for knowledge of the disease.

Of interest to health educators, mental health professionals and social scientists.

379. GABAY, Edwin Daniel. "Public fear of AIDS: AIDS-phobia, homophobia and locus of control." Ph.D. dissertation, The Wright Institute, Berkeley, 1986.

AIDS-phobia was studied in 54 males and 59 females of varying age, education, and marital status. Data were also available on 116 subjects studied in 1985.

Research

Findings from the combined subject pools (N=229) include significant positive correlations between AIDS-phobia and both homophobia and external locus of control. In 1985, subjects showed greater fear of contracting AIDS through contaminated food and an increased awareness that transmission is mediated by blood and sexual contact The implications for intervention are discussed.

Of interest to health educators, psychologists, and mental health professionals.

380. GREGG, Larry J. "Public school administrators' knowledge of acquired immunodeficiency syndrome (AIDS) and their attitudes toward working with a carrier of the disease in the school setting." Ed.D. dissertation, University of Kansas, 1988.

A study with a two-fold purpose: 1) to investigate Kansas City public school administrators' knowledge of AIDS and their attitudes toward working with a person with AIDS, a person who is showing symptoms of ARC, or a person who is a known asymptomatic carrier of the HIV; and 2) to determine the correlation between the administrators' attitudes and levels of knowledge with selected demographic data.

Research

Kansas City public school administrators had a fairly high level of knowledge regarding AIDS, and their attitudes toward working with a person with AIDS, an ARC patient, or a known asymptomatic carrier of HIV were positive. The magnitude of the correlation between the level of knowledge of AIDS and attitude toward working with a person with AIDS was very small. Levels of knowledge of AIDS and attitude towards working with a person with AIDS varied significantly between levels of administration, districts with or without AIDS policies, and between districts which have provided different amounts of information to their employees regarding AIDS.

Of interest to health educators, school administrators, and public policymakers.

2. ETHICAL ISSUES

a. Articles

381.   ADLER, Michael W. "Patient safety and doctors with HIV infection." *British Medical Journal* 295 (1987): 1297-1298.

Discusses legal and ethical issues regarding patient safety and the responsibility of the HIV infected physician.

Editorial

Suggests that a recent court opinion upholding the right to confidentiality of the HIV infected physician is appropriate. Describes reasonable safeguards for patients that are incumbent in standard medical practice.

Appropriate for a general audience.

382.   ———, and Anne M. Johnson. "Contact tracing for HIV infection." *British Medical Journal* 296 (1988): 1420-1421.

Discusses the arguments for and against the use of contact tracing in the control of HIV infection.

Commentary

Contact tracing is used to break the chain of disease transmission by early identification and treatment of exposed people and has been vital in controlling sexually transmitted diseases in which there is a symptomatic phase of infection, a short incubation period, and effective treatment that confers a clear benefit. Few, if any, of these characteristics are true of HIV infection; the long incubation period and uncertain infectious period of HIV infection make the logistics of contact tracing daunting and raise questions about its effectiveness. While the Centers for Disease Control and the U.S. Surgeon General recommend contact tracing for HIV, and the American Secretary of Education has suggested that positive test results be reported to the sexual partners of those tested, others argue that contact tracing would be difficult and ineffective, violate confidentiality, and tend to drive the disease underground. In the absence of effective treatment for HIV infection, and the likelihood of stigmatization and discrimination of the identified infected, valid arguments exist on both sides of this issue.

Of general interest.

383. BADER, Diana, and Elizabeth McMillan. *AIDS: Ethical Guidelines for Healthcare Providers.* St. Louis, MO: The Catholic Health Association of the United States, 1987.

Provides a set of summary guidelines for use by administrators and health workers in the hospital, the long term care setting, and in other places in the continuum of care.

Guidebook

This booklet discusses the care and treatment of AIDS patients (quality care, treatment decisions, decision making, and privacy and confidentiality) and the perspective of health care workers. Sections are provided on institutional policies, such as testing and screening for HIV, and on corporate relations and social policy: the institution's posture toward the community and the institutional role in shaping public policy. A brief glossary and lists of readings and resources are included.

Of use to health professionals.

384. BAYER, Ronald. "AIDS and the duty to treat: Risk, responsibility, and health care worker." *Bulletin of the New York Academy of Medicine* 64 (1988): 498-505.

A discussion of the risks to and responsibilities of health care workers in the treatment of AIDS patients.

Discussion

Not everyone will bear the same burden of risk in this epidemic. Not everyone will be called upon to assume similar responsibilities. Those who chose to become medical professionals and workers have chosen unique social roles; with those roles come unique social responsibilities. Professional societies, as well as the broader community, must make it clear that refusals to treat are antithetical to the practice of a socially responsible medicine. By education, persuasion, counseling, intraprofessional and institutional regulation, and by statute, if necessary, it will be critical to underscore the shared commitment to those in need of care.

Of interest to all health professionals.

385. ———. "Gays and the stigma of bad blood." *Hastings Center Report* 13, no. 2 (1983): 5-7.

Discusses the controversy, which arose from the U.S. Public Health Service (PHS) recommendation that sexually active homosexual and bisexual men with multiple partners be prohibited from donating or selling their blood.

Commentary

Promiscuous gay and bisexual men are at increased risk for AIDS, which is transmitted by blood and blood products. The National Hemophilia Foundation, alarmed because hemophiliacs were becoming inadvertent victims of a contaminated blood supply, pressed for a ban against blood donations by "sexually active gays and bisexuals with multiple partners." The organized gay community, fearing that stigmatization would accompany the assumption that all gays were a potential source of "bad blood," resisted the ban, creating a moral dilemma over the extent to which the increased risk of those in need of blood ought to override the interests of the majority of gays. The author discusses the rationale behind the PHS recommendation for the screening of donors as a temporary measure; the need for cooperation and honesty if the PHS policy is to work; and the fact that the success of the measure, and the well-being of all who are in need of blood, are dependent on the courage and altruism of gay men.

Of interest to ethicists and historians.

386. ———. "Screening and AIDS: The limits of coercive inter-vention." *Annals of the New York Academy of Sciences* 530 (1988): 159-162.

Discusses the ethical problems raised by voluntary HIV testing and whether HIV screening should be mandatory.

Essay

The protection of confidentiality is central to the goals of public health. If antibody testing, in conjunction with counseling, is to be encouraged, a system of publicly funded anonymous testing sites must be maintained. Those who are antibody positive must be encouraged to notify past sexual partners or, if unable to undertake this task, to provide the names of those whom they might have infected. This will require the strictest regulations regarding the confidentiality of both infected persons and the contacts they name. Routine screening of specified populations is not necessary to provide public health officals with the information they need to plan strategies for intervention; epidemiological surveillance by screening blood samples drawn for other reasons and unlinked to personal identifiers will serve this function. The modification of individual behavior will come only from a public commitment to the kind of sexual education that will place life above morality.

Of interest to medical ethicists and public health professionals.

387. ———, Carol Levine, Thomas H. Murray. / "Guidelines for confidentiality in research on AIDS." *IRB: A Review on Human Subjects Research* 6, no. 6 (1984): 1-7.

Presents guidelines designed to provide a basis for cooperation between the research community and the subjects of AIDS research.

Descriptive

Persons with AIDS and others who might be research subjects recognize that research is essential to understand, treat, and prevent this disease, but are concerned that information divulged for research purposes might be used in ways that are detrimental to their interests. Unless they have confidence in the system designed to protect their privacy and in the people to whom information is divulged, they may provide invalid or incomplete data. A set of guidelines, developed by a multidisciplinary group representing professional, public, and social interests, recommend changes that are deemed necessary to afford the fullest degree of protection for confidentiality compatible with sound scientific research.

Addressed to research institutions, individual researchers, institutional review boards, and public health departments.

388. ———, Carol Levine, Susan M. Wolf. "HIV antibody screening: An ethical framework for evaluating proposed programs." *Journal of the American Medical Association* 256 (1986): 1768-1777.

Focuses on the use of blood tests to identify individuals who have been infected with HIV.

Discussion

The authors believe that the greatest hope for stopping the spread of HIV infection lies in the voluntary cooperation of those at higher risk and their willingness to undergo testing and to alter their personal behavior and goals in the interest of the community. This voluntary cooperation can be expected only if the legitimate interests of these groups and individuals are protected from discrimination by legislators, professionals, and the public.

Of interest to the general public.

389. BELL, Nora Kizer. "AIDS and women: Remaining ethical issues." *AIDS Education and Prevention* 1, no. 1 (1989): 22-30.

Addresses important ethical issues relating specifically to women with AIDS.

Discussion

It is predicted that, by 1991, the number of documented cases of AIDS among women will nearly equal that among men now diagnosed with the disease. Future public health policy will have to take seriously the central role of women in the future of AIDS. There seem to be important public policy reasons for attempting to reshape attitudes about mortality and sexual responsibility where they concern AIDS

transmission, to advocate that there are certain things that morally
and sexually responsible people just don't do, and to pursue a variety
of programs that teach both safe sex and safer sex practices. Women
must be helped to protect themselves by the creation of a moral
climate in which there is no stigma attached to AIDS testing, men
respect women's rights to remain healthy, and it can be taken for
granted that partners will not expose each other to AIDS.

Of interest to health educators and public health officials.

390.   BREMNER, Marie N., and Leslie B. Brown.   "Learning to care
       for clients with AIDS--the practicum controversy."   *Nursing
       and Health Care* 7 (1986): 250-253.

Discusses the question of whether nursing students have the right to
refuse to care for clients with AIDS.

Discussion

AIDS creates an ethical dilemma for educators who must decide whether
to assign students to care for clients with the disease.   Nursing
faculty members, before deciding whether to assign students to care
for AIDS patients, should ask themselves whether the curriculum has
prepared the students to care for AIDS patients, what level of
sophistication the students are functioning at in terms of psychomotor
skills, and whether the assignment will help the students meet the
clinical/course objectives.   They should consider the potential risks,
the risk/benefit ratio, and the potential for litigation of having the
students care for AIDS patients.   An institutional forum that allows
nursing faculty members to consider and discuss the ethical and legal
implications of teaching students to care for clients with a disease
they will undoubtedly encounter in practice is suggested.

Of interest to nurses and nursing educators.

391.   CHRISTAKIS, Nicholas A.   "The ethical design of an AIDS
       vaccine trial in Africa."   *Hastings Center Report* 18, no. 3
       (1988): 31-37.

Discusses the ethical issues in conducting AIDS vaccine trials in
Africa.

Theoretical

Calls for a reevaluation of a uniform, international view of research
ethics.   Presents the need for cultural sensitivity in designing AIDS
vaccine trials in Africa.

Should interest clinical investigators, policymakers, and medical
ethicists.

392.   CLOSEN, Michael L., and Scott H. Isaacman.   "Notifying
       private third parties at risk for HIV infection: What is the
       role of doctors and other health care providers?"   *Trial* 25,
       no. 5 (1989): 50-55.

Discusses the role of health care providers in notifying third parties at risk for HIV infection.

Descriptive

Health care providers regularly confront the dilemma of honoring patient confidentiality or warning their patients' sexual or needle-sharing partners about the risk of HIV infection. With regard to most other diseases, compliance with a state or national reporting law discharges the provider's obligation to warn third parties of their risk of infection; the situation is more complicated with HIV. The author recommends that a provider document, in the medical record, that the patient was asked to identify current sexual or needle-sharing partners and counseled to inform such partners of their risk of infection, and, if the patient could not be trusted to refrain from risk behavior and inform partners of their risk, that steps were taken to notify endangered third parties.

Of interest to physicians and medical administrators.

393. COMMITTEE for the Protection of Human Participants in Research, American Psychological Association. "Ethical issues in psychosocial research on AIDS." *IRB: A Review of Human Subjects Research* 8, no. 4 (1986): 8-10.

An application of the *APA Ethical Principles of Psychologists* to assist anyone conducting or planning research on the medical, psychological, and social aspects of AIDS.

Discussion

Current research on the psychological aspects of AIDS raises acute ethical dilemmas. Despite considerable pressure to "bend the rules" in regard to confidentiality and premature disclosure of data, researchers must consider the welfare of participants and guard their civil rights. Investigators should consider carefully the relative risks and benefits of possible research on AIDS, and deliberate personally and in consultation with peers and the public in deciding whether and how to undertake such research. Participants in a study should be carefully debriefed and followed up appropriately. Researchers should avoid reporting data for which conclusions cannot be obtained; carefully determine whether the potential benefits of disclosing preliminary data outweigh any harm which may result if it should prove erroneous; and conscientiously report the limitations of a study, emphasizing points of uncertainty and alternative interpretations.

Of interest to psychosocial and clinical researchers.

394. CONDIT, Douglas, and Robert W.M. Frater. "Human immunodeficiency virus and the cardiac surgeon: A survey of attitudes." *Annals of Thoracic Surgery* 47 (1989): 182-186.

All of the known board-certified cardiac surgeons in the United States were polled by questionnaire to determine their willingness to perform open cardiac procedures on HIV carriers and AIDS patients.

Research

Fifty-three percent of the surgeons responded. Two-thirds said they would operate on HIV carriers needing a cardiac operation, but regarded the presence of AIDS as a contraindication to cardiopulmonary bypass. Those who said they would not operate on HIV carriers appeared to be motivated by fear of contagion rather than by moral judgments concerning the patients. Almost all surgeons (95%) believed that high-risk patients should be tested, and a substantial majority (73%) wanted all patients to be tested.

Of interest to physicians caring for AIDS patients.

395. COUNCIL on Ethical and Judicial Affairs, American Medical Association. "Ethical issues involved in the growing AIDS crisis." *Journal of the American Medical Association* 259 (1988): 1360-1361.

Outlines the physician's ethical responsibility to his patients and to society in light of the AIDS epidemic.

Report/Recommendations

A physician has an ethical responsibility to treat any patient within his realm of competence, and to do so with compassion and respect for human dignity, regardless of personal risk. If unable to provide the services required by AIDS patients, appropriate referrals should be made. The physician has an ethical obligation to respect the rights of privacy and of confidentiality of AIDS patients and seropositive individuals. However, a physician who knows that a seropositive individual is endangering a third party must first attempt to persuade the patient to cease his threatening behavior, then, if persuasion fails, notify public health authorities, and finally, if no action is taken, notify the endangered party. A physician who knows that he or she is seropositive or has AIDS must refrain from any activity that creates a risk of transmission to others and should consult colleagues as to which activities the physician can pursue without creating a risk to patients.

Important guidelines for all health professionals.

396. CRISP, Roger. "Autonomy, welfare and the treatment of AIDS." *Journal of Medical Ethics* 15 (1989): 68-73.

Examines six important areas in which HIV infection and AIDS raise problems for the individual doctor, and proposes a methodology for approaching practical moral questions.

Philosophical

The moral principles of autonomy and welfare often seem to be in conflict with one another, counseling inconsistent courses of action and giving rise, in particular cases, to moral dilemmas. Many of us feel attracted by both principles, but the liberal tends to exaggerate the value of autonomy, while the utilitarian ignores it. Both have an impoverished conception of welfare. By seeing autonomy as part of welfare, doctors can think more directly about such issues as paternalism, confidentiality, and consent. The author uses simplified case studies, illustrating conflicts regarding paternalism, the right to ignorance, confidentiality, the rights of practitioners, consent, and the rights of patients, to illustrate his point, presenting the liberal and utilitarian positions regarding each case. He then discusses a more balanced approach for ethical and moral decision-making regarding each case in point.

Of interest to physicians and medical ethicists.

397. DAN, Bruce B. "Patients without physicians: The new risk of AIDS." *Journal of the American Medical Association* 258, no. 14 (1987): 1940.

A commentary on the attitude of physicians in taking on the responsibility of treating patients with HIV infection.

Commentary

Author advocates that physicians put the patients' welfare ahead of their own and reaffirm their vow to serve their fellow man.

Of particular interest to physicians.

398. DAVIS, Dena. "Children with AIDS in the public schools: The ethical issues." *Journal of Medical Humanities and Bioethics* 8 (1987): 101-109.

Addresses the question of whether parents should send their healthy children to school with children who have AIDS.

Essay

Parents face conflicting commitments in deciding whether to allow their children to attend school with a child who has AIDS: the commitment to minimize their children's risk of infection, and the commitment to avoid further burdening a sick child with ostracism and isolation. Similarities exist between this issue and that of proxy consent for children to participate in low-risk, non-therapeutic research. The author concludes that parents of healthy children should accept the presence of children with AIDS in the public schools.

Of interests to ethicists, teachers, school administrators, and parents of school children.

399. DOYAL, Len, and Brian Hurwitz. "The recent BMA ruling on AIDS: The patient's right to informed consent versus the doctor's right to protection." *Practitioner* 231 (1987): 1217-1222.

Discusses the pros and cons of HIV antibody testing without first
obtaining informed consent.

Editorial

The British Medical Association's decision to support the right of
general practitioners to test for HIV antibodies without necessarily
obtaining the patient's consent raises two important ethical
questions: To how much danger are doctors morally obligated to expose
themselves in the patient's behalf, and what should doctors do when
measures taken for their own protection conflict with the rights of
the patient? A hypothetical case is offered for consideration, and
the pros and cons of the BMA ruling are debated.

Of interest to physicians, lawyers, and medical philosophers.

400. EMANUEL, Ezekial J. "Do physicians have an obligation to
        treat patients with AIDS?" *New England Journal of Medicine*
        3118 (1988): 1686-1690.

A discussion of the question, "Are physicians obligated to treat
patients with AIDS?"

Commentary

Three points about the physician's obligation to treat patients with
AIDS need emphasis. This obligation depends on viewing medicine as a
profession, not as a commercial enterprise. Physicians who join the
profession assume an obligation to care for the ill, even at some
reasonable personal risk. Because of this inclusive obligation,
physicians have a specific obligation to patients with AIDS. This
obligation can be limited by several factors, especially excessive
personal risk, although it appears that a few physicians are assuming
excessive risk in treating their patients with AIDS. Because medicine
is committed to caring for the sick, physicians must care for patients
with AIDS.

Of interest to physicians and other health professionals.

401. FOWLER, Marsha D.M. "Acquired immunodeficiency syndrome
        and refusal to provide care." *Heart and Lung* 17 (1988):
        213-215.

Identifies and discusses ethical dilemmas in the care of AIDS
patients.

Commentary

When a patient's need is great and the refusal to care is likely to
result in harm, the duty to care is great. There is, however, no duty
to care when that care will not benefit the patient: needless sacri-
fice is not warranted. A general duty to care, conditioned by the
level of risk to the professional, exists wherever care will meet
need, prevent harm, and prove efficacious.

Of interest to all health professionals caring for AIDS patients.

402. FREEDMAN, Benjamin, and the McGill/Boston Research Group. "Non-validated therapies and HIV disease." *Hastings Center Report* 19, no. 3 (1989): 14-20.

Proposes the designation of authorized investigational units to preserve the integrity of clinical trials for new AIDS drugs, protect patients, and enhance clinicians' flexibility.

Commentary

It is proposed that certain AIDS centers be granted the authority to prescribe restricted investigational drugs, free of charge, on a compassionate basis. This would give physicians in the designated centers greater latitude in making treatment decisions, provide patients with rapid access to new treatments, and insure sound evaluation. Natural incentives for drug companies to complete testing would be retained since the costs of research and development could not be recovered until completion of the approval process. Although prior approval would not be required, regulatory agencies would monitor the use of the drugs, acting as a retrospective control.

Of interest to drug company executives, regulatory officials, medical researchers, physicians, legislators, and patient advocates.

403. GALLAGHER, Morris. "AIDS and HIV infection: Ethical problems for general practitioners." *Journal of the Royal College of General Practitioners* 38 (1988): 414-417.

Discusses ethical problems that general practitioners are likely to encounter in dealing with patients who are HIV positive or who have AIDS.

Theoretical

The duty to care, informed consent, and patient confidentiality are the ethical issues most likely to confront general practitioners working with patients who have AIDS or HIV infection. Case studies illustrate the use of fundamental ethical principles in resolving problems.

Of particular interest to primary care physicians.

404. GRAY, Lizbeth A., and Anna K. Harding. "Confidentiality limits with clients who had the AIDS virus." *Journal of Counseling and Development* 66 (1988): 219-223.

Reviews the medical background of AIDS, legal limits, and ethical tenets of confidentiality.

Review

A position supporting breach of confidentiality is taken and specific suggestions for counseling the client are offered.

Of interest to counselors and mental health professionals.

405. HAGEN, Michael D., Klemens B. Meyer, Stephen G. Pauker. "Routine preoperative screening for HIV: Does the risk to the surgeon outweigh the risk to the patient?" *Journal of the American Medical Association* 259 (1988): 1357-1359.

Argues against preoperative screening of low-risk patients for HIV.

Commentary

Routine preoperative screening could be even more socially destructive than a program to screen the general population. Privacy would be extensively compromised, and the specificity of serological tests might be somewhat lower, potentially giving rise to many false-positive results. The authors demonstrate that the risk of HIV infection to surgeons, nurses, and technicians is of the same magnitude as the risk to an uninfected person in "safer" sexual contact (e.g., using a condom) and argue that as long as we eschew screening in low-risk heterosexual populations, we should not recommend it for low-risk patients awaiting surgery. Screening low-risk patients before surgery implies that preventing HIV infection in health professionals is more important than preventing the infection in others, which is neither rational nor ethical.

Of particular interest to surgeons, operating room nurses, technicians, and health policymakers.

406. HALPERIN, Edward C. "The right to privacy and the duty to protect." *Southern Medical Journal* 81 (1988): 1286-1290.

Examines the conflicts between the patient's right to privacy and the physician's duty to protect persons who may be injured by contact with the patient.

Theoretical

Privacy and confidentiality are not absolutes in the practice of medicine. The duty to protect overrides the right to privacy if 1) the physician is mandated to provide information to authorities or 2) the patient places others at risk by failing to comply with disease control measures. Litigation and experience will help in determining where to draw the line between privacy and duty.

Of interest to physicians who treat HIV-infected persons, ethicists, and policymakers.

407. HENRY, Keith, Karen Willenbring, Kent Crossley. "Human immunodeficiency virus antibody testing: A description of practices and policies at U.S. infectious disease-teaching hospitals and Minnesota hospitals." *Journal of the American Medical Association* 259 (1988): 1819-1822.

A questionnaire asking about policies that concern the use of HIV antibody tests was sent to 200 hospitals in the United States that conduct infectious disease fellowship training and to 171 short-term-care Minnesota hospitals in January 1987.

Research

Information was received from 189 (94.5%) of the U.S. infectious disease hospitals and from 160 (94%) of the Minnesota hospitals. Only 49% of the U.S. hospitals and 37% of the Minnesota hospitals had an HIV antibody-test ordering policy; 47% of the U.S. hospitals and 39% of the Minnesota hospitals had a specific educational program for physicians about the HIV antibody test; and 62% of the U.S. hospitals and 41% of the Minnesota hospitals had an HIV autopsy policy. There was marked variety in approaches to handling test results, obtaining patient consent, and providing risk-reduction information among the hospitals. These data suggest the need for consensus on the optimal use of HIV antibody testing at hospitals.

Of particular interest to hospital administrators and public health professionals.

408. HOWE, Edmund G. "Ethical aspects of military physicians treating patients with HIV/Part one: The duty to warn." *Military Medicine* 153, no. 1 (1988): 7-11.

Addresses ethical issues military physicians confront when they acquire epidemiological data from service persons with HIV infection.

Discussion

Analyzes ethical issues and emphasizes how important it is that military physicians make an attempt to maximize service persons' autonomy by telling them, beforehand, what will be done with the information they disclose.

Of particular interest to physicians and health professionals in military and government services.

409. ————. "Ethical aspects of military physicians treating patients with HIV/Part two: The duty to take initiative." *Military Medicine* 153 (1988): 72-76.

Explores ethical aspects of several initiatives military physicians might take in an attempt to improve the clinical care of service persons with HIV.

Descriptive

Initiatives discussed include maximizing gay service persons' opportunities for counseling, enhancing the options of service persons to refuse unwanted interventions and to make advance directives, protecting patients from early knowledge that HIV is impairing their mental functioning, and furthering these patients' interests when medical resources are limited.

Of interest to health professionals in the military services.

410.   ———. "Ethical aspects of military physicians treating patients
       with HIV/Part three: The duty to protect third parties."
       Military Medicine 153 (1988): 140-144.

Addresses ethical conflicts military physicians may face when HIV
infected service persons will not tell their sexual partners of their
condition or appear likely to engage in unsafe sex.

Discussion

Legal and ethical aspects of these situations in civilian and
military settings are compared, and practical approaches for military
physicians are emphasized.   The author suggests that   military
physicians consider three things before making decisions   regarding
these patients: the physician's potential for influencing behavior
change in these service persons, the suffering these persons are
already undergoing as a result of HIV infection, and the possibility
that the physician's judgment has been affected by prejudice against
these patients.

Of particular interest to military physicians and counselors.

411.   JONSEN, Albert R., Molly Cooke, Barbara A. Koenig. "AIDS
       and ethics."   *Issues in Science and Technology* 2, no. 2
       (1986): 56-65.

Describes how medical practitioners in San Francisco have dealt with
ethical problems regarding AIDS.

Descriptive

Outlines the ethical principles that should guide public policy when
diseases such as AIDS threaten both public health and personal
liberties.

Of interest to health professionals and public health officials.

412.   KAPP, Marshall B., and Eric E. Fortess. "Screening for AIDS:
       Ethical and legal issues."   *New England Journal of Human
       Services* 6, no. 4 (1986): 19-23.

An analysis of the issues that underlie procedures to screen donated
blood for AIDS virus antibodies.

Analytic

After analyzing the issues, the authors reached the following
conclusions.   The best results will be attained for donors and for
society if guidelines for managing donations are based on
truth-telling and respect for individuals.   Because of the magnitude

of the task of screening millions of donations annually, it is
unlikely that the blood supply will ever be absolutely AIDS-free; the
risk to blood recipients will remain low, but the few who contract
AIDS will face catastrophic consequences. The utility of AIDS test
results depends on the context; how to use the results will remain a
value judgment. Public policy regarding AIDS screening should be
formulated on the basis of broad, interdisciplinary participation by
experts in medicine, ethics, law, economics, and policy, and by representatives of high-risk groups.

Of interest to blood bank personnel, hospital administrators,
ethicists, lawyers, and public policymakers.

413. KELLY, Jeffrey A., Janet S. St. Lawrence, Steve Smith, Jr.,
     Harold V. Hood, Donna J. Cook. "Stigmatization of AIDS
     patients by physicians." *American Journal of Public Health*
     77 (1987): 798-791.

A randomly selected sample of physicians in three large cities were
given vignettes to read describing a patient who differed only in his
identification as having either AIDS or leukemia. They then completed
a set of objective attitude measures eliciting their reaction to the
patient.

Research

Harsh attitude judgments and much less willingness to interact, even
in routine conversation, were associated with the AIDS portrayals.
Since increasing numbers of AIDS patients will be seeking medical
attention all over the country, it will be important for the health
care professions to develop programs to counter unreasonable stigma
and prejudicial attitudes.

Of interest to medical and other health professions educators, social
and behavioral scientists, and members of the helping professions.

414. KELLY, Kevin. "AIDS and ethics: An overview." *General
     Hospital Psychiatry* 9 (1987): 331-340.

A discussion of the ethical questions and problems arising from the
AIDS epidemic.

Review

The ethical questions concerning AIDS generally fall into familiar
categories for which established ethical principles apply. However,
new considerations are required for certain features of this epidemic,
and the calculation of competing values is affected by the mystery,
uncertainty, lack of definitive treatment, social stigma, and
psychological effects of the disease. There is little ethical
justification, except in specific limited situations, for infringing
on the civil rights of individuals, violating confidentiality, or
permitting discrimination against AIDS patients or against persons who
are at risk.

Of interest to physicians, public health professionals, public
policymakers, insurance underwriters, and members of the research
community.

415. KIM, Jerome H., and John R. Perfect. "To help the sick: An
     historical and ethical essay concerning the refusal to care for
     patients with AIDS." *The American Journal of Medicine* 84
     (1988): 135-138.

A discussion of the historical and ethical issues in refusing to care
for patients with AIDS.

Essay

The authors conclude that we are impelled, ethically, and are not
excused, scientifically, to participate in the care of patients with
HIV disease. The decision is a personal one, but should acknowledge
both moral responsibility and the improbability of personal risk.

Of interest to all health care professionals.

416. KOOP, C. Everett. "Challenge of AIDS." *American Journal of
     Hospital Pharmacy* 45 (1988): 537-540.

The Surgeon General describes the ethical challenges of AIDS.

Speech to Pharmacists

Given the high cost of care of AIDS patients, the question of whether
the nation can pay for the best possible care for every patient must
be dealt with. Also, the right of an individual to confidentiality
must be balanced against risk to the community. To deal compas-
sionately and justly with AIDS, courageous leadership and serious
discussion of ethical issues are needed.

Of interest to the general public.

417. LEVINE, Carol, and Joyce Bermel (Eds.).   "AIDS: The
     emerging ethical dilemmas." *Hastings Center Report* 15,
     Supplement (August 1985): 1-32.

A series of seven essays on the social and ethical issues surrounding
AIDS.

Special Supplement

Covers topics such as blood screening, the epidemiological investigation of AIDS, clinical care and research in AIDS, AIDS and public
health, public policy and AIDS, and media responsibility in AIDS.

Of interest to health professionals, laymen, and professionals in law,
ethics public health, and social science.

418. LOEWY, Erich H. "AIDS and the human community." *Social Science and Medicine* 27 (1988): 297-303.

Examines ethical behavior in the face of the threat of AIDS from the vantage point of: different ways of looking at communal structure; notions of justice and of rights that develop from different ways of looking at community; and views of the natural lottery and of self-causation linked to attitudes towards community, justice, and rights.

Discussion

Concludes that most look at community as constituted by more than the minimal obligations of refraining from harm to one another and include beneficence among the moral obligations. The incompatibility of freedom as a moral obligation is stressed. The medical community bears a special obligation for dispassionate examination of the facts in light of its special training, as well as for a compassionate analysis in light of its tradition of compassion towards the ill.

Of interest to philosophers, counselors, ethicists, and persons in the humanities.

419. ————. "Duties, fears and physicians." *Social Science and Medicine* 22 (1986): 1363-1366.

AIDS is used as a paradigm in dealing with the physician's fear of contagion.

Review

The author examines the concepts of duty, fear, and courage in their medical setting; deals with the historical aspects of the problem; analyzes the role of social contract and professionalism; and develops a viewpoint of the physician's obligation based on these considerations. He concludes that the physician has an enduring social contract with his/her community, which has been profitable for both. If medicine honors its contract, it is deserving of honor; if it breaks its contract, it will, instead, be deserving of infamy.

Of interest to physicians, historians, and medical ethicists.

420. MELTON, Gary B., and Joni N. Gray. "Ethical dilemmas in AIDS research: Individual privacy and public health." *American Psychologist* 43 (1988): 60-64.

Discusses the dilemmas involved in balancing individual rights with social welfare when conducting psychosocial research in AIDS.

Commentary

Significant legal threats to confidentiality are matched inadequately by legal means of protecting privacy. Researchers are advised to request certificates of confidentiality from the Public Health Service. A privilege statute is needed to protect the privacy of participants in research on AIDS.

Of interest to AIDS researchers.

421. MELTON, Gary B., Robert J. Levine, Gerald P. Koocher,
      Robert   Rosenthal,   William   C.   Thompson.   "Community
      consultation in socially sensitive research: Lessons from
      clinical trials of treatments for AIDS." *American Psychologist*
      43 (1988): 573-581.

Discusses dilemmas in socially sensitive research, especially ongoing
clinical trials of medications to treat AIDS.

Commentary

Although the investigator and relevant regulatory bodies are not
absolved of responsibility by community consultation, such a procedure
may help to create a partnership between the investigator and
participants, consistent with ethical duties of respect for persons,
beneficence, and fidelity.   Community consultation may also dampen
participants' anxiety and increase the perceived justice of decisions
about the research.   Such a procedure has the potential to mitigate
ethical problems in research involving a wide variety of socially
sensitive topics and in randomized clinical trials of treatments for
conditions other than AIDS.

Of interest to social and behavioral scientists engaged in research on
AIDS.

422. MITCHELL, Christine, and Laureen Smith. "If it's AIDS, please
      don't tell." *American Journal of Nursing* 87 (1987): 911- 914.

Discusses the ethical dilemma faced by nurses who have been asked   to
withhold information about a patient's condition.

Case Study

Uses the case history of a hemophiliac who tested positive for HIV to
illustrate the ethical dilemma of nurses, placed in the uncomfortable
position of having to evade questions or answer dishonestly, who are
torn between the obligation to respect the patient's wishes and
protect him and his family from possible stigma and discrimination and
the obligation to tell the truth and protect others from accidental
HIV infection.   The ethical questions involved in disclosure dilemmas
are identified.

Of interest to health care providers and medical ethicists.

423. MORRISON, Constance F.   "AIDS: Ethical implications for
      psychological   intervention."   *Professional   Psychology:
      Research and Practice* 20 (1989): 166-171.

Explores some of the ethical issues likely to arise for psychological
practitioners responding to the AIDS epidemic.

Descriptive

Duty to treat is examined with a consideration of homophobia and biases about IV drug abusers. Confidentiality is discussed in the context of record keeping, in cases of conflict with duty to warn, and in cases of suicide. Psychologists are urged to consider possible ethical dilemmas before they arise, in order that the best decisions might be made.

Of interest to psychologists, other mental health professionals, and physicians.

424. NOLAN, Kathleen. "Ethical issues in caring for pregnant women and newborns at risk for HIV infection." *Seminars in Perinatology* 13 (1989): 55-65.

Examines ethical issues related to perinatal care.

Discussion

Mandatory neonatal screening is rejected, primarily on the grounds that the benefits do not justify overriding parental autonomy and family values. Testing is warranted for children whose medical care might be enhanced by the knowledge of seropositivity, for those who might infect others in day care centers or schools by biting or uncontrolled bodily secretions, and for those who are to be adopted or placed in foster care. Although prenatal testing for HIV should be offered, it should not be required; the risk to the fetus of HIV infection is not 100%, and there is an uneven geographic and racial distribution of HIV infection among women of childbearing age. The most effective means of reducing perinatal transmission is to decrease the number of infected women in a community. This can be accomplished by offering incentives to decrease needle sharing, by increasing the availability of methadone and drug treatment, and by encouraging the use of condoms.

Will interest medical ethicists and public health officials.

425. ———, and Ronald Bayer (Eds.). "AIDS: The responsibilities of health professionals." *Hastings Center Report* 18, no. 2, Supplement (1988): S1-S32.

A series of articles present and discuss the dilemmas troubling health professionals in light of the AIDS epidemic.

Special Journal Supplement

The five articles in this special supplement deal with the following topics: health care workers and the risk of HIV transmission; a note on history regarding the politics of physicians' responsibility in epidemics; AIDS and the duty to treat; health professions, codes, and the right to refuse to treat HIV-infected patients; and legal risks and reponsibilities of physicians in the AIDS epidemic.

Of interest to health professionals, lawyers, ethicists, and the general public.

426. NOVICK, Alvin. "At risk for AIDS: Confidentiality in research and surveillance." *IRB: A Review of Human Subjects Research* 6, no. 6 (1984): 10-11.

Discusses current and projected research projects concerning the AIDS epidemic, related surveillance, the importance of such data collection, and the privacy and confidentiality of research subjects.

Commentary

The appropriate product of surveillance and research on AIDS is knowledge, leading to containing the epidemic, first by understanding it and then by reducing transmission. Education and counsel concerning risks are necessary and proper tools. Persons at risk for AIDS and their advocates fear that the products of surveillance and research on AIDS may be social and political oppression as well as personal exposure and its consequences. Research, upon which our knowledge depends, depends upon voluntary cooperation. To assure that cooperation, the rights of the research subjects to privacy and confidentiality must be assured by law and regulation, by social expectation, and by greatly enhanced sensitivity. AIDS researchers must be especially vigilant in honoring and protecting these rights.

Of interest to AIDS researchers.

427. ———, Nancy Neveloff Dubler, Sheldon H. Landesman. "Do Research subjects have the right not to know their HIV antibody test results?" *IRB: A Review of Human Subjects Research* 8, no. 5 (1986): 6-9.

Discusses the controversy that has arisen in the context of AIDS over whether an individual has the right not to know certain information that may be profoundly disturbing.

Commentary

An individual who is seropositive is presumed to be infectious, able to transmit the virus to others sexually or through shared needles or blood. Knowledge about seropositivity, therefore, brings into conflict principles of beneficence and respect for persons with that of preventing harm. The question then arises as to whose is the locus of moral responsibility for protecting others; does it lie with the seropositive individual or with the researcher? The three authors, respectively, present their views regarding why burdensome knowledge need not be imposed, treating research subjects fairly, and the ethical obligations of research subjects to be informed of their HIV status.

Of particular interest to researchers and ethicists.

428. PERRY, Samuel W. "Pharmacological and psychological research
on AIDS: Some ethical considerations." *IRB: A Review of
Human Subjects Research* 9, no. 5 (1987): 8-10.

Calls attention to some specific ethical issues that have arisen
during the course of conducting federally funded pharmacological and
psychological research related to AIDS.

Descriptive

Despite precautions to ensure confidentiality, breaches in confidentiality can occur if 1) the research setting permits implicit
identification by association; 2) requests for laboratory procedures
identify the subject as a participant in an HIV study; or 3)
psychosocial interventions are conducted using a group format.
Institutional Review Boards need to be alert to ethical problems that
may require special consideration.

Of interest to researchers, ethicists, and members of Institutional
Review Boards.

429. RATZAN, Richard M., and Henry Schneiderman. "AIDS,
autopsies, and abandonment." *Journal of the American
Medical Association* 260 (1988): 3466-3469.

Discusses the arbitrary and capricious refusals of some pathologists
to perform autopsies on AIDS patients.

Discussion

The medical profession has an obligation to ensure that autopsy is as
available for AIDS patients as it is for others. Inappropriate
avoidance of autopsies causes potential harm to the decedent's
reputation; the loss of all benefits derived from autopsies,
potentially causing harm to other persons; and harm to the professional status of physicians. Although most practicing physicians,
since the advent of antibiotics, have enjoyed a comparatively
risk-free occupation, the advent of AIDS should serve to remind them
that to be a physician is to take personal risks.

Of interest to all health professionals.

430. REAMER, Frederic G. "AIDS and ethics: The agenda for social
workers." *Social Work* 33 (1988): 460-464.

A discussion of ethical issues for social workers regarding: testing
for AIDS; confidentiality of information related to AIDS; and the
delivery of services to persons with AIDS, their families, and their
partners.

Discussion

Social workers must lobby vigorously to ensure that the rights and
special needs of high risk populations are not jeopardized because of

gratuitous or counterproductive testing. They must support efforts to
ensure confidentiality of all written and oral communications related
to AIDS. Social workers must be especially vigilant in their efforts
to ensure that persons with AIDS are not denied services and resources
to which they are entitled.

Of special interest to social workers.

431. ROSS, Michael W.   "Psychosocial ethical aspects of AIDS."
      Journal of Medical Ethics 15 (1989): 74-81.

Discusses ethical considerations of the psychological and social
aspects of AIDS.

Descriptive

The ethical dilemmas arising from AIDS relate, not primarily to the
medical aspects of the disease, but to the issues dealing with a
pathogen that is predominantly affecting minority groups subject to
stigmatization.   The author argues that ethical judgments of
persons infected by or at risk of HIV can have adverse
psychological effects on the subjects of such judgments, and that
negative ethical judgments about HIV and associated infections can
actually harm the common good by increasing rather than reducing the
spread of HIV within the community.   He concludes that the
psychosocial aspects of HIV infection impose ethical psychological,
as well as medical, obligations to reduce harm and prevent the spread
of infection.

Of interest to health professionals and medical ethicists.

432. ROY, D.J., and C. Tsoukas.   "AIDS and clinical ethics:
      Honoring the patients' dignity."   *Dimensions in   Health
      Service* 63, no. 7 (1986): 32-33.

Discusses the ethical issues associated with AIDS.

Commentary

AIDS challenges us to critically review the foundations of
social, professional, and personal ethics. Although homosexual and
bisexual men and intravenous drug users still comprise the largest
segment of AIDS victims, sexual partners of those having AIDS,
prisoners, prostitutes, recipients of contaminated blood and blood
products, people from Central Africa and Haiti, and children of all
these people have also contracted the disease. AIDS is not and never
was simply a "homosexual" disease. Nevertheless, the danger exists
that prejudice and panic may shape behavior towards AIDS victims as
some people transfer their fear of the disease and of death and their
repugnance against homosexuality and drug abuse to persons afflicted
with AIDS. The primary ethical challenge is to perceive the sufferer
as greater than his disease and disability, possessing a human dignity
incalculably superior to the behavior others may scorn. The ethical
tragedy occurs when the disease becomes the identity of the sufferer
in his own eyes and those of others.

Of interest to a general audience.

433.   SHARP, Sanford C.   "The physician's obligation to treat AIDS
       patients."   *Southern Medical Journal* 81 (1988): 1282-1285.

Discusses the physician's professional obligation to treat persons
with AIDS.

Theoretical

Five arguments, based on professional traditions, formal ethical
codes, the dependent nature of the patient, the social contract, and
medicine, support the contention that a physician is obligated to
treat all who can benefit from his care, even if the treatment puts
him at risk of infection. Medical students who are unwilling to treat
patients with AIDS are advised either to seek other careers or to
choose specialties with low patient contact.

Of interest to physicians and medical students.

434.   SIMON, Robert I. (Ed.).   "Ethical treatment of patients with
       AIDS." *Psychiatric Annals* 18 (1988): 555-605.

The eight articles in this special issue address the ethical dilemmas
surrounding AIDS that are faced by medical practitioners and their
institutions.

Special Journal Issue

Addressed are: the psychiatrist's ethical and legal duty to stay
abreast of new knowledge about AIDS; HIV related diseases and the
future of the delivery of psychiatric care; confidentiality versus the
duty to protect; AIDS, ethics, and psychiatry; evolving law and
liability regarding psychiatric patients with AIDS; ethical and legal
issues surrounding the AIDS patient on the psychiatric unit; psychiatric reflections on AIDS education; and AIDS, psychiatry, and
euthanasia.

Useful to all physicians, especially psychiatrists.

435.   STEELE, Shirley M.   "AIDS: Clarifying values to close in on
       ethical questions."   *Nursing and Health Care* 7 (1986):
       247-248.

Adapts the values clarification process for nurses caring for persons
with AIDS.

Descriptive

Values clarification involves determining alternatives, choosing the
most appropriate one, and acting on it. Heterosexual nurses, faced
with caring for homosexual patients with AIDS, must clarify their own
values so that they can deal in a rational manner with the social and
ethical dilemmas brought about by AIDS and can help their colleagues
and others to clarify their values.

Of interest to nurses.

436. STEINBROOK, Robert, Bernard Lo, Jill Tirpak, James W.
      Dilley, Paul A. Volberding. "Ethical dilemmas in caring for
      patients with the acquired immunodeficiency syndrome."
      Annals of Internal Medicine 103 (1985): 787-790.

Three cases illustrate the ethical dilemmas and stresses of caring for
patients with AIDS.

Case Histories

Caring for patients with AIDS raises ethical dilemmas concerning the
provision of life-sustaining treatments. Many patients become
mentally incompetent and unable to participate in making decisions.
Lovers or friends, unless they have been legally designated to do so,
cannot make decisions for them. Because caring for patients with AIDS
is stressful, decision-making guidelines may be difficult to
implement.

Of interest to physicians, counselors, and other caregivers of persons
with AIDS.

437. SWARTZ, Martha S. "AIDS testing and informed consent."
      Journal of Health Politics, Policy and Law 13 (1988): 607-621.

Examines the issue of informed consent for HIV testing in hospitals.

Discussion

The author argues that specific consent for an HIV test should be
obtained from the patient. When the test is ordered to protect health
care workers, the patient should be told of its true purpose. If the
patient is not properly informed, the physician and/or hospital may be
liable for claims of fraud or duress. Testing of patients to protect
health care workers should be discouraged; the use of universal
precautions for handling blood and body fluids provides adequate
protection for hospital staff.

Of interest to physicians, hospital administrators, and health care
workers.

438. WACHTER, Robert M., John M. Luce, Bernard Lo, Thomas A.
      Raffin. "Life-sustaining treatment for patients with AIDS."
      Chest 95 (1989): 647-652.

Reviews studies of the prognosis for AIDS patients requiring intensive
care and provides ethical principles for decision making regarding
therapy for the terminally ill.

Review/Discussion

AIDS patients admitted to an ICU for reasons other than respiratory
failure had a survival rate to hospital discharge ranging from 20 to
43%. The survival rate for those with respiratory failure was 86 to
100% in eight studies and 50 to 58% in two studies. The authors
recommend that patients with AIDS be encouraged, within a short time

of diagnosis, to provide directives regarding life-sustaining treatments or to designate surrogates to make such decisions in the event
of mental incompetence. Although physicians should use alternatives
to the ICU when the prognosis for recovery is minimal, arbitrary
policies denying intensive care to AIDS patients are not warranted.

Of interest to persons with AIDS, physicians, hospital administrators,
and medical ethicists.

439. WALTERS, LeRoy. "Ethical issues in the prevention and treat-
      ment of HIV infection and AIDS." *Science* 239 (1988):
      597-603.

Discusses how the ethical principles of beneficence, justice, and
respect for autonomy relate to the AIDS epidemic.

Discussion

Both health care workers and the health care system have a moral
obligation to provide care to people with HIV infection, but heroic
self-sacrifice should not be required, provided that infection control
precautions are observed. Patients with neurological involvement and
terminally ill patients will benefit from statutes allowing recognition of advance directives about preferred modes of care or
nontreatment. There is a moral imperative to perform intensive
research directed toward the understanding, treatment, and prevention
of HIV infection and AIDS.

Of interest to laymen and health professionals.

440. YOUNG, Ernlé W.D. "AIDS: Emerging moral questions."
      Journal of American College Health 34 (1986): 240-242.

Examines some of the moral questions that AIDS poses for homosexual
and bisexual men, for medical caregivers, and for society at large.

Descriptive

Raises questions for those at risk for AIDS or actually infected with
it about honesty and love in sexual relationships. For caregivers, it
raises questions about the nature of their professional obligations.
And for society at large, it raises questions about confidentiality
and scapegoating.

Of interest to philosophers, theologians, and pastoral counselors.

441. ZUGER, Abigail. "Professional responsibilities in the AIDS
      generation. AIDS on the wards: A residency in medical
      ethics." *Hastings Center Report* 17, no. 3 (1987): 16-20.

A personal account of the education in medical ethics received by an
internal medicine resident working on the AIDS wards at New York's
Bellevue Hospital.

Essay

In addition to the ethical issues that occur in the medical care of any patients who are critically ill, the care of AIDS patients involves a number of "physician-oriented" ethical issues. For example, the medical profession is currently divided about what a physician's responsibility is regarding the acceptance of patients with AIDS. Many physicians are reluctant to care for AIDS patients for a variety of reasons besides the fear of AIDS. However, residents caring for AIDS patients develop a facility for dealing with dying patients and their families, a familiarity with most of the ethical dilemmas that face physicians, and an insight into their own conceptions about the duties of a physician in plague time. Residencies would be greatly improved by the provision of counseling and formal instruction in medical ethics by experienced AIDS physicians, available to guide and advise.

Of interest to medical educators, medical ethicists, and hospital administrators.

442. ———, and Steven H. Miles. "Physicians, AIDS, and occupa-
      tional risk: Historic traditions and ethical obligations."
      Journal of the American Medical Association 258, no. 14
      (1987): 1924-1928.

A discussion of the reluctance of some physicians to care for patients with acquired immunodeficiency syndrome.

Commentary

A new professional ethic is needed to guide physicians in the immunodeficiency syndrome pandemic. This ethic cannot be derived entirely from the right of these patients to health care, which is primarily a claim against society rather than individual practition-ers. A professional duty to treat human immunodeficiency virus-infected persons could be based on the understanding of medicine as a moral enterprise.

Of interest to physicians and medical philosophers and historians.

3. PUBLIC HEALTH AND PUBLIC POLICY ISSUES

a. Books

443. *AIDS and the Third World: The Impact on Development.*
      Hearing Before the Select Committee on Hunger, House of
      Representatives, One Hundredth Congress, Washington, DC,
      June 30, 1988. Serial No. 100-29. Washington, DC: U.S.
      Government Printing Office, 1988.

House of Representatives Hearing on the impact of AIDS in the Third World.

Proceedings

Contains prepared statements, letters, and other information from representatives of the World Health Organization, the United Nations, and various African organizations.

Of interest to the general public and to public health professionals.

444.   BAYER, Ronald.   *Private Acts, Social Consequences: AIDS and the Politics of Public Health.*   New York: Free Press, 1989.

Discusses the challenge of AIDS to the political community of America.

Text

Like epidemics of the past, AIDS has the potential for generating social disruption, challenging the fabric of social life, and inspiring rash and oppressive measures, especially since it has been marked in the United States by the social position of those most affected by the disease in its formative period.   Because it is transmitted in the context of the most intimate social relationships, or in contexts that have proven refractory to effective social control, HIV has forced a confrontation with the problem of how to respond to private acts that have critical social consequences. Public health officials, in the face of escalating tension between the rights of privacy and the demands of public health, must pursue those policies most likely to contribute to the emergence of a culture of restraint and responsibility among people whose life circumstance make the prospect for such a culture problematical.   An understanding of the history and legacy of the epidemic and the forces called into play by AIDS will be critical if the challenges of the epidemic are to be met and important social values preserved.

Of interest to public health officials, policymakers, and laymen.

445.   BLANCHET, Kevin D. (Ed.).   *AIDS: A Health Care Management Response.*   Rockville, MD: Aspen, 1988.

Deals with the difficult issues faced by hospital personnel in the midst of the AIDS epidemic from the perspective of the health care administrator.

Book of Readings

Offers a general overview of the disease and then enters into such issues as hospital infection control, public relations, legal issues, developing AIDS services, and the cost of care.   Contains information on the diagnosis, virus, and epidemiology of AIDS; infection control; nursing care; management of the psychosocial aspects of AIDS; the role of the social work department in the care of AIDS patients; and the challenge presented by AIDS to public relations and legal professionals in the hospital environment.

Useful to hospital administrators, physicians, nurses, social workers, public relations professionals, and legal professionals working in hospitals.

446.   BROWN, Raymond Keith.   *AIDS, Cancer and the Medical Establishment.*   New York: Robert Speller, 1986.

Presents three interwoven, unorthodox, and controversial themes regarding the nature, treatment, and politics of AIDS.

Monograph

Presents evidence that the AIDS virus is primarily an additional and catalytic cofactor precipitating disease in individuals whose body defenses are already compromised or defective; that cell wall deficient (pleomorphic) organisms that appear to bridge the gap between bacteria and viruses have been found in patients with AIDS and cancer; and that the tensions and conflicts between the philosophies of the medical establishment and of those who use alternative health and medical approaches to disease, as well as the inflexibility of our medical institutions, have resulted in the unavailability in the United States of many therapies pertinent to the treatment of AIDS. Argues that scientific medicine must reestablish a working alignment with the biologic aspects of health oriented medicine, as the capabilities of both are optimum when they work together and are allied to the concepts of holistic medicine, emphasizing mind, spirit, and biologic energies.

Of interest to physicians, researchers, and medical philosophers.

447. FALCO, Mathea, and Warren J. Cikins (Eds.).   *Toward a National Policy on Drug and AIDS Testing.* Washington, DC: The Brookings Institution, 1989.

This volume in the *Brookings Dialogues on Public Policy* is the product of two Brookings conferences on AIDS and drug-testing.

Conference Proceedings

Summarizes the discussions held at two meetings sponsored by the Brookings Institution to examine the critical issues raised by drug and AIDS testing. Participants in these meetings addressed the legal and political concerns, medical and public health concerns, private sector perspectives, and public policy implications of mandatory testing.

Of interest to public policymakers, public opinion analysts, and political scientists.

448. GRIGGS, John (Ed.).   *AIDS: Public Policy Dimensions.*   New York: United Hospital Fund of New York, 1987.

Based on the proceedings of a two-day national conference to respond to public policy issues raised by the AIDS epidemic held in New York City in January 1986 under the co-sponsorship of the United Hospital Fund of New York and the Institute for Health Policy Studies of the University of California, San Francisco School of Medicine.

Book of Readings

Following the introduction, 24 chapters provide an overview of the AIDS epidemic and information on the politics of AIDS, AIDS and the schools, AIDS and the blood supply, acute medical services, community care services, financial perspectives, and a long-term view of AIDS policy. Three appendices provide a case definition of AIDS; a statistical update, surveys, and projections; and a list of resources and organizations. The authors assess both the most effective approaches to dealing with the problems of AIDS and the implications the epidemic holds for our society.

Of interest to social scientists, public health professionals, and public policymakers and planners.

449. HUMMEL, Robert F., William F. Leavy, Michael Rampolla, Sherry Chorost (Eds.). *AIDS: Impact on Public Policy. An International Forum: Policy, Politics, and AIDS*. New York: Plenum Press, 1986.

Proceedings of a conference, co-sponsored by the New York State Department of Health and the Milbank Memorial Fund in New York City on May 26-28, 1986, to promote a wider understanding of the social, medical, and economic issues surrounding AIDS and the role of governments in responding to them.

Conference Proceedings

The three keynote addresses deal with the fear and reality of heterosexual transmission of AIDS; AIDS as a classical public health problem in modern guise; and AIDS in the United Kingdom. The five conference sessions address the health, social, and ethical perspectives on public health and private rights; international cooperation and competition in research; treatment modes and impact on the health care system; enhancing public understanding and fostering disease prevention; and an international perspective on AIDS and economics.

Of particular interest to health care administrators, health educators, public health professionals, government officials, legislators, and public policymakers.

450. INSTITUTE of Medicine, National Academy of Sciences. *Confronting AIDS: Directions for Public Health, Health Care, and Research*. Washington, DC: National Academy Press, 1986.

Reports on a study initiated to develop recommendations about the best course of action for dealing with the problems raised by the AIDS epidemic.

Committee Report

The committee's rationale for its major recommendations, which are abstracted at the end of the book, is underscored in seven chapters: summary and recommendations for confronting AIDS; understanding of the disease and dimensions of the epidemic; the future course of the epidemic and available national resources; opportunities for altering the course of the epidemic; care of persons infected with HIV; future research needs; and international aspects of AIDS and HIV infection. Included among the appendices are chapters on the clinical manifestations of HIV infection, serologic and virologic testing, and the risk of HIV transmission from blood transfusions as well as a list of public and private resources for fighting AIDS, the Center for Disease Control's surveillance definition of AIDS, the CDC classification system for HIV infections, and the Public Health Service plan for prevention and control of AIDS and the AIDS virus.

Intended for government officials, members of the research community, physicians and other health care workers, corporate leaders, and members of the general public.

451. ———. *Confronting AIDS: Update 1988*.   Washington, DC: National Academy Press, 1988.

This is an update of *Confronting AIDS: Directions for Public Health, Health Care, and Research*, which was published in 1986. It does not duplicate, but supplements, the material in the original report.

Text

This volume presents the findings and recommendations of the AIDS Activities Oversight Committee of the Institute of Medicine/National Academy of Sciences. It highlights new information or events that have given rise to the need for new directions. It also focuses on recommendations from the earlier report that deserve re-emphasis. The chapters deal with HIV infection and its epidemiology; understanding the course of the epidemic; altering the course of the epidemic; care of persons infected with HIV; the biology of HIV and biomedical research needs; international aspects of AIDS and HIV infection; and a national commission on HIV infection and AIDS.

Of interest to epidemiologists, health care providers, public health officials, and researchers concerned with HIV and AIDS.

452. McKUSICK, Leon (Ed.).   *What to Do About AIDS: Physicians and Mental Health Professionals Discuss the Issues*.   Berkeley and Los Angeles: University of California Press, 1986.

Papers from a conference convened in San Francisco, September 13-14, 1985, by the AIDS Clinical Research Center at the University of California, San Francisco.

Book of Readings

Provides a background of basic medical information, including neuropsychiatric developments, and describes: mental health aspects of the epidemic; the specific impact of AIDS on gay men, drug users, newly seropositive individuals, women, and bereaved survivors; and the administrative strategies developed in San Francisco in efforts to serve the medical and psychosocial needs imposed by AIDS.

Of interest to physicians, nurses, and other health care providers, mental health professionals, health educators, public health officials, and public policymakers.

453. MILLER, Norman and Richard C.Rockwell (Eds.). *AIDS in Africa: The Social and Policy Impact.* Lewiston, NY: The Edward Mellen Press, 1988.

Brings together working papers and resource material from authors in Africa, North America, and the United Kingdom.

Book of Readings

Seeks to clarify the health and social realities in Africa, to pose questions and concepts for understanding the problem, and to provide bibliographic resources needed by instructors and researchers who would take up the AIDS challenge. The volume is designed to move from epidemiologic assessments of the problem, through historic and ecological issues, to longer sections that address the management and policy questions and, thereafter, the social and educational questions. The final section of the book is designed as a resource guide that addresses the question, "Where do we go from here?"

Of interest to social scientists, historians, political analysts, and epidemiologists.

454. PANEM, Sandra. *The AIDS Bureaucracy.* Cambridge, MA: Harvard University Press, 1988.

Centers on the AIDS bureaucracy—the institutions on which we most rely during a health emergency.

Text

The discussion of the various agencies shows how the lack of communication within and among the various groups exacerbated the effort to manage the AIDS epidemic. The federal budget process is examined to show the vital role politics plays in determining fiscal priorities. The public relations and communications aspects, particularly how the media affected public perceptions and misconceptions about the disease, is discussed. The book concludes with suggestions of ways to improve the management of future novel health emergencies. Public policy options that might facilitate crisis management are explored.

Of interest to the general public.

455. PETRICCIANI, J.C., I.D. Gust, P.A. Hoppe, H.W. Krijnen (Eds.). *AIDS: The Safety of Blood and Blood Products.* Chichester: John Wiley & Sons, 1987.

Proceedings of a World Health Organization meeting to review and discuss the current global situation regarding the safety of blood and blood products and issues related to donor antibody screening in order to formulate updated WHO recommendations for member states on the safety of blood and blood products in relation to AIDS.

Conference Proceedings

Divided into five sections: overview of infection with the AIDS virus, transmission of AIDS by blood and blood products, screening for antibodies to the AIDS virus, donor notification issues, and policy issues and screening strategies.   An appendix contains the newly formulated WHO recommendations.

Of interest to public health professionals, government policymakers, health care providers, laboratory personnel, and anyone who works with blood and blood products.

456. PIERCE, Christine, and Donald Vandeveer (Eds.).   *AIDS: Ethics and Public Policy.* Belmont, CA: Wadsworth, 1988.

Examines the ethical and public policy aspects of society's controversies over AIDS in an attempt to answer the question, "What should we do about AIDS?"

Book of Readings

Provides a broad overview of the AIDS epidemic, focusing on the factual aspects of AIDS and the ways in which it may be viewed (societal conceptions of the issues).   Identifies and examines the leading moral grounds purporting to justify restrictions on liberty; explores specific policy or legislative proposals for dealing with various aspects of the AIDS crisis and the concerns they raise regarding privacy, use of test data, job discrimination, and funding for health care for persons with AIDS; and examines the consequences of a general, widespread tendency to associate AIDS with sexually immoral behavior.

Of interest to public health officials, to legislators and public policymakers, and to concerned laypersons.

457. *REVIEW of the Public Health Service's Response to AIDS.* Washington, DC: U.S. Congress, Office of Technology Assessment, OTA-TM-H-24, February 1985.

Reviews the recent and proposed activities of the Public Health Service in response to AIDS, and evaluates the planning, resources, and staffing of PHS's efforts to control AIDS.

Review/Critique

Examines both technical aspects of research and related issues of public health policy, and addresses related issues of science and public policy.   Particular attention is paid to the adequacy, suitability, and direction of AIDS research encouraged and supported by PHS, including the efforts to develop vaccines against the disease; the adequacy and timeliness of the distribution of new knowledge and information among researchers and regulators; and the adequacy of PHS resources to support the activities needed to yield the best chances for immediate results in the prevention and treatment of AIDS.

Of particular interest to public health professionals and AIDS researchers.

458. ROWE, Mona, and Caitlin Ryan. *AIDS, A Public Health Challenge: State Issues, Policies and Programs. Volume 1: Assessing the Problem.* Washington, DC: U.S. Department of Health and Human Services, Public Health Service, October 1987.

This first of three volumes, providing a comprehensive review, for public policymakers, of the policy issues with which AIDS confronts the states, deals with the general assessment of the problem.

Sourcebook

The introduction to this volume contains a medical overview of AIDS and a list of major policy questions. It is followed by chapters on the administration and organization of AIDS-related programs, screening and testing for AIDS, surveillance of HIV infection, protecting the individual's right to confidentiality while protecting the public health, and reducing the potential for discrimination.

Intended for public policymakers for the states.

b. Articles

459. "AIDS and public health." *American Journal of Public Health* 78 (1988): Entire Issue.

A collection of articles focusing on the impact of AIDS on local and state health departments.

Special Journal Issue

This special issue contains 17 articles, which begin with a review of AIDS in historical perspective, and of lessons from the past in the control of venereal disease. The current impact of AIDS on state and local health departments is examined; the needs and priorities for epidemiologic research regarding the prevention of AIDS and HIV infection are reviewed; specific issues confronting public health departments and current responses are examined and analyzed; and future directions for public policy are discussed.

Of interest to all health professionals dealing with AIDS as well as public health professionals.

460. ADAM, Barry D. "The state, public policy, and AIDS disease." *Contemporary Crises* 13 (1989): 1-14.

Probes the "deep structure" of perceptions of AIDS and the ensuing public policy trends.

Descriptive

From 1981 to 1983, public talk about AIDS was virtually taboo. Since 1983, the massive proliferation of AIDS discourse has led to the development of an "official story," common in the press and clear in the presumptions underlying recent state policies in the United States, Canada, and the United Kingdom. These policies have favored state control of sexual speech and education, as well as control of people "blamed" for HIV infection, while community-based groups have sought to empower people to affirm their sexuality while avoiding viral transmission.

Of interest to public policymakers and public health officials.

461. ALDERMAN, Michael H., Ernest E. Drucker, Alan Rosenfield, Cheryl Healton. "Predicting the future of the AIDS epidemic and its consequences for the health care system of New York City." *Bulletin of the New York Academy of Medicine* 64 (1988): 175-183.

Utilizes existing data to develop a plausible scenario of AIDS on the health care system of New York City.

Analytical

HIV infected people now occupy 4.5% of the city's hospital beds. Projections of more inpatient beds consumed by HIV will produce bitter competition for space. Alternative methods of providing care can unburden the system, but the alternative care available in San Francisco does not exist elsewhere. Home care, hotels, clinics, day care hospitals, hospices, and the manpower to manage these services do not emerge by accident. The authors call for communal leadership to assess need and identify, plan, and implement schemes that will require new facilities and manpower.

Of interest to public health officials.

462. ARNO, Peter S. "AIDS: A balancing act of resources." *Business and Health* 4, no. 3 (1986): 20-24.

Discusses the federal response to the AIDS crisis, highlighting flaws in the public policy process and the health care system.

Discussion

Federal funds were not directly allocated to AIDS until two years after its recognition, hampering the biomedical and public health community's response and raising questions about the government's role and responsibility in protecting public health and providing medical care. Claims of racism, leveled at the health care system, blamed the government's initial lethargy on the fact that the first major risk groups were stigmatized minorities. Controversies arose regarding allocation of funds which, until recently, were targeted at basic biomedical studies and clinical drug trials rather than education and patient care. The financial burden of care has fallen on patients, their families and friends, and state and local governments, pointing out the need for an equitable system to finance general and catastrophic illness. Community-based organizations, which evolved to provide needed social support and health care services, have received generous local support in the form of money and volunteer labor. Their integrated approach to patient care provides a constructive model for the management of catastrophic illness.

Of interest to health professionals, policymakers, and laypersons.

463. BARNISH, Michael, and David V. Condoluci. "New Jersey's approach to AIDS." *Journal of the American Osteopathic Association* 88 (1988): 1091-1094.

Describes New Jersey's efforts to curb the AIDS problem.

Descriptive

In the last two years, New Jersey has quadrupled its spending on AIDS research and prevention to $8.2 million yearly. A network of services for local management is being coordinated by state legislators and public and private health groups throughout New Jersey. The AIDS program is divided into six areas: education and prevention, surveillance, testing and counseling, treatment and community support, home health care, and laboratory services.

Of interest to health professionals, public officials, and laymen.

464. BECKER, Marshall H. "AIDS and behavior change." *Public Health Reviews* 16 (1988): 1-11.

Suggests avenues for future intervention programs.

Review

The author paints a picture of a multi-faceted and complex set of behavioral problems that require serious and sustained interactions at the individual, community, and societal levels. The next series of planned interventions to change risky practices must take into account, tested principles of human behavior.

Of interest to social and behavioral scientists and health educators.

465. BENJAMIN, A.E. "Long-term care and AIDS: Perspectives from experience with the elderly." *Milbank Quarterly* 66 (1988): 415-443.

The author argues that with respect to the organization, financing, and delivery of health care services to persons with AIDS, there is another body of knowledge and experience on which we may draw, long-term care for the elderly.

Descriptive/Analytical

Despite the differences between the young adult population afflicted
with AIDS and the frail elderly with chronic illness, there are
important similarities between the problems facing these two
populations and the broad solutions available to them. Findings from
research on the elderly raise important issues relevant to AIDS and
may provide a basis for the development of service models for the care
of persons with AIDS. It seems essential, with respect to AIDS, to
study the disease course in terms of the needs and preferences of
family members, friends, volunteers, and nonmedical professionals, and
to identify specific circumstances in which medical intervention may
be necessary. Data on situational preferences is needed before
estimates can be made of the demand for nursing home and other
services.

Of interest to social scientists, public policy analysts, and health
care planners and policymakers.

466.   BOLAND, Mary G., Theodore J. Allen, Gwendolyn I. Long,
       Mary Tasker.   "Children with HIV infection: Collaborative
       responsibilities of the child welfare and medical communities."
       Social Work 33 (1988): 504-509.

Describes the collaborative efforts between the New Jersey Department
of Human Services and the Children's Hospital AIDS Program of New
Jersey.

Descriptive

The multiple social, ethical, legal, and medical issues related to HIV
infection suggest that the child welfare and health care communities
have a responsibility to work together and ensure that comprehensive
and coordinated services are available for children and their
families.

Of interest to social workers, child welfare workers, and
pediatricians.

467.   BRENNAN, Troyen A.   "Ensuring adequate health care for the
       sick: The challenge of the acquired immunodeficiency
       syndrome as an occupational disease." *Duke Law Journal* 1
       (1988): 29-70.

Explores the legal and ethical issues involved in requiring health
professionals to care for HIV-infected persons, and suggests ways to
encourage the provision of adequate care.

Analytical

Legal action based on patient abandonment, the Hill-Burton Reconstruction Act, anti-discrimination statutes, and/or a sense of duty
will cause some institutions and professionals to provide adequate
care for HIV-infected persons. It is proposed that a more effective
way of ensuring care would be to provide governmental incentives to
hospitals to become AIDS centers and generous compensation plans for
professionals with occupationally acquired HIV infections.

Of interest to health care professionals, public health officials, public policymakers, and legislators.

468. CARLSON, Gregory A., Michael Greeman, Thomas A. McClellan. "Management of HIV-positive psychiatric patients who fail to reduce high risk behaviors." *Hospital and Community Psychiatry* 40 (1989): 511-514.

Describes the clinical and legal dilemmas faced by psychiatric staff involved in providing inpatient care to HIV carriers who continue to practice high risk behaviors.

Discussion

Staff were unsure of their obligation to report the patients under a state law giving the Commissioner of Health the discretion to limit the freedoms of HIV-infected individuals who continue to practice high risk behaviors. Treatment of the patients also raised concerns about the appropriateness of treating noncompliant HIV-infected patients in traditional psychiatric settings and the lack of suitable aftercare facilities. The authors advocate a specialized treatment approach for noncompliant HIV-infected patients and provide recommendations that might serve as the foundation for such an effort.

Of interest to mental health professionals, public health officials, and lawyers.

469. CARLSON, Gregory A., and Thomas A. McClellan. "The voluntary acceptance of HIV-antibody screening by intravenous drug users." *Public Health Reports* 102 (1987): 391-394.

An investigation of interest in HIV antibody screening and extent of exposure among intravenous drug abusers in a methadone program.

Research

A group of intravenous drug abusers in a Minnesota methadone program were offered HIV antibody screening. All were aware of AIDS and the risk of exposure through the sharing of injection paraphernalia. Thirty-nine (85%) were willing to be tested. Factors associated with acceptance of testing were: patient awareness of high seropositivity rates, indifference to potential negative social consequences of positive status, and the voluntary nature of the testing. None of the patients tested were positive.

Of interest to public health officials and mental health professionals involved in drug abuse programs.

470. "CONSENSUS Conference. The impact of routine HTLV-III antibody testing of blood and plasma donors on public health." *Journal of the American Medical Association* 256 (1986): 1778-1783.

A conference of biomedical investigators, blood bank specialists, clinicians, consumers, and representatives from public interest groups to consider questions regarding HTLV-III antibody testing.

Conference Summary

A procedure should be adopted by all blood banks to allow donors to indicate confidentially that their blood should not be transfused. A policy of protection of the individual donor's privacy should be vigorously pursued; however, blood banks must be responsible for properly informing the individual and arranging for counseling. Better methods of discouraging possibly infected donors and handling the psychosocial problems occurring in those with positive test results must be discovered through sound research projects.

Of interest to health professionals in general.

471.   COUGHLIN, Thomas A. III.   "AIDS in prisons: One correctional
       administrator's   recommended   policies   and   procedures."
       Judicature 72 (1988): 63-70.

Documents the steps necessary to meet the emerging crisis of AIDS in the correctional setting and demonstrates the importance of developing an integrated approach to administering equitable, judicially sanctioned AIDS policies and procedures.

Descriptive

The author draws upon his experience in dealing with AIDS issues in New York. He discusses program development, the identification and movement of prisoners with AIDS or ARC, placement and programming, educational efforts, testing, condoms and IV needles, and legal and confidentiality issues.

Of interest to correctional administrators.

472.   FALLONE, Edward A.   "Preserving the public health: A
       proposal to quarantine recalcitrant AIDS carriers."   *Boston
       University Law Review* 68, no. 2 (1988): 441-505.

Addresses the public safety and civil rights issues that must be weighed in formulating an effective response to the AIDS epidemic.

Theoretical

Quarantine of recalcitrant AIDS carriers is the most effective way to protect the health of the public. An existing statute can be amended to include AIDS in the list of diseases quarantinable under state law, or a new law can be enacted. Isolation of carriers should be used only as a last resort. Quarantine powers should include such options as surveillance, occupational restrictions, and orders to modify behaviors that transmit the virus. Quarantine legislation can survive judicial testing if it addresses the problems of procedural and substantive due process and equal protection.

Of interest to lawyers, legislators, and public health officials.

473. FAUCI, Anthony S. "The scientific agenda for AIDS." *Issues in Science and Technology* 4, no. 2 (1988): 33-39.

A description of the direction and role of the National Institutes of Health in combatting AIDS.

Commentary

The urgency of AIDS forced NIH to modify its traditional practice of letting investigator-initiated research guide scientific programs. NIH has funded a large number of government-directed contracts and issued many specific requests for grant applications. More recently, NIH has allocated a greater proportion of its funds to collaborative agreements. As more investigators become interested in AIDS research and more institutions develop the capability of treating AIDS patients, the program is slipping back toward investigator-initiated research. Central to NIH's policies on AIDS is support of basic research.

Of interest to health professionals and public health officials.

474. FOX, Daniel M. "AIDS and the American Health Polity: The history and prospects of a crisis in authority." *The Milbank Quarterly* 64, Supplement 1 (1986): 7-33.

Discusses how a crisis of authority was transforming the U.S. polity.

Discussion

Changing priorities between infectious and chronic diseases, community and individual responsibility for health, and comprehensive services and cost control created a fragmented health polity, leaderless and ill-prepared to address the AIDS epidemic. The U.S. health polity may best serve the public interest when institutions within it do not accept fragmentation as the goal and the norm of health affairs.

Of interest to public policy makers, political scientists, and public health officials.

475. FREUDENBERG, Nicholas, Jacalyn Lee, Diana Silver. "How black and Latin community organizations respond to the AIDS epidemic: A case study in one New York City neighborhood." *AIDS Education and Prevention* 1, no. 1 (1989): 12-21.

Investigators, to determine what specific roles community-based orga- nizations are playing in AIDS prevention and how such efforts are changing their activities and perceived goals, are examining how community groups in two black and Latino neighborhoods in New York City are responding to local and prevention campaigns. Preliminary data from one community are presented and discussed.

Research

Many community-based organizations have already defined a role for themselves in AIDS prevention, supporting the view that neighborhood groups can play a vital role in AIDS prevention. However, community action for AIDS prevention is not a substitute for significant government involvement in the AIDS control effort. Neighborhood groups, even when they understand the threat posed by the AIDS epidemic, need training, administrative and staff support, and financial resources if they are to be able to take on AIDS prevention. Public health officials seeking to encourage community organizations to become active need to understand that AIDS is just one more stress among a wide variety of problems and must learn how to integrate AIDS prevention into a larger community agenda.

Of particular interest to public health officials.

476. GARRISON, Jean (Ed.). "AIDS and adolescents: Exploring the challenge." *Journal of Adolescent Health Care* 10, no. 3 Supplement (May 1989): Entire issue.

Outgrowth of the first national conference focusing on AIDS as it affects adolescents, convened in New York City on March 27 and 28, 1988, to focus attention on the adolescent population as an at risk group with distinct needs and problems, facilitate information sharing, and develop a set of recommendations that could serve as the basis for a national agenda to address the AIDS epidemic as it relates to adolescents.

Special Journal Issue

Includes articles and excerpts from addresses on adolescents and AIDS; AIDS in adolescence: exploring the challenge; and ethical and legal issues in research and intervention; as well as the recommendations of the four work groups, focusing on AIDS prevention and education, services and treatment issues, AIDS policies on youth, and AIDS testing and epidemiology for youth.

Of interest to health professionals and researchers concerned with adolescent medicine.

477. GERBERDING, J. Louise, and David K. Henderson. "Design of rational infection control policies for human immunodeficiency virus infection." *Journal of Infectious Diseases* 156 (1987): 861-864.

Describes some of the current issues and controversies that must be addressed by practitioners who are responsible for developing institutional infection control policies for HIV.

Review

Dispute has arisen regarding the role of testing for HIV infection. Two national trends have recently become apparent: 1) increased demand for HIV testing as a prerequisite for assigning infection control procedures, and 2) increased commitment to universal precautions regarding blood and body fluids from all patients, regardless of HIV test results. The relative advantages and disadvantages of screening for HIV infection and of universal precautions are discussed.

Of interest to physicians, public health officials, and hospital administrators.

478. GINZBURG, Harold M., Patricia Leehan Fleming, Kirk D. Miller. "Selected public health observations derived from the Multicenter AIDS Cohort Study." *Journal of Acquired Immune Deficiency Syndromes* 1 (1988): 2-7.

Reviews selected findings from the Multicenter AIDS Cohort Study (MACS) of homosexual/bisexual men, and addresses high risk sexual behaviors, the use of drugs/alcohol, condom use, and behavior change.

Review

Educational programs and those that focus on behavior modification are potentially significant strategies for public health intervention. Until a realistic timetable for vaccine availability and more effective chemotherapy exist, the MACS will provide the opportunity to continue to study the effects of behavior change on the AIDS epidemic.

Of interest to epidemiologists and public health officials.

479. GOEDERT, James J. "What is safe sex? Suggested standards linked to testing for immunodeficiency virus." *New England Journal of Medicine* 316 (1987): 1229-1342.

Urges widespread voluntary testing of sexually active adults for HIV and the development of standards for safe sex.

Editorial

Although the influence of testing on the medical, psychological, social, and economic consequences of HIV infection are real and important concerns, the benefits of widespread voluntary testing to seropositive, as well as seronegative persons, may well outweigh the potential harms. Testing, in conjunction with counseling and unequivocal "standards" for safe sex, provides an important first step in meeting the public health challenges posed by AIDS. Sensitive and specific HIV-antibody testing can be used as a tool for scientifically defining rational standards for sexual partners that will eliminate the further sexual spread of HIV.

Of particular interest to public health professionals.

480. GOSTIN, Larry, and William J. Curran (Eds.). "AIDS: Law and policy." *Law, Medicine and Health Care* 15, nos. 1-2 (1987): Entire issue.

This second part of a two-issue special symposium on AIDS touches on
each of the major legal and ethical issues facing the U.S. government
nationally and WHO internationally.

Special Journal Issue

The essays in this issue cover criminal, civil, public health, and
anti-discrimination law. They demonstrate the legislative dimensions
of AIDS, analyzing available public policy options to slow the spread
of the disease; demonstrate the legal and practical problems involved
in criminalizing transmission; explain the legal theories and possible
defenses that inform civil litigation for transmission of HIV; show
why personal control measures would achieve no clear public health
objective,   while   trampling   on   human   rights;   consider   the
constitutional implications of state AIDS policies; set forth the
public health strategy for combatting AIDS; probe the limits of the
law in search of a remedy for discrimination against persons with HIV;
and review the scientific and legal challenges of getting an AIDS
vaccine to the market.

Of interest to health professionals, public health officials, lawyers,
legislators, and public policymakers.

481. ——— (Eds.). "AIDS: Science and Epidemiology." *Law,
      Medicine and Health Care* 14, nos. 5-6 (1986): Entire issue.

Brings together the research of physicians, epidemiologists, and
social scientists who have been at the forefront of devising a medical
and public health response to AIDS.   Addresses the major public
controversies surrounding the disease.

Special Journal Issue

A series of nine essays, which address a public health strategy in
response to the epidemic, epidemiologic predictions, research on
experimental drugs, intravenous drug abusers, screening, treatment,
and worldwide strategies.

Of interest to health professionals, social and behavioral scientists,
lawyers, and epidemiologists.

482. ———.   "AIDS screening, confidentiality, and the duty to
      warn." *American Journal of Public Health* 77 (1987): 361-365.

General criteria for assessing compulsory screening of persons with
antibodies to HIV.

Descriptive

Testing for the presence of HIV antibodies can provide a clear focus
for public education and counseling as a foundation for behavior
change. The cost free and timely availability of professional testing
for persons vulnerable to HIV is an essential part of the public
health strategy to impede the spread of the infection. In order to

protect the privacy of high-risk groups and be fair to clinicians, statutory confidentiality protection with specific exceptions for foreseeable harm to others would be an important adjunct to this strategy.

Of interest to lawyers, public policymakers and public health officials.

483. ———. "Control measures for AIDS: Reporting requirements, surveillance, quarantine, and regulation of public meeting places." *American Journal of Public Health* 77 (1987): 214-218.

Discusses reporting, surveillance and contact tracing, personal control measures, and regulation of public meeting places.

Descriptive

Public policymakers can be virtually assured of judicial and political support for compulsory public health measures to control the spread of AIDS that are carefully based upon the current state of scientific understanding.

Of interest to public policymakers, public health professionals, and lawyers.

484. GOSTIN, Larry, and Andrew Ziegler. "A review of AIDS-related legislative and regulatory policy in the United States." *Law, Medicine and Health Care* 15 (1987): 5-16.

Presents a survey of U.S. public health statutes and regulations to control the spread of AIDS, using data collected by the Harvard School of Public Health and the Governmental Health Policy Project at George Washington University.

Research

The statutes are classified according to their broad public health function or purpose. It is argued that public health law need not be restrictive or punitive; rather, the law can make a rich contribution to public health efforts by setting standards, mandating education and services, funding research, and safeguarding individual privacy and rights.

Of interest to lawyers, public policymakers, and health care administrators.

485. GOSTIN, Larry O. "Public health strategies for confronting AIDS." *Journal of the American Medical Association* 261 (1989): 1621-1630.

Categorizes and reports on AIDS-related legislative and regulatory policy in the United States.

Descriptive

This review of AIDS legislation throughout the country reveals a mixed record. Most states have come to accept the health service research that has shown the sometimes remarkable efficacy of well-targeted education and counseling and the promise of pharmaceutical research. There has been a wide acceptance of the critical public health importance of confidentiality and guarantees of antidiscrimination. Ensuring the privacy and equal treatment of persons with HIV infection is essential to the success of epidemiologic studies, testing, outreach programs, and treatment for IV drug users. While legislatures have responded well to health service research, they have also been highly susceptible to the attitude that the primary modes of HIV transmission are immoral, even criminal. Political pressures on legislatures to use coercive powers of the state to combat the epidemic are unmistakable. The use of coercive powers, far from accomplishing the objective of impeding the AIDS epidemic, could well fuel it.

Of interest to public health officials, legislators and lawyers.

486. GOSTIN, Lawrence O., William J. Curran, Mary E. Clark. "The case against compulsory casefinding in controlling AIDS-testing, screening and reporting." *American Journal of Law and Medicine* 12 (1987): 7-53.

Proposes criteria for evaluating compulsory testing and screening programs.

The fairness and accuracy of compulsory screening programs depend upon the reliability of medical technology and the balancing of public health and individual confidentiality interests. There must be a fully planned distribution of test sites in areas with high infection rates, infected individuals must be identified on a voluntary basis, and a comprehensive program of focused education and counseling provided. States must enact statutes to protect the confidentiality of sensitive information obtained during testing, counseling, and contact tracing. Voluntary identification, education, and counseling of infected persons in an atmosphere of trust will encourage the behavior changes necessary to halt the spread of AIDS.

Of interest to public health professionals and public planners and policymakers.

487. HENRY, Keith. "Setting AIDS priorities: The need for a closer alliance between public health and clinical approaches toward the control of AIDS. *American Journal of Public Health* 78 (1988): 1210-1212.

A summary of the author's experience with AIDS as a physician and public health official.

Commentary

Three suggestions are made: additional studies about the biology of HIV in the genital tract need to be conducted; clinical trials studying drug therapy of HIV infection need to assess the effect of HIV in the genital tract; and clinicians involved in studies and the care of HIV infection need to implement educational strategies minimizing transmission of HIV from their patients. More interaction between public health and clinical approaches to AIDS is needed.

Of interest to public health officials.

488. HERRING, L.W. "The increasing role of constituencies of a federal public health agency: A case study on acquired immunodeficiency syndrome (AIDS)." *International Journal of Public Administration* 10 (1987): 235-254.

Examines the effect of constituencies on the programs and policies of a public health agency using AIDS as a case study.

Case Study

The influence of constituencies and the effect of public opinion on development, implementation, and administration of public sector programs is well illustrated in the confrontation with the threat of AIDS to the public health. These constituencies are a major element in which public agencies carry out their business. Appropriate and timely press releases, informational materials directed to targeted audiences, sensitive and informed telephone response to public inquiries, and a conscious effort to present information in a direct, meaningful manner are challenges and mandates for public administrators. Agencies must continue to get the message to the media to answer the fears and questions raised by AIDS, to combat hysteria, and to change behaviors that promote the transmission of AIDS.

Of interest to public health officials.

489. JOSEPH, Stephen C., Stephen Schultz, Rand Stoneburner, Peggy Clarke. "AIDS policy and prevention in New York City." *Bulletin of the New York Academy of Medicine* 63 (1987): 659-672.

Describes projections on the AIDS epidemic in New York City and nationally; analyzes current and evolving policy in New York City; presents the epidemic's epidemiology; and outlines specific issues of prevention.

Descriptive

The AIDS epidemic over the next five to ten years will persist as a medical, social, and political problem in New York City. Public policy must reflect current knowledge of disease transmission and, at the same time, be flexible enough to accommodate important discoveries relevant to the etiology and biology of AIDS.

Of general interest to health professionals and laymen.

490. KASTNER, Theodore A., Mary Lu Hickman, Dennis
     Bellehumeur. "The provision of services to persons with
     mental retardation and subsequent infection with human
     immunodeficiency virus (HIV)." *American Journal of Public
     Health* 79 (1989): 491-494.

Discusses the implications of HIV infection in their clients for
agencies which provide services to mentally retarded persons.

Commentary

The first reported cases of individuals with mental retardation who
have subsequently become infected with HIV are presented. While the
mentally retarded do not constitute a high risk group for HIV
infection, deficits in social judgement, combined with high-risk
behavior, can increase the risk of HIV infection. The medical,
social, ethical, and political implications of this finding for
agencies which provide services to persons with mental retardation are
described. The authors propose that, where conflicts arise, ethical
review committees provide consultation to service agencies who must
ultimately determine how they will provide for the needs of their
clients.

Of interest to mental health professionals.

491. KERR, Dianne L. "AIDS update: The Canada Youth and AIDS
     Study." *Journal of School Health* 59 (1989): 86.

Summarizes findings from a survey of 30,000 Canadians, 11 to 21 years
of age, about their knowledge, attitudes, and behaviors relating to
AIDS and other sexually transmitted diseases.

Research

Findings demonstrate that although most Canadian youth know what AIDS
is and how it is transmitted, they continue to take behavioral risks.
Street youth, who do not have money to buy condoms, are most at risk
because of their sexual and needle-sharing activities. Many Canadian
youth have the same feelings toward people with HIV infection as they
have toward homosexuals.

Of interest to social scientists, health educators, and public health
officials.

492. KLATT, Edward C., and Thomas T. Noguchi. "The medical
     examiner and AIDS: Death certification, safety procedures,
     and future medicolegal issues." *The American Journal of
     Forensic Medicine and Pathology* 9, no. 2 (1988): 141-148.

Outlines an approach to handling AIDS deaths based upon case
definition, diagnosis by available information and procedures, and
proper infection control.

Descriptive

The authors have worked with HIV infected cases for over eight years and have performed over 200 AIDS autopsies without transmission of HIV or other infectious agents to themselves or their employees. Accurate documentation of findings and certification of deaths through attention to detail has enabled the authors to deal with medicolegal issues with minimal problems.

Of interest to physicians, especially pathologists.

493. KLEIMAN, Mark A.R. "AIDS, vice, and public policy." *Law and Contemporary Problems* 51 (1988): 315-368.

This essay first examines transmission and transmission prevention, interventions and the way individuals can be expected to react to changes in risk, and the technical ramifications and political implications of testing and identification devices and then applies those general concepts to specific populations and problems.

Essay/Descriptive

Policy analysis has something to say about the AIDS epidemic and how to limit it. It can allow rough calculations of efficacy and rough comparisons of cost effectiveness across the choices to be made given current knowledge and techniques. By illuminating crucial areas of ignorance, it can guide future research efforts. Analysis shows that people who say that the AIDS problem will be solved by education are either using the term extremely broadly or are badly oversimplifying the problem.

Of interest to public policy analysts, lawyers, and social scientists.

494. KRUSKALL, Margot S., and Joel Umlas. "Acquired immunodeficiency syndrome and directed blood donations: A dilemma for American medicine." *Archives of Surgery* 123 (1988): 23-25.

A discussion of recipient-orchestrated (directed) blood donations as a method of improving the safety of blood transfusions.

Commentary

Blood banks should discourage the use of directed blood donations, and physicians should work to educate the public about the lack of benefit of directed donations and their potential risk.

Of interest to all health professionals and public health officials.

495. KULLER, Lewis H., and Lawrence Kingsley. "The epidemic of AIDS: A failure of public health policy." *The Milbank Quarterly* 64, Supplement 1 (1986): 56-78.

The AIDS epidemic was introduced on a substantial and rising epidemic of sexually transmitted diseases. Complex social, political, and professional factors are examined based on previous studies with a single risk group--homosexual men--to illuminate the continuing failure to combat the epidemic.

Commentary

Selective traditional public health measures, applied vigorously and objectively with a new legal framework, are still appropriate.

Of interest to public policy makers and health care administrators.

496.   LEE, Philip R., and Peter S. Arno.   "The federal response to the AIDS epidemic." *Health Policy* 6 (1986): 259-267.

The response of the U.S. government to the AIDS epidemic is reviewed within the context of health policy making in the U.S.

Review

This review, which involves multiple levels of government, addresses the relationship of government to the private sector, the diffusion of authority within a federal system, the long delays in policy implementation because of the absence of mechanisms to deal with emergency situations, and the tendency to fund the response to AIDS from reallocation of appropriated funds, thereby creating financial distress for existing programs. The federal response to AIDS is considered uncoordinated, insufficient, and inadequate, particularly with respect to the support of public health education and the financing of health care for AIDS patients.

Of interest to health professionals, public officials, and the lay public.

497.   LEVINE, Carol, and Joyce Bermel (Eds.).   "AIDS: Public health and civil liberties." *Hastings Center Report* 16, Supplement (December 1986): 1-36.

A series of five essays weave together themes from law, public health, and ethics in analyzing 19th century public health responses to infectious disease.

Special Supplement

The conclusions suggest that calls for a wide-ranging compulsory public health response, in the form of screening, reporting of HIV seropositivity, isolation, and quarantine, are unjustified on scientific, legal, or ethical grounds. However, limited, carefully planned and implemented programs, with adequate protections for individuals, can be effective under some circumstances.

Of interest to health professionals, laymen, and professionals in law, ethics, and public health.

498.   LOVICK, Lloyd F.   "New York State in the AIDS epidemic." *Bulletin of the New York Academy of Medicine* 63 (1987): 692-712.

Describes projections for the future incidence of AIDS in New York State and outlines actions necessary to retard the growth of this epidemic.

Descriptive/Analytical

Surveillance data amply demonstrate the occurrence of HIV infection in growing numbers. Further spread will make intervention even more difficult. If this is the scope of the problem, the solution is to educate and encourage behaviors among the public that will interrupt the transmission. Focusing on risk groups will continue to be necessary, but this is a community-wide problem in which the entire population must be aware of risky behaviors, consequences, and reduction techniques. The New York State Department of Health will continue to gather and to improve surveillance data, to offer counseling and screening, and to provide a coordinated care system for patients.

Of particular interest to health professionals in New York and other eastern states.

499. MEJTA, Cheryl L., Evelyn Denton, Mary Ellen Krems, Rebecca A. Hiatt. Acquired immunodeficiency syndrome (AIDS): A survey of substance abuse clinic directors' and counselors' knowledge, attitudes, and reactions." *Journal of Drug Issues* 18 (1988): 403-419.

Two surveys of the drug abuse treatment system in the Chicago area were conducted to acquire information about the willingness of drug abuse treatment providers to work with those at risk for or with AIDS and their attitudes and reactions toward this client population.

Research

Across clinics, policies and practices were found to be inconsistent, frequently incomplete, inadequate, and, at times, questionable. Many directors would not admit or were uncertain if they would admit persons with AIDS for treatment. Most had incomplete AIDS infection control policies, a few had questionable policies, and several had none. Clearer, nondiscriminatory federal and state AIDS guidelines need to be established and implemented at the clinic level. Counselors, like the general population, have apprehensions concerning AIDS.

Of interest to drug or substance abuse counselors and mental health professionals.

500. MEYER, Klemens B., and Stephen G. Pauker. "Screening for HIV: Can we afford the false positive rate?" *New England Journal of Medicine* 317 (1987): 238-241.

Discusses the possible impact on the general public of widespread HIV-antibody testing.

Commentary

Plans to test low-risk populations for HIV antibody generally ignore the possibility of false positive results. Before adopting a public policy of widespread screening, we should consider whether testing that is justified in the blood bank is justified in other settings. Screening a population in which the prevalence of HIV is relatively low, while the possibility of false positive results exists, will unavoidably stigmatize and frighten many healthy people, especially those unfortunate individuals who are incorrectly identified as infected. It is not certain that widespread screening will affect the course of the AIDS epidemic, and serious consideration must be given to the fact that the benefits of identifying infected persons may not justify the personal and social burden of false positive results.

Of particular interest to public health officials, legislators, and health policymakers.

501. MIRAMONTES, Helen.   "Needed: Effective national policy on
      AIDS/HIV infection."   *Nursing Outlook* 36 (1988): 262-263.

Cites the continued lack of leadership after seven years of the AIDS epidemic.

Commentary

Reviews three major areas of controversy--routine testing of blood and body chemistries, education, and allocation of services--and appeals for a national policy to deal with AIDS.

Of general interest to health professionals.

502. MORIN, Stephen.   "AIDS in one city."   *American Psychologist*
      39 (1984): 1294-1296.

An interview with Mervyn Silverman, Director of Health for San Francisco, California.

Commentary

Chronicles the public health department's efforts to address the many problems of the AIDS epidemic. Calls upon representatives of the health establishment to be consistent in their messages and policy statements about AIDS.

Will interest a general audience.

503. O'HARA, Joseph J., and Gary J. Stangler.   "AIDS and the
      human services."   *Public Welfare* 44, no. 3 (1986): 7-13.

A discussion of the process by which policies regarding AIDS were formed in State Departments of Corrections and Departments of Mental Health.

Discussion

Human service administrators must be aggressively proactive and develop appropriate policies and procedures, train necessary staff, and mount suitable public information programs before a situation becomes a confrontation.

Of interest to state human services administrators.

504. OSBORN, June E. "AIDS: Politics and science." *New England Journal of Medicine* 318 (1988): 444-447.

Discusses inappropriate political responses to AIDS.

Commentary

Because much has been determined about the causes, transmission, and effective means of prevention of HIV infection, policymakers have the opportunity to respond without panic and without resorting to extreme measures. However, few are taking advantage of the opportunity for rational action and, instead of endorsing public education, some politicians are espousing such inappropriate actions as mandatory testing and quarantine. Policies dominated by overreaction have the effect of victimizing the sick rather than making use of available scientific insights to protect the public health.

Of general interest.

505. QUINTON, Anthony. "Plagues and morality." *Social Research* 55 (1988): 477-489.

Discusses the interrelationship of plagues and morality.

Opinion

Epidemics historically provoke responses, based on moral beliefs, that involve the rights of the infected and non-infected, social policy, and personal responsibility. The author advocates the segregation of HIV-infected prisoners, discharge of seropositive military personnel, and antibody screening of insurance applicants. He suggests that physicians should inform patients of their infection and that HIV-infected persons should take precautions against infecting others.

Of interest to ethicists, public health officials, and public policymakers.

506. "REPORT of the second Public Health Service AIDS Prevention and Control Conference." *Public Health Reports* 103, Supplement no. 1 (1988): Entire issue.

Results from a conference of AIDS experts, assembled by the Public Health Service in Charlottesville, VA on June 1-3, 1988, to examine the current dimensions of the HIV problem, assess our progress to date, and plan for the future.

Report/Special Journal Issue

The full report of the 1988 Charlottesville meeting identifies more than 100 issues, 200 goals, and 500 objectives as priority areas for Public Health Service efforts in controlling the AIDS epidemic. The report is divided into ten sections, corresponding to the nine major areas of activity on AIDS and HIV within the Public Health Service, and to the HIV epidemic as it affects women, minorities, and children.

Of interest to all health professionals and public officials.

507. RICHARDS, Edward P. "Communicable disease control in Colorado: A rational approach to AIDS." *Denver University Law Review* 65, no. 2-3 (1988): 127-179.

Provides practical information to Colorado professionals dealing with communicable diseases, including AIDS, and gives persons outside Colorado an overview of the legal premises and practical details of the Colorado AIDS control law.

Descriptive

As a society, we must reappraise our economic, political, and intellectual commitment to public health. HIV is a human tragedy, but it is also a warning. Shifting patterns of urbanization, transportation, and class stratification will disrupt the dormancy of traditional plagues and set the stage for new disease agents and vectors. HIV has demonstrated that we are not prepared to meet these challenges.

Of interest to public policymakers, legislators, and lawyers.

508. SCHOUB, B.D. "The AIDS test." *South African Medical Journal* 74 (1988): 97-98.

Discusses the need for control of laboratory testing for HIV seropositivity in South Africa.

Editorial

The author expresses concern about the quality of HIV tests carried out by non-specialist laboratories in South Africa using newly marketed commercial tests. According to a recent report from the U.S. Army, on at least one occasion, more than half of the laboratories using such kits that applied for contracts with the army could not analyze test samples to a level of 95% accuracy and had to be rejected. Because of the potential social and personal consequences of misdiagnosis, it is suggested that the issue of controlling HIV testing by non-specialist laboratories be considered.

Should interest laboratory personnel, physicians, and health policymakers.

509. SCHULMAN, Lawrence C., and Joanne E. Mantell. "The AIDS crisis: A United States health care perspective." *Social Science and Medicine* 26 (1988): 979-988.

Examines the organizational impact and responses to the AIDS crisis in urban U.S. health care institutions with particular emphasis on New York City agencies, which have treated 1/3 of the cases.

Descriptive

Eleven recommendations for a comprehensive, coordinated health services delivery network are presented. Alternatives to an acute care locus for persons with AIDS are explored.

Of interest to social and behavioral scientists.

510. SMITHSON, R.D. "Public and health staff knowledge about AIDS." *Community Medicine* 10 (1988): 221-227.

A postal questionnaire was sent to 1,000 members of the public and 1,000 Health Authority employees in Walsall prior to the DHSS leaflet and TV advertising campaign to ascertain knowledge about AIDS.

Research

The survey showed good knowledge in both groups about how AIDS is transmitted. There was some uncertainty about ways in which it is not transmitted, particularly amongst the public and older age groups. Especially worrisome was the number of people, both public and health staff, who thought they could catch AIDS from donating blood.

Of interest to public health officials and health educators.

511. STAWAR, Terry L., Diane Goroum, Linda Brooks. "AIDS and infection control in community mental health agencies." *Perceptual and Motor Skills* 65 (1987): 786.

Provides an overview of the current effect of AIDS on infection control in community mental health agencies.

Survey

Results suggest that, nationally, as of 1986, community mental health agencies had not responded to AIDS, to any appreciable degree, with the development of infection control procedures or specialized services. Model infection control procedures for AIDS and other contagious diseases have generally called for blood-borne disease precautions similar to those for hepatitis B. These precautions may be problematic for outpatient and nonhospital based community mental health programs because facilities and resources are inadequate.

Of particular interest to mental health professionals.

512. SULLIVAN, Kathleen M., and Martha A. Field. "AIDS and the coercive power of the state." *Harvard Civil Rights-Civil Liberties Law Review* 23 (1988): 139-197.

Discusses quarantine and criminalization with respect to AIDS.

Review/Discussion

Four coercive devices for confining AIDS carriers or punishing AIDS transmission were discussed: status-based quarantine, behavior-based quarantine, traditional criminal laws, and possible new AIDS-specific criminal laws. If criminalization imposed no social harms, it might be a useful reinforcement of education and the dictates of undivided conscience, but any determination that criminal enactment might add to uncertainties that already exist is not worth the disadvantages of using the criminal law as a tool to contain the AIDS epidemic. Criminalization, like quarantine, would encourage some people to avoid voluntary testing. Moreover, punishing AIDS transmission would threaten the privacy of sexual relationships ranging beyond those that transmit AIDS. It would be a mistake to enact either criminal measures or quarantine to deal with the problem of transmission of AIDS.

Of particular interest to lawyers and public health officials.

513. TEMOSHOK, Lydia, David M. Sweet, Jane Zich. "A three city comparison of the public's knowledge and attitudes about AIDS." *Psychology and Health* 1 (1987): 43-60.

A survey was administered simultaneously in New York, San Francisco, and London to investigate how knowledge, beliefs, and attitudes about AIDS may be influenced by social and cultural contexts as well as by disease epidemiology.

Research

General fear of AIDS and anti-gay attitudes were significantly negatively correlated with knowledge about AIDS across all samples of the general public (excluding risk group members) in the three cities, and were significantly and positively associated with both sexual and health behavior change in London. In the New York sample, only sexual behavior change was significantly correlated with general fear of AIDS and anti-gay variables, while neither was significantly associated with behavior change of any kind in San Francisco. Data support the need for specific programs aimed at the general public that take into account the sociocultural and epidemiologic differences in the target populations.

Of interest to public health professionals, health professionals, health educators, public policy planners, and social and behavioral scientists.

514. VALDISERRI, Ronald O. "The immediate challenge of health planning for AIDS: An organizational model." *Family and Community Health* 10, no. 4 (1988): 33-48.

Proposes a model for health planning for AIDS to be used by health care facilities, and discusses the implications of AIDS for patient care.

Discussion

Making a commitment to planning is the most important step in the planning process. Adequate resources should be allocated to educating the staff about the psychosocial, epidemiologic, and medical issues related to AIDS. Policies, which address patient care, occupational exposure to AIDS, and HIV testing and confidentiality, should be developed. Patient education should include the protection of sexual and needle-sharing partners. The development of practical and psychosocial services should depend largely on the local incidence of AIDS. If the health facility's mission includes community outreach, education of community members should emphasize the fact that AIDS is a problem to be faced by the entire community.

Of interest to health care administrators, health educators, counselors, and social workers.

515. VERNON, Thomas M. "Colorado's promising 'model' for AIDS control." *Denver University Law Review* 65, no. 2-3 (1988): 109-116.

Describes the decisions made by Colorado's political and public health leadership to control AIDS.

Descriptive

The traditional disease control interventions adopted by Colorado do not constitute the entirety of an AIDS control program, but its successful contribution is testimony that a balance can be found for public health interactions, which protects the public's health as well as individual rights and confidentiality.

Of interest to politicians, legislators, lawyers, and public policymakers.

516. WEINBERG, David S., and Henry W. Murray. "Coping with AIDS: The special problems of New York City." *New England Journal of Medicine* 317 (1987): 1469-1473.

Presents an overview of the current AIDS situation in New York City with particular emphasis on the problems posed by the drug-abusing population.

Review

Approximately 500,000 persons in the New York metropolitan area were estimated to be infected with HIV in May 1987, and 10,322 cases of AIDS had been reported within the city, more than 25% of all the cases of AIDS reported nationwide. New HIV acquisition rates seem to have slowed among homosexuals, but they are increasing among IV drug abusers and are likely to continue doing so. Efforts to reach, educate, and motivate this population have had little success. The future need for hospital beds within the city may well be staggering, threatening the capacity of the city's entire system of acute hospital care, compromising the care of other acutely ill patients, and affecting the training of medical students and housestaff. The problem is exacerbated by the lack of a flexibly designed program for long-term home, hospice, or foster care. Projections of the magnitude of the epidemic over the next five years are made and suggestions offered for alleviating its possible consequences.

Of particular interest to public health officials, health policymakers, and legislators.

517. WINDOM, Robert E. "Current status of public health service efforts to cope with acquired immunodeficiency syndrome (AIDS) on a national basis." *Journal of the American Academy of Dermatology* 18 (1988): 743-743.

An overview of AIDS as related to dermatology.

Editorial

Dermatologic research is rapidly emerging as one of the most important potential avenues of study for gaining insight into the clinical management and character of this disease. Recent studies show that the many skin conditions associated with HIV infection and AIDS may bear some direct relation to the course of the disease.

Of interest to dermatologists.

518. ———, (Ed.). "The response to AIDS." *Public Health Reports* 103 (1988): Entire Issue.

Experts in a variety of fields share their perspectives on the battle against AIDS and the problems and prospects for progress in their particular areas.

Special Journal Issue

The nineteen articles in this collection present information on the various public health and public policy issues raised by the AIDS epidemic; the role of various governmental and private agencies in response to AIDS; the efforts to prevent and control HIV infection and AIDS through information, education, and research; the response of the medical community to AIDS, its efforts to combat the disease and to educate health professionals about exercising proper precautions while providing quality care; formulating AIDS policy; meeting the needs of persons with AIDS; and dealing with the ethical and economic concerns that arise from the AIDS epidemic.

Of interest to public health officials, health professionals, social service professionals, and public policymakers.

c. Chapter

519. KATZ, A.J., P.D. Cummings, S.G. Sandler, A. Berkowitz. "The impact of AIDS on the voluntary blood donor system: A preliminary analysis." *In* Irving J. Selikoff, Alvin S. Teirstein, Shalom Z. Hirschman (Eds.). *Acquired Immune Deficiency Syndrome.* New York: New York Academy of Sciences, 1984.

An assessment of the potential impact of AIDS on blood donor selection policy, blood collections, inventory levels, and distributions.

Review

The effectiveness of changes in blood donor screening await long-term observation because of the lack of baseline data on members of high risk groups and because collaborative efforts and education have led to deferral of donation prior to presentation at a blood collection center. Distribution changes of whole blood and red blood cells may relate to more conservative blood use by physicians due to sensitivity to AIDS, or to increasing cost consciousness.

Of interest to blood banking personnel and public health officials.

4. ECONOMIC ISSUES

a. Books

520. EDEN, Jill, Laurie Mount, Lawrence Miike. *AIDS and Health Insurance: An OTA Survey.* Washington, DC: Health Program, Office of Technology Assessment, United States Congress, February 1988.

Reports on a survey by the Office of Technology Assessment to collect basic information on underwriting practices and the use of medical screening by health insurers and to document how health underwriters are responding to the AIDS epidemic.

Research

The survey, which was an attempt to provide a view of HIV testing in the context of other routine tests required by health insurers, was sent to 88 commercial insurers who comprise 70% of the commercial individual health insurance market; to 15 of the 77 Blue Cross/Blue Shield plans; and to the 50 largest local and national HMOs in the U.S. The overall response rate was 83%. Included in this report are a summary of the OTA study, an introduction, and the survey results. Two appendices provide a copy of the survey questionnaire and a list of abbreviations and glossary of terms.

Of interest to health economists, public health officials, public policymakers, and legislators.

521. FOUNDATION Center. *AIDS: A Status Report on Foundation
      Funding.* The Foundation Center, 1987.

The Foundation Center monitors private foundation activity and trends
in foundation giving through its systems of data collection and
analysis. During the period July 15 through August 15, 1987 the
Center surveyed 568 foundations regarding funding for AIDS-related
programs.

Report

In the body of the report, and in the statistical tables provided,
information is given regarding the reporting of 253 grants awarded by
85 foundations in the amount of $18,612,738. The main body of the
report consists of descriptions of foundations that reported
AIDS-related grants, along with corresponding lists of grants that
include information about the recipients, the amounts and dates of the
awards, and the purposes to be served.

Of special interest to AIDS researchers.

522. ROWE, Mona, and Caitlin Ryan. *AIDS, A Public Health
      Challenge: State Issues, Policies and Programs.* Volume 2:
      Managing and Financing the Problem. Washington, DC: U.S.
      Department of Health and Human Services, Public Health
      Service, October 1987.

The second of three volumes, which provide a comprehensive review, for
public policymakers, of the policy issues with which AIDS confronts
the states, this book deals with the administration and financing of
state sponsored AIDS-related programs.

Sourcebook

Examines the financing options available to help states respond to the
AIDS crisis; how appropriate policies and programs might be developed
to accommodate HIV-infected patients when scientific understanding
about the disease is changing; the kinds of support services required
for short- and long-term planning in high-, moderate-, and
low-incidence areas, and how these services should be coordinated;
the type of AIDS education programs that should be implemented, and
how they should be funded; and whether funding AIDS research should be
a state responsibility and, if so, why, what type, and to what extent.

Intended for public policymakers for the states.

b. Articles

523. ANDRULIS, Dennis P., Virginia S. Beers, James D. Bentley,
      Larry S. Gage. "State Medicaid policies and hospital care for
      AIDS patients." *Health Affairs* 6, no. 4 (1987): 110-118.

This study, using data from a national survey of AIDS inpatient care
in U.S. hospitals during 1985, examines the relationship and characteristics of treating AIDS patients in states with liberal and
restrictive programs.

Research

This analysis suggests that major differences in AIDS inpatient revenues and payer sources are related to the status of state Medicaid programs. Where Medicaid eligibility levels are such that fewer patients are covered, hospital revenues tend to be lower and the number of charity-care patients, higher.

Of particular interest to hospital administrators, public health officials, and health policymakers.

524. BERGER, Randy. "Cost analysis of AIDS cases in Maryland." *Maryland Medical Journal* 34 (1985): 1173-1175.

This report is the first cost analysis of AIDS cases in Maryland.

Analytical

If, in 1985, there are 150 newly diagnosed cases of AIDS, with an estimated 2.5 hospital admissions per case and an average length of stay of 20 days per admission, the total cost of these patients would be $4,125,000. The estimated cost per patient in Maryland is $27,500. The figure does not take into account out-of-hospital costs, such as home nursing care and the indirect cost of lost wages.

Of interest to public health officials.

525. BLOOM, David E., and Geoffrey Carline. "The economic impact of AIDS in the United States." *Science* 239 (1988): 604-609.

The economic impact that will result from the spread of AIDS is discussed.

Analytical

This analysis of several previous studies of the cost of AIDS suggests that the lifetime cost of medical care per patient will not exceed $80,000, an amount similar to the cost of treating other serious illnesses. If current projections of future AIDS cases are accurate, the cumulative lifetime costs of 270,000 cases diagnosed between 1981 and the end of 1991 will not exceed $22 billion. This amount is small compared with total U.S. medical spending.

Of interest to health economists, public health officials, and public policymakers.

526. BRENNAN, Troyen A. "The acquired immunodeficiency syndrome (AIDS) as an occupational disease." *Annals of Internal Medicine* 107 (1987): 581-583.

Discusses the issue of compensation for work-related AIDS in health care workers.

Editorial

Hospitals and leaders in medicine must develop plans for dealing with
the compensation of health care workers who develop AIDS as a result
of workplace exposure if they wish to ensure available care for AIDS
patients and protect seronegative patients from the risk of exposure
resulting from the care provided by seropositive workers who are
concealing their condition. State and federal governments must
realize the further increase in the enormous cost of AIDS that will
result from such plans, and not expect the hospitals to carry the
burden.

Of interest to health administrators, legislators, and economists.

527. CLIFFORD, Karen A., and Russel P. Inculano. "AIDS and
     insurance: The rationale for AIDS-related testing." *Harvard
     Law Review* 100 (1987): 1806-1825.

The authors argue in favor of the continued use by insurers of
AIDS-related testing to determine insurability.

Commentary

Begins with an explanation of some fundamental principles of
insurance, explaining how these principles might apply to individuals
at risk for developing AIDS. Reviews the legal and medical rationales
behind testing by insurers, and sets forth actions by several
jurisdictions that have prohibited AIDS-related testing for insurance
purposes. Concludes that such actions present potential dangers to
both insurers and the insurance-buying public. Finally, suggests an
alternative means of financing the AIDS-related costs of individuals
who are denied insurance.

Of interest to health economists, insurers, lawyers, legislators, and
public health officials.

528. DRUMMOND, Michael, and Linda Davies. "Treating AIDS: The
     economic issues." *Health Policy* 10 (1988): 1-19.

Reviews the evidence on the costs of treating AIDS, comparing European
data with those from the U.S. Also investigates the reasons for
variations in cost estimates.

Discussion/Analysis

This review showed that despite the public concern about AIDS, very
little is known about the cost-effectiveness of treatment practices.
More economic analysis of the costs and effects of treatment for AIDS,
which consider a broad range of costs, including that of ambulatory
care, should be undertaken in the future. The frequency and length of
spells of inpatient care should be recorded from the time of diagnosis
of an AIDS-related condition until death; data on the social and
physical functioning of AIDS patients should be collected; economic
analyses should be undertaken jointly with clinical studies; and
results of cost-effectiveness analyses of AIDS treatment should be
compared with those of other health care interventions.

Of interest to economists, public policymakers, and health administrators.

529. "The ECONOMIC impact of AIDS: Research methodology."
Health Policy 11, no. 2 (April 1989): Entire issue.

Papers presented at a Johns Hopkins School of Public Health conference, convened in Baltimore in September 1988 with the goal of increasing the precision of cost of AIDS projections.

Special Journal Issue

The seven papers in this special issue focus on conceptual issues in estimating the economic impact of AIDS; present three different approaches to projecting the cost of AIDS; review the direct and indirect costs of medical care, support services, and prevention programs for AIDS; discuss the evolution of AIDS economic research; and present an agenda for AIDS economic research.

Of interest to health economists, public health officials, and public policymakers.

530. HARRIS, Jeffrey E. "The AIDS epidemic: Looking into the 1990s." *Technology Review* 90 (1987): 58-64.

Discusses the future of AIDS and its social and economic implications.

Theoretical

The author estimates that the toll of the AIDS epidemic in the U.S. will reach 250,000 cases by 1991, placing a severe burden on our health care and insurance systems as well as on society at large. As insurance companies and employers feel the pressure to exclude people at risk for AIDS, the government will have to step in with public funding of all AIDS care. To have a fair, efficient system of financing in place by the 1990s, it is important that we start now to work out the details.

Of interest to health economists, insurers, legislators, and government policymakers.

531. HATZIANDREU, Evridiki, John D. Graham, Michael A. Stoto.
"AIDS and biomedical funding: Comparative analysis."
Reviews of Infectious Diseases 10 (1988): 159-167.

Although many citizens might prefer that expanded funding of AIDS-related research might come from a reduction in nuclear armaments or an increase in taxes, the political reality is that the trade-offs are likely to be made with other health research programs. The authors discuss and analyze this question.

Review/Discussion

The Centers for Disease Control's projection of AIDS cases for 1991 could prove to be too low or too high. Risk-related behavior seems to be changing at the same time recognition of the prevalence and consequences of the disease is increasing. The ground rules for the diagnosis of AIDS are changing, as are the ground rules for informing and treating patients. The rapidly changing situation suggests a need to reevaluate, periodically, the priority given to AIDS research.

Of interest to health professionals and policy analysts.

532. HELLINGER, Fred J. "National forecasts of the medical care costs of AIDS: 1988-1992." *Inquiry* 25 (1988): 469-484.

Forecasts, for 1988 through 1992, the personal medical care costs of persons diagnosed with AIDS.

Analytical

Based on an estimate of $60,000 per patient remaining stable between 1988 and 1992, the analysis forecasts the cumulative lifetime medical care costs of treating all patients diagnosed with AIDS to be about $2.6 billion in 1988, $3.5 billion in 1989, $4.7 billion in 1990, $6.0 billion in 1991, and $7.5 billion in 1992.

Of interest to public health officials, medical economists, hospital administrators, and health policymakers.

533. HERLITZ, Claes, and Bengt Brorsson. "The AIDS epidemic in Sweden: Estimates of costs, 1986, 1987 and 1990." *Scandinavian Journal of Social Medicine* 17 (1989): 39-48.

This study calculates the cost of medical care during the different stages of HIV infection, from the asymptomatic period to a confirmed diagnosis. The authors have also estimated the total cost of taking specimens and performing tests related to HIV, and the cost of information and research.

Analytical

Medical costs were based on estimates of the average cost per day and the total number of days at the various stages of HIV infection. The cost estimates for testing include costs related to taking specimens, analyzing samples, managing test results, etc. The cost outlook until 1990 is discussed, using different assumptions concerning incidence, survival, and the level of preventive efforts. The total estimated costs for medical care, HIV tests, etc. doubled between 1986 and 1987. During 1987, costs totaled 313 million Swedish kroner. The costs discussed in this study will probably increase by at least 50% by 1990.

Of interest to public health officials and medical economists.

534. KRIEGER, N. "AIDS funding: Competing needs and the politics of priorities." *International Journal of Health Services* 18 (1988): 521-541.

Criticizes the Reagan administration for excess spending on defense, and calls for a national health program to decrease the competition for funds between health programs.

Theoretical/Editorial

Despite the Department of Health and Human Services' 1983 claim that AIDS is the nation's "number one health priority," funding for AIDS research, prevention, and treatment remains inadequate. Funds have been diverted from sexually transmitted disease and prenatal care programs and transferred to AIDS programs. To decrease competition for funds, activists for AIDS and other health programs must argue that defense spending must be decreased; spending for health research and services increased; and a national health program implemented.

Of interest to public policymakers and legislators.

535. LEE, Philip R. "AIDS: Allocating resources for research and patient care." *Issues in Science and Technology* 2, no. 2 (1986): 66-73.

Examines the allocation of federal resources for AIDS research and patient care.

Descriptive

The author finds that the inadequate federal response was heavily influenced by efforts of the Reagan administration to reduce spending on domestic social programs, to shift federal responsibilities to state and local governments, and to encourage greater competition and an expanded private sector role in health care.

Of interest to public health officials, public policymakers, and health care administrators.

536. ———, and Andrew R. Moss. "AIDS prevention: Is cost-benefit analysis appropriate?" *Health Policy* 8 (1987): 193-196.

The authors suggest that cost-benefit analyses may be useful in determining what policies to adopt in response to the HIV/AIDS epidemic.

Commentary

The focus of policies to prevent the spread of HIV infection should be on the development of scientifically, socially, and culturally sound interventions based on current knowledge of HIV transmission and AIDS. How this is done, and what resources can be applied to the task, will differ among countries, but the basic goal and principles remain the same.

Of interest to policymakers, public health officials, and health administrators.

537. OHI, Gen, Ichiro Kai, Yasuki Kobayashi, Tomonori Hasegawa,
      Nobuyuki Takenaga, Syo Takata, Fumimara Takuku, Hiroshi
      Yoshikura, Takeshima Yoshimura. "AIDS prevention in Japan
      and its cost-benefit aspects." *Health Policy* 8 (1987): 17-27.

A cost-benefit analysis of preventive medicine programs for AIDS in
Japan.

Analytical

The magnitude of the imminent AIDS epidemic in Japan was estimated,
using the Delphi technique, and the economic performance of preventive health programs was analyzed. The annual incidence of AIDS in
the years 1988, 1991, and 1996 was predicted to be 100, 450, and 950,
respectively. Preventive programs based on the counseling and
education of homosexual men are highly cost-effective, but screening
of blood donors in the metropolitan areas would yield a net loss under
the predicted epidemiological circumstances.

Of interest to public health professionals, economists, and health
policy planners and legislators.

538. OPPENHEIMER, Gerald M., and Robert A. Padgug. "AIDS and
      health insurance: Social and ethical issues." *Public Policy
      Journal* 2 (1987): 11-14.

Discusses challenges that the AIDS epidemic poses to the U.S. health
care system, particularly its financial mechanisms.

Discussion

It is contended that the health insurance industry is a mixture of
private profit-making systems and social welfare purposes. It is
generally conservative, unable to cope with esoteric diseases or
groups of people who utilize higher than average levels of health care
services. AIDS threatens the private health insurance system by
striking directly at its basic principles, particularly that of "sound
underwriting."

Of interest to health economists and health care administrators.

539. ——. "AIDS: The risk to insurers, the threat to equity."
      Hastings Center Report 16, no. 5 (1986): 18-22.

Can we provide adequate health care to all who need it and still meet
the financial requirements of the private health insurance industry?

Commentary

More insurance carriers are turning to antibody testing in order to
eliminate poor risks from non-group, direct-pay pools. Some cost-
conscious employers have attempted to fire AIDS patients summarily or
to exclude AIDS coverage from group insurance policies. Various
remedies are available for spreading the financial risks of the

epidemic, such as covering persons with AIDS under Medicare or in state-sponsored health insurance pools. Ethical questions about cost and access may also rekindle the debate about the need for national health insurance.

Of interest to health economists, public health officials, and health care administration.

540. SCITOVSKY, Anne A. "The economic impact of AIDS in the United States." *Health Affairs* 7, no. 4 (1988): 32-45.

Reviews the principal studies and estimates, to date, of the personal health care costs of persons with AIDS, how these costs compare with those of some other diseases, and the expected impact of the epidemic on hospitals.

Review

After very brief sections on the estimates of direct nonpersonal costs of the epidemic and of direct personal costs, the author discusses the limitations of estimates of the personal health care costs of persons with AIDS that have been made to date and the major data gaps that make more accurate estimates difficult. Concludes with some suggestions regarding the type and content of future studies of the costs of AIDS.

Of interest to hospital administrators, health economists, and public health officials.

541. ———, and Dorothy P. Rice. "The cost of AIDS." *Issues in Science and Technology* 4 (1987): 61-70.

A very readable and thorough discussion of the various cost para-meters of AIDS in the United States.

Review

A discussion of the costs of the loss of productive years, personal medical care costs, nonpersonal costs such as research, screening services, and support services provided by local government, and the costs of illness and premature death. The authors estimate $8.5 billion in medical care costs alone due to AIDS in 1991.

Of general interest to health professionals and laymen.

542. ———. "Estimates of the direct indirect costs of acquired immunodeficiency syndrome in the United States, 1985, 1986, and 1991." *Public Health Reports* 102 (1987): 5-17.

Presents estimates of the direct and indirect costs of the AIDS epidemic in the U.S. in 1985, 1986, and 1991 based on prevalence estimates provided by the Centers for Disease Control.

Research

Personal medical care costs of AIDS will rise from $630 million in
1985 to $1.1 billion in 1986 to $8.5 billion in 1991. Costs for
research, screening, education, and general support services are
estimated to rise from $319 million in 1985 to $542 million in 1986 to
$2.3 billion in 1991.

Of interest to health professionals, laymen, and public policy
analysts.

543. SEAGE, George R., III, Stuart Landers, Kenneth H. Mayer,
      Anita Barry, George A. Lamb, Arnold M. Epstein. "Medical
      costs of ambulatory patients with the AIDS-related complex
      (ARC) and/or generalized lymphadenopathy syndrome (GLS)
      related to HIV infection, 1984-85." American Journal of
      Public Health 78 (1988): 969-970.

To develop cost estimates of treating AIDS related complex and
generalized lymphadenopathy syndrome, the authors studied inpatient
and outpatient health care utilization for a cohort of patients with
ARC/GLS.

Analytical

Findings suggest that the medical management of ARC and GLS did not
require significant financial resources for individual patients.
Previous studies of AIDS patients, using a similar methodology, have
estimated their annual medical costs to range from $31,900 to $46,505
per patient with an incidence of hospitalization of 3.3 per patient
per year. Evaluation of 28 patients in this study found the average
cost to be $489 per patient per year. None of the patients in this
study were hospitalized and none progressed to AIDS. No specific
treatment, such as AZT, was available when this study was completed.

Of interest to medical economists and hospital administrators.

544. SISK, Jane. "The costs of AIDS: A review of the estimates."
      Health Affairs 6 (Summer 1987): 5-19.

A comprehensive review of the cost estimates that have been made
regarding AIDS and related infections.

Review

Analyzes the reasons for the tremendous variation in cost estimates
regarding AIDS and related diseases, identifies specific factors that
have accounted for differing cost estimates in 18 studies, discusses
problems in predicting costs associated with AIDS, and raises issues
relating to future cost estimates.

Useful to health care providers, legislators, planners, and policymakers as well as economists.

545. STOTO, Michael A., David Blumenthal, Jane S. Durch, Penny H. Feldman. "Federal funding for AIDS research: Decision process and results in fiscal year 1986." *Reviews of Infectious Diseases* 10 (1988): 406-419.

Focuses on the role that the federal government plays in setting priorities for AIDS research.

Analytical

On the basis of this analysis, two recommendations are made: the director of the National Institutes of Health and the heads of other U.S. Public Health Service agencies should have discriminatory funds to use for AIDS activities; and better channels of communication between Congress, the Public Health Service, and outside biomedical researchers should be established for consultation on priorities for AIDS research.

Of interest to all health professionals.

546. THOMPSON, Velma Montoya. "AIDS testing: An economic assessment of evolving public policy." *Economic Inquiry* 27 (1989): 259-269.

Considers issues in the economics of property rights raised by the introduction of the AIDS antibody test and the efficient government response.

Analytical

The author applies a recent theorem from the economics of property rights to consider whether laissez faire should prevail regarding the private-market supply of the AIDS antibody test and to assess the legal and economic effects of rules guaranteeing strict confidentiality of test results. She concludes that the optimal policy regarding the AIDS antibody test differs according to whether individuals are at low risk or high risk, and that rules guaranteeing strict confidentiality of test results are unjustified. They also are unjustified on traditional legal grounds.

Of interest to health economists, lawyers, legislators, and public policymakers.

547. WELLS, James A. "Foundation funding for AIDS programs." *Health Affairs* 6 (1987): 113-123.

Examines patterns of giving for AIDS programs by private foundations.

Essay

Discusses trends in the number of grants given over the period from 1981 to early 1987, the categories in which the awards have been made, and the foundations participating in AIDS giving. Examines three specific grants to illustrate giving in the area of AIDS, and discusses some problems in giving to AIDS and prospects for future foundation participation in AIDS giving.

Of interest to AIDS researchers.

548. ———, Andrea Zuercher, John Clinton. "Foundation funding for AIDS education." *Health Affairs* 7, no. 5 (1988): 146-158.

Reviews the status of philanthropic responses to AIDS in the United States and the evaluation of AIDS/HIV educational projects supported by philanthropic foundations.

Essay

A total of $51.6 million has been awarded by 157 private foundations to almost 600 AIDS/HIV programs, including medical care, medical research, and public health programs. The Robert Wood Johnson Foundation has contributed about half of the funds. There is a trend for corporations and foundations to join coalitions to deal with the epidemic on a local level. Few foundation-supported AIDS education programs have included an evaluation component because of lack of expertise and time among grantees, expense, lack of generalizability to other groups at risk, and the belief that evaluation is the duty of the public sector.

Of interest to philanthropic foundation members, public policy officials, educators, and researchers.

549. WHYTE, Bruce M., David B. Evans, Esther J. Schruers, and David A. Cooper. "The costs of hospital-based medical care for patients with the acquired immunodeficiency syndrome." *Medical Journal of Australia* 147 (September 21, 1987): 269-272.

This study measures the direct costs of hospital care for AIDS patients in Australia. Projections of potential costs to 1990 are also made.

Research

The mean cost for hospital-based care was $A22,332 (range $4,229 to $58,398). The mean cost of care of those who presented with an opportunistic infection was significantly higher than that of those who presented with a malignancy, but there was no difference according to the age at the time of diagnosis. If the predictions of 3,000 AIDS cases in Australia by 1991 are realized, such cases will represent, conservatively, an additional cost to the community of $58.5 million.

Of interest to health professionals and laymen.

550. WILKIE, P.A. "Life assurance, HIV seropositivity and hemophilia." *Scottish Medical Journal* 119-121.

Discusses problems encountered by hemophiliacs in acquiring life insurance and other services.

Review

Reviews the medical issues of HIV seropositivity and AIDS, and discusses several approaches to risk pooling, rate/premium relationships, and public participation in providing life insurance coverage for hemophiliacs. Case reports are used to illustrate several ethical issues associated with the problems of obtaining life insurance for hemophiliacs.

Intended for public policymakers for the states.

551. WINKELWERDER, William, Austin R. Kessler, and Rhonda M. Stolec. "Federal spending for illness caused by the human immunodeficiency virus." *New England Journal of Medicine* 320 (1989): 15598-15603.

Reports total federal spending related to HIV from 1982 through 1989. In addition, the authors project the level of such spending through 1992.

Analytical

In all, $5.5 billion will have been spent on HIV-related illness during 1982-1989 by the federal government. Federal spending on HIV-related illness in 1989 will reach $2.2 billion, representing over one third of all estimated national (public and private) HIV expenditures, and tripling state expenditures. In 1992, federal spending on the epidemic will reach an estimated $4.3 billion. Federal spending for HIV research and prevention is similar to funding for other major diseases.

Of interest to all health professionals, public policymakers, and laymen.

5. LEGAL ISSUES

a. Books

552. DALTON, Harlon L., Scott Burris, and the Yale AIDS Law Project (Eds.). *AIDS and the Law: A Guide for the Public.* New Haven: Yale University Press, 1987.

Addresses and communicates, in language that laypersons can understand, the law as it relates to AIDS.

Book of Readings

Divided into six sections: the medical background, government responses to AIDS, private sector responses to AIDS, AIDS and health care, AIDS in institutions, and the problems of special groups. Illustrates how the law both frames and is shaped by society's response to the AIDS epidemic.

Useful and of interest to anyone who may have a personal or professional need to confront the legal issues spawned by the AIDS epidemic.

553. DAVIS, Margaret L., in consultation with Robert S. Scott. *Lovers, Doctors, and the Law: Your Legal Rights and Responsibilities in Today's Sex-Health Crisis.* New York: Harper & Row, 1988.

Shows the reader and his/her lover how to share their most intimate secrets, how to communicate with frankness about his/her sexual and health history, and how to keep those promises made in the dark.

Text

Examines, in detail, the legal risks inherent in transmitting STDs to others. Explains basic legal concepts and state by state laws dealing with STDs. The book also includes a state by state legal guide of relevant statutes and medical review charts for various STDs.

Of interest to the lay public and to members of the legal and medical professions.

554. DORNETTE, William H.L. (Ed.). *AIDS and the Law.* New York: John Wiley & Sons, 1987.

Explains the medical background of infections with the AIDS virus and the associated legal issues to members of the medical and legal professions, and to non-professionals, and attempts to provide the reader with a better insight into the rights of persons on both sides of disputed issues.

Book of Readings

Reviews the changing climate in law and medicine as it affects those infected with or exposed to the AIDS virus. The 15 chapters cover: the medical background, introduction to the law, AIDS in the workplace, educating the infected child, housing the AIDS victim, AIDS and the family, discrimination against the handicapped, negligence and intentional torts, criminal sanctions and quarantine, AIDS and the criminal justice system, health insurance, life insurance, blood products and tissue transplants, health care issues, and confidentiality issues.

Of interest to physicians, lawyers, and concerned laypersons.

555. SLOAN, Irving J. *AIDS Law: Implications for the Individual & Society.* New York: Oceana, 1988.

A monograph about the legal aspects of AIDS.

Monograph

The ten chapters cover topics such as: tort and criminal liability for the sexual transmission of AIDS; liability for transmission of AIDS through the blood supply; AIDS discrimination in the workplace; AIDS and health care providers' liabilities; school children and AIDS; insurance and AIDS; the military and AIDS; immigration and AIDS; and AIDS in prison. Appendices of resource lists of legal organizations and various statutes and summaries of legislation are included.

A good legal resource in nontechnical language for the layman.

b. Articles

556. ANNAS, George M. "Not saints, but healers: The legal duties of health care professionals in the AIDS epidemic." *American Journal of Public Health* 78 (1988): 844-849.

Explores the legal framework within which health care professionals must work as "healers" in the AIDS epidemic, and suggests ways in which the law can reinforce an ethic of professionalism in this modern plague.

Essay

This analysis suggests that health providers in private practice have no legal duty to treat except in specific situations. Health care professionals do have special legal obligations because they have been granted special privileges by society. In motivating health care workers to care for AIDS and HIV-infected patients, reasonable steps must be taken to address fear of death and grief as key shared values of contemporary society.

Of interest to all types of health professionals.

557. APPLEBAUM, Paul S. "AIDS, psychiatry, and the law." *Hospital and Community Psychiatry* 39 (1988): 13-14.

A sampling of legal problems related to AIDS that have occurred in mental health facilities.

Review

Discusses such issues as protecting third parties from HIV carriers, duty to warn, detention and admission of HIV positive persons in mental health facilities, etc.

Of interest to lawyers and mental health professionals.

558. BECKHAM, Joseph. "The AIDS dilemma: Recent court decisions place a burden of persuasion on public schools." *National Association of Secondary School Principals Bulletin* 70, no. 489 (April 1986): 91-95.

An analysis of recent court decisions that will affect schools' employee policies on AIDS.

Commentary

Recent decisions in three court cases (Arline vs. School Board of Nassau County, New York Association of Retarded Children vs. Carey, and Doe vs. New York University) have placed a burden of persuasion on school boards to justify exclusions based on concern for the health and safety of students and coworkers. They indicate that the courts will review administrative processes to determine whether grounds exist for exclusion and evaluate the extent of the risk to public safety that the exclusionary policy seeks to avoid. Without a strong factual basis for a discriminatory policy, courts are likely to infer that the school board's safety concerns merely mask stereotypical or unreliable fears about the person's health conditions.

Of concern to school officials and attorneys.

559. BODINE, Margot R. "Opening the schoolhouse door for children with AIDS: The Education for all Handicapped Children Act." *Boston College Environmental Affairs Law Review* 13, no. 4 (1986): 583-641.

Focuses on the applicability of the Education for All Handicapped Children Act (EAHCA) of 1975 to AIDS as legislative protection for a child excluded from school because of AIDS.

Review/Discussion

A child with AIDS may litigate his/her case more effectively if classified as handicapped under the EACHA as well as the Rehabilitation Act of 1973. EACHA protects the rights of handicapped children to free appropriate education in classrooms with their peers unless their "handicaps" prevent satisfactory education in this environment, even with supplemental aids or services. Its application to the child with AIDS entitles him/her to a variety of federally mandated procedural safeguards. Application of EACHA avoids constitutional litigation and encourages a speedy resolution by local administrative bodies. In addition, it provides a handicapped child with a right of action to the federal courts once administrative remedies have been exhausted.

Of interest to school administrators, parents of children with AIDS, and attorneys.

560. BRICKLEY, Kathleen M. "AIDS: A university's liability for failure to protect its students." *Journal of College and University Law* 14 (1987): 529-530.

Discusses the measures universities should and should not take to protect themselves from potential liability in the event a student transmits AIDS to another student.

Note

Presents a general overview of AIDS in light of current medical knowledge; analyzes the risks inherent in university policies designed to keep AIDS victims off campus entirely; and discusses other methods of safeguarding the student body from contracting AIDS. Concludes that a university can possibly shield itself from liability by educating all of its students about AIDS, maintaining a comprehensive AIDS policy, and, in the event the university becomes aware of an AIDS victim on campus, providing monitoring and counseling.

Of interest to university administrators and lawyers.

561. BROCKMAN, Leslie N. "Enforcing the right to a public education for children afflicted with AIDS." *Emory Law Journal* 36, no. 2 (Spring 1987): 603-648.

Examines the nature of acquired immune deficiency syndrome, and determines whether a child with AIDS should be permitted to attend public school.

Analytical

Allowing children with AIDS to attend public school, with certain precautions based on present medical knowledge, is both logical and simple in its application. Research has shown that AIDS is not transmitted through casual contact. Apprising parents of this research would go a long way towards alleviating the fear of AIDS. Once the fear has dissipated, the protests and lawsuits from parents who do not want their children exposed to classmates with AIDS will be a thing of the past.

Of particular interest to lawyers, public school officials, and parents with school-age children.

562. CLOSEN, Michael L., Susan Marie Connor, Howard L. Kaufman, Mark E. Wojcik. "AIDS in America: Death, privacy, and the law." *Human Rights* 14, no. 3 (1987): 26-29, 48-51.

A review and analysis of the legal rights of persons with HIV, ARC, and AIDS.

Discussion/Analysis

A discussion of the Rehabilitation Act of 1973, constitutional law, procedural due process, the right to privacy, and other issues related to AIDS.

Of interest to lawyers, the general public, and policymakers.

563. ———. "AIDS: Testing democracy--irrational responses to
     the public health crisis and the need for privacy in sero-
     logic testing." *John Marshall Law Review* 19 (Summer 1986):
     835-928.

A discussion of the medical background, legal background, and legal
directions that relate to AIDS testing.

Review

Much of the crisis deals with personal choices, which individuals
should be encouraged to make after appropriate education in the
medical aspects of transmission. Since the modes of transmission
have been medically identified as limited to exchanges of blood and
semen, any discrimination based on misinformation or conjecture must
be eliminated or prohibited. No one has the right to make another
person the victim of his or her ignorance. Until the ultimate goals
of successful public education and medical research are achieved,
constitutional guarantees, including the right of privacy, must be
utilized to protect individual rights. Legislation should concentrate
on protection of victims of irrational discrimination.

Of special interest to lawyers and policymakers.

564. ———. "The test: Is it accurate? Is it legal?" *Human Rights*
     14, no. 3 (1987): 30-32.

A discussion of the HTLV-III test, its purpose, indications, limitations, and legal implications.

Discussion

The HTLV-III antibody test, though frequently misnamed as an "AIDS
test," must be thought of only as an antibody screening test. The
test does not directly detect the presence of the HTLV-III virus, but
rather antibodies thought to be induced by the virus. While this is
considered to be adequate for screening purposes, there are major
flaws in utilizing such a test for any other purpose.

Of interest to laymen and health professionals.

565. CURRAN, William J. "The impact of legal issues on the practice
     of infectious disease: National survey of AIDS legislation."
     Bulletin of the New York Academy of Medicine 63 (1987):
     569-581.

Discusses legislation at both state and national levels due to the
AIDS epidemic, as well as some more general legal issues applicable to
infectious disease control.

Review

The AIDS epidemic presents a great challenge in the field of infectious disease control under law in our society. The legal issues are complex, and serious obstacles often stand in the way of implementation. Early legal developments and general results of the 1986 legislative sessions are examined; legislative action is analyzed; fundamental constitutional issues and the potential for backlash on inactivity are discussed; and speculations about future legislative and regulatory proposals are presented.

Should interest lawyers, legislators, policymakers, and public health professionals.

566. DICKENS, Bernard M. "Legal limits of AIDS confidentiality." *Journal of the American Medical Association* 259 (1988): 3449-3451.

Discusses the issues surrounding AIDS confidentiality in the medical or health care setting.

Essay

Reliance cannot be placed on the law to restrict breaches of confidentiality of HIV-infected persons' identities. Too much in the law, itself, compels, justifies, and excuses disclosure of information. Patients exposed to humiliation, stigmatization, and ostracism cannot confidently seek legal remedies for harmful disclosures when the law requires or tolerates publicity of their medical condition.

Of general interest to health care professionals.

567. ——. "Legal rights and duties in the AIDS epidemic." *Science* 239 (1988): 580-585.

An overview of some major areas of legal concern in which the AIDS epidemic is having an impact.

Descriptive

The rights of infected individuals to testing, treatment, and confidentiality are reviewed, and emphasis is given to their claims to nondiscrimination regarding access to health care, employment, housing, education, insurance, and related interests. Infected persons' duties to contain transmission of AIDS are outlined under principles of criminal and civil law, including liability for provision of contaminated blood products. Uninfected people's general rights to protection are considered, and health professionals' and authorities' rights and duties are given attention.

Of interest to lawyers and public policymakers.

568. FONTANA, Vincent R. "The ramifications of the AIDS crisis for local governments." *Tort and Insurance Law Journal* 23 (1987): 195-214.

A review of AIDS as a disease; governmental, legal, and economic implications; rights, protection, and due process.

Review

The trend of the law concerning AIDS has been to recognize the rights of AIDS patients and to interpret the law to help AIDS patients. This trend can be expected to continue so long as no evidence develops that the disease can be spread by casual contact.

Of particular interest to lawyers, city officials, and public health officials.

569. FORD, Nancy L., and Michael D. Quam.   "AIDS quarantine:
      The legal and practical implications."   *Journal of Legal
      Medicine* 8 (1987): 353-396.

Discusses the legal and practical issues of AIDS quarantine.

Review/Analytical

Discusses the nature of AIDS, comparison with other epidemics, legality of state isolation and quarantine laws, AIDS quarantine under current state laws, and implications for public health policy.

Of special interest to lawyers, public health officials, and public policymakers.

570. GIRARDI, John A., Robert M. Keese, Lynn Bonilla Traver,
      David R. Cooksey. "Psychotherapist responsibility in
      notifying individuals at risk for exposure to HIV." *Journal
      of Sex Research* 25 (1988): 1-27.

Delineates the legal risks of psychotherapists who know of a patient's HIV or AIDS diagnosis, but fail to warn the patient's sexual partners.

Debate

Attorneys from two prominent Los Angeles law firms debate the responsibility of a psychotherapist to notify individuals at risk of exposure to AIDS. A fictional case, initial arguments, and rebuttals are presented.

Of interest to psychotherapists, lawyers, and physicians.

571. HAMMET, Leah.   "Protecting children with AIDS against
      arbitrary exclusion from school."   *California Law Review* 74
      (1986): 1373-1407.

Proposes a federal statute that will allow states to establish administrative boards to decide whether a child with AIDS may attend school.

Review/Discussion

The history of quarantine and isolation as methods of curbing the spread of disease is traced, and early cases limiting the states' power to restrict individual liberty are summarized. The author argues that the judgment regarding whether a child with AIDS presents a danger to others at school should be made by a board of physicians, not by the school board. Although the article focuses on AIDS, non-fatal diseases that are more easily transmitted than AIDS are also discussed.

Of interest to school administrators, educational policymakers, and legislators.

572. JENNER, Robert K.   "Identifying HIV-infected blood donors: Who is John Donor?"   *Trial* 25, no. 6 (1989): 47-55.

Examines the pros and cons of permitting the identification of HIV-infected blood donors.

Review

In a review of transfusion-associated AIDS litigation, the author examines the competing interests of blood banks in fulfilling the public demand for blood versus those of the public in receiving blood that is not HIV-infected. He concludes that donor disclosure would foster a safer blood supply by discouraging persons at risk from giving blood and encouraging more diligent screening of potential donors.

Of interest to blood bank administrators, hospital administrators, and attorneys.

573. KERMANI, Ebrahim J.   "Handicapped children and the law: Children afflicted with AIDS."   *Journal of the American Academy of Child and Adolescent Psychiatry* 27 (1988): 152-154.

Children with AIDS have recently been determined by the courts to be entitled to rights under statutes protecting the handicapped.

Discussion

Child psychiatrists and mental health professionals who work with handicapped children should be aware of the new developments in law, legislation, and court rulings in order to give adequate and appropriate guidance to the AIDS-affected, their families, and their communities.

Of general interest, especially to educators.

574. ——, and Bonnie A. Weiss.   "AIDS and confidentiality: Legal concept and its application in psychotherapy."   *American Journal of Psychotherapy* 43 (1989): 25-31.

Persons with HIV infection appear to have the same right to confidentiality as other medical psychiatric patients.

Descriptive

The ethical and legal duties of practitioners who learn that their HIV positive patients are endangering others is discussed. The essential policies of CDC, AMA, and APA are reviewed along with the current legal situation. One conclusion is that applying the Tarasoff doctrine to warn/protect a third party, if that party may already be infected, is useful only when the third party is moral and sensible enough to cease behavior that would spread the disease to others.

Of interest to lawyers, mental health professionals, and counselors.

575. KIRBY, M.D.   "AIDS legislation--turning up the heat?" *Journal of Medical Ethics* 12 (1986): 187-194.

Examines the catalogue of legislative and other legal responses to the spread of AIDS; analyzes the AIDS condition in its historical context; and categorizes the responses of lawmakers to the condition, according to the approach taken.

Analytic

The author contrasts the hysteria accompanying AIDS with the similar hysteria associated with other epidemics experienced in Australia over the last 200 years and suggests that the appropriate legislative and other legal responses should depend upon such factors as the present magnitude of the condition, its likely course, the availability of cures and protections against its spread, and objectives being sought in intervention. Unless these factors are taken into account, gross overreaction can occur, causing social disruption and much personal injustice.

Of interest to lawyers, legislators, public policymakers, and public health officials.

576. KIRKLAND, Martin, and Dean Ginther.   "Acquired immune deficiency syndrome in children: Medical, legal, and school-related issues." *School Psychology Review* 17 (1988): 304-310.

Reviews several biological/medical, legal, and psychological/educational issues associated with AIDS in a school setting.

Review

Schools should adopt procedures for handling AIDS-related issues whether or not AIDS students presently are in attendance. In order for schools to develop an adequate policy on AIDS, the biological/medical, legal, and psychological issues should be addressed. Administrators, psychological and medical personnel, teachers, and community representatives should all be involved in the development of a comprehensive policy on AIDS.

Of interest to educators, lawyers, and school administrators.

577. KIRSH, Marla S. "AIDS: Anonymity in donation situations--where public benefit meets private good." *Boston University Law Review* 69 (1989): 187-212.

Analyzes arguments for and against the discoverability of blood donors' names in cases involving HIV transmission.

Review/Commentary

Rule 26(c) of the Federal Rules of Civil Procedure empowers courts to limit the broad rules of discovery where good cause exists. In cases where the identity of a blood donor in an AIDS-related case is at issue, the court must balance the litigant's interest against both the donor's rights and the general public interest. The author concludes that, when the interests of all parties are considered, blood donors' privacy rights and societal interests tip the scales in favor of non-disclosure.

Of interest to blood bank officials, attorneys, judges, and ethicists.

578. LEWIS, Hilary E. "Acquired immunodeficiency syndrome: State legislative activity." *Journal of the American Medical Association* 258, no. 17 (November 6, 1987): 2410-2414.

Discusses AIDS-related legislation that has been enacted by state governments since 1983, focusing on ten major subject areas--antibody testing, blood and blood products, confidentiality, employment, housing, informed consent, insurance, marriage, prison population, and reporting--that have become matters of state law.

Review

State regulations, which generally carry the force of the law, constitute one means by which policymakers have responded to the AIDS crisis. Over 450 bills on the subject of AIDS were introduced in state legislatures in 1987, reflecting the serious public health concerns raised by this disease in every part of the country.

Of general interest.

579. MacFARLANE, Maureen Anne. "Equal opportunities: Protecting the rights of AIDS-linked children in the classroom." *American Journal of Law and Medicine* 14 (1989): 377-430.

Discusses section 504 and equal protection analyses used by the courts.

Analytical

The author concludes that both section 504 and the equal protection clause ensure that AIDS-linked children will not be barred from the classroom unless the presence of additional factors increases the risk of these children transmitting the virus to others.

Of interest to lawyers, public school administrators, and teachers.

580. MAHON, Nancy B. "Public hysteria, private conflict: Child
     custody and visitation disputes involving an HIV infected
     parent." *New York University Law Review* 63 (1988):
     1092-1141.

Argues that a court's use of a parent's HIV infection as per se
evidence of parental unfitness contravenes the best interests
standard.

Legal Note

Part I details current medical knowledge on the diagnosis, transmission, and symptoms of HIV infection. Part II explores the psychological literature on a child's response to parental divorce and
possibly fatal parental illness and concludes that cutting a child off
from its HIV infected parent is detrimental to the child's emotional
growth. Part III then explores how these standards should be applied
to disputes in which one parent is HIV infected. Part IV analyzes
disputes involving an HIV positive parent in light of limitations
legislators and courts have placed on the consideration of parental
handicap, parental behavior, and community bias in custody and
visitation cases. Part V offers guidelines courts should employ to
factor HIV infection into such determinations.

Of interest to pediatricians, lawyers, and public policymakers.

581. MARTIN, Andrew Ayers. "Title VII discrimination in biochemi-
     cal testing for AIDS and marijuana." *Duke Law Journal* 1
     (1988): 129-153.

Discusses the implications of the disparate impact doctrine of Title
VII for employment testing for marijuana and AIDS.

Review

The author argues that the prohibition in Title VII of the 1964 Civil
Rights Act against disparate employment practices that have an impact
on persons of a particular race, national origin, sex, or religion
applies to employers who require biochemical tests or establish hiring
policies that discriminate against persons testing positive for HIV or
marijuana. To demonstrate non-discrimination, employers must use high
cutoff scores and confirmation tests to ensure accuracy and must
validate employment policies by external guidelines.

Of interest to employers, managers, and lawyers.

582. MERRITT, Deborah Jones. "Communicable disease and constitu-
     tional law: Controlling AIDS." *New York University Law
     Review* 61, no. 5 (1986): 736-799.

Discusses the legal dilemmas created by the delicate balance between
the protection of public health and the defense of individual liberty
in attempts to control the spread of AIDS.

Analytical

After examining the constitutionality of three controversial proposals for controlling AIDS, the author concludes that legal precedent and current equal protection jurisdiction are inadequate to deal with the AIDS problem. Many proposed public health measures, although they may be constitutional in certain circumstances, violate the equal protection clause. A new method of equal protection analysis is proposed.

Of interest to public health professionals and public policymakers and legislators.

583. NANULA, Peter J. "Protecting confidentiality in the effort to control AIDS." *Harvard Journal on Legislation* 24 (1987): 315-344.

Focuses on the urgent need for protecting the confidentiality of potential and confirmed AIDS carriers and victims to facilitate the public health effort to control the disease. Then examines possible sources of legal protection of confidentiality, evaluating the prospects and suggesting reforms.

Commentary

Expansion of the common law duties of doctors and other health care personnel to maintain confidentiality is desirable but should not be expected. Courts faced with constitutional challenges to AIDS reporting and testing laws should recognize the confluence of interests present and pay primary attention to confidentiality. Legislative solutions to this unique and pressing problem are, perhaps, the most promising, though attempts to implement them have only just begun. Legislatures must recognize the strategic need for protecting confidentiality and guide public policy in that direction.

Of interest to lawyers, legislators, and public opinion analysts.

584. NORTHROP, Cynthia E. "Rights versus regulation: Confidentiality in the age of AIDS." *Nursing Outlook* 36 (1988): 208.

Describes a legal case in which a hospital was sued for discrimination and violation of confidentiality.

Descriptive

A pharmacist sued a hospital for discrimination because he was rejected for employment on the basis of a positive HIV test. The role of the nurse who revealed the test results to the examining physician is examined and the ethical considerations discussed.

Of particular interest to nurses and other health professionals who have access to patient records.

585. ORR, Alistair. "Legal AIDS: Implications of AIDS for British
      and American law." *Journal of Medical Ethics* 15 (1989):
      61-67.

Examines how British and American law might compromise in the areas of
medico-legal matters, criminal and tort law, employment, insurance,
and education to simultaneously protect the public and the individual.

Discussion

In its approach to HIV and AIDS, the law must recognize both the right
of the public to be protected against the disease and the right of the
individual not to be unfairly restricted by having or being at risk of
the disease. Some compromise must be reached, which will protect the
public health while protecting the individual so that he/she will feel
free to seek available treatment. In this way, prevention of further
spread of the disease will be encouraged.

Of interest to lawyers, judges, legislators, and public policymakers.

586. PASCAL, Chris B. "Selected legal issues about AIDS for drug
      abuse treatment programs." *Journal of Psychoactive Drugs* 19
      (1987): 1-12.

The purpose of this article is to sensitize drug abuse treatment
program personnel to the legal issues surrounding AIDS, with special
emphasis on matters of confidentiality and disclosure.

Discussion

In trying to comply with the law and limit its legal liabilities, the
drug treatment program should keep abreast of the latest scientific
and medical knowledge on the causation and treatment of AIDS and
implement treatment programs based on that knowledge. The program
should also be aware of the legal issues involved in the use and
disclosure of AIDS information and of the legal duties it may owe its
patients, staff, and others. Although there is no one best method for
reconciling the conflicting interests of those various parties, being
aware of the federal, state, and local laws and being knowledgeable
about the latest scientific and medical information about AIDS greatly
increases the likelihood of sound, defensible decision-making and,
consequently, reduces the potential for legal liability.

Of interest to substance abuse program administrators and personnel.

587. PERKINS, Nancy. "Prohibiting the use of the human immunode-
      ficiency virus antibody test by employers and insurers."
      Harvard Journal on Legislation 25 (1988): 275-315.

Analyzes the costs and benefits of HIV antibody testing by employers
and insurers and proposes a four-part legislative solution to the
screening problem.

Commentary

The author recommends that states: 1) prohibit both employers and insurers from inquiring into the results of HIV antibody tests voluntarily taken in the past by current or potential employees or by applicants for insurance, 2) either prohibit the use of test results to determine eligibility for employment or, as an alternative, declare persons who test HIV-positive handicapped for purposes of handicap discrimination laws, 3) prohibit the use of test results to determine eligibility for health insurance, and 4) permit the use of test results to determine life insurability only under strict regulatory guidelines. Also recommends that states establish health insurance pooling organizations, to which all insurers within each state be required to belong, that will provide insurance to all persons considered uninsurable by individual companies.

Of interest to public health officials, employers, and public policymakers.

588. PIORKOWSKI, Joseph, Jr. "Between a rock and a hard place: AIDS and the conflicting physician's duties of preventing disease transmission and safeguarding confidentiality." *The Georgetown Law Journal* 76 (1987): 169-202.

Briefly reviews the relevant scientific data about AIDS, examines the potential liability of physicians to at-risk third parties for failing to warn them about the risk of acquiring HIV infection, and examines the possibility that a physician who provides a warning to a third party may then be liable for breach of a common law or statutory duty to maintain patient confidentiality.

Note

Concludes with a discussion of the need for legislative action to guide physicians regarding their legal duty to third parties who are foreseeably at risk of requiring HIV infection from an AIDS patient.

Of interest to physicians, lawyers, and legislators.

589. REINER, Joseph. "AIDS discrimination by medical care providers: Is Washington law an adequate remedy?" *Washington Law Review* 63 (1988): 701-724.

Recommends banning the common forms of medical care discrimination and requiring heightened HIV testing standards as an important step towards creating effective AIDS antidiscrimination law.

Review/Analysis

Three recommendations are offered for statutory charges regarding AIDS: that health care providers shall not discriminate against AIDS or HIV patients; that procedures shall be implemented to assure HIV test results do not become a part of the patient's routine medical record; and that AIDS plaintiffs bringing actions under chapter 49.60 or chapter 70.24 of the Revised Code of Washington need not exhaust administrative remedies, and a court may order educational counseling of persons or institutions found guilty of violating either chapter.

Of particular interest to lawyers.

590. RUBINSTEIN, William B.   "Law and empowerment: The idea of
     order in the time of AIDS."   *Yale Law Journal* 98 (1989):
     975-997.

Explores the way in which *AIDS and the Law: A Guide for the Public*
struggles to order the uncertainty of AIDS-related law.

Essay

The tension between order and uncertainty in applying existing laws to
AIDS and enacting new laws in the United States is compared to the
struggle of people with AIDS (PWAs) to overcome victimization and take
control of their own lives.   An analogy is drawn between the legal
system's efforts to order the epidemic and PWAs' efforts to empower
themselves to act.   The indeterminacy, anxiety, and confusion of the
AIDS crisis are embodied in AIDS-related legal discourse.   The author
recommends that efforts to order that discourse not minimize the
turbulence of AIDS, but ensure that it continues to inform those
efforts.

Of particular interest to lawyers, judges, and legislators.

591. SCHEPARD, Andrew.   "AIDS and divorce."   *Family Law
     Quarterly* 23 (1989): 1-42.

Explores the impact of AIDS on divorce law, highlighting fundamental
questions about the purposes of divorce law and procedure.

Commentary

Unless a spouse has engaged in morally blameworthy conduct, increasing
the risk of transmission to his family, an AIDS-related divorce should
be treated like any other divorce.   This premise promotes public
health policy, cooperation between spouses, and the children's
welfare.   Courts have, thus far, demonstrated the capacity to separate
fact from fiction in AIDS-related divorces.   Legislatures should
ensure the continuation of this capacity by creating mechanisms for
updating the courts on AIDS.   They should also review aspects of
divorce law that encourage moral condemnation of HIV-infected persons.
In most divorce cases, an AIDS-infected person should be treated as a
spouse and parent with an illness, not as a pariah.

Of interest to divorce lawyers and legislators.

592. SMITH, David Randolph.   "Medicine and law: AIDS, constitu-
     tional challenges to tort reform and medical malpractice."
     Tort and Insurance Law Journal 23 (1988): 370-404.

Examines the topics of AIDS, constitutional challenges to tort reform,
and medical malpractice.

Review

Explores significant and developing legal issues related to AIDS in the areas of discrimination, criminal law, tort liability, and insurance. Analyzes the constitutionality of recent tort reform laws, particularly under emerging principles of state constitutional law. Discusses medical malpractice liability with a focus on trends in the law of informed consent, emotional distress, and hospital liability for premature transfer of uninsured patients.

Of interest to physicians, hospital administrators, and lawyers.

593. SMITH, Mark D. "AIDS and its legal ramifications." *The Journal of Legal Medicine* 9 (1988): 341-347.

Reviews two books on AIDS and the law that cover many of the same subjects—the medical facts of AIDS, legal precedent regarding workplace discrimination against persons with AIDS, housing law, tort law, and the use of the criminal justice system to deal with infected persons who knowingly put others at risk—and discusses the necessity for such books.

Book Review

The books often cite the same cases and reach the same conclusions. Both agree that the fears of coworkers do not justify a discriminatory policy toward a person with AIDS by an employer; stress the importance of education about AIDS in the workplace, schools, and other settings; and make the point that the best solution to AIDS-related conflicts lies in avoiding litigation and seeking common-sense, negotiated solutions acceptable to the various interests affected. Despite their similarities, the books have different approaches and are targeted to different audiences. Both contain useful glossaries, a wealth of references, and bibliographic material and would make valuable desk references.

Of interest to lawyers and to the lay public.

594. SOTTO, Lisa J. "Undoing a lesson of fear in the classroom: The legal recourse of AIDS-linked children." *University of Pennsylvania Law Review* 135 (1986): 193-221.

Argues that children facing AIDS-related discrimination are protected by several federal laws that prohibit discrimination against disabled individuals, as well as by the equal protection clause of the 14th amendment to the constitution.

Commentary

There appears to be absolutely no risk of spreading AIDS by casual contact, such as that which occurs in the classroom. In addition, the risk that a child diagnosed as having AIDS will contract a potentially harmful disease from his/her peers in school should be assessed on an individual basis. School administrators who arbitrarily segregate all AIDS-linked children from their classmates are yielding to the pressure of uninformed public fear. Proper authorities should separately assess each AIDS-linked child to determine the appropriate educational placement for that child.

Of interest to lawyers and school administrators.

595.   TURNER, Ronald. *"Arline, Chalk,* The Civil Rights Restoration
       Act and the AIDS handicap." *Labor Law Journal* 40 (1989):
       3-11.

Assesses the impact of the decisions in the Arline and Chalk court
cases and the Civil Rights Restoration Act (CRRA) on employment-re-
lated AIDS law.

Review

Legal precedent and legislation have confirmed AIDS as a handicap
within the meaning of the 1973 Rehabilitation Act, Section 504.
However, questions remain including that of whether individuals with
AIDS are handicapped on the basis of physical impairment or contagion.
It is not known either how the requirements for reasonable accommo-
dations will apply to persons with AIDS or how much protection the
CRRA amendment will provide persons with AIDS. Employers to whom the
Rehabilitation Act applies should recognize that employees with or
regarded as having AIDS may rely upon the act's prohibition of employ-
ment discrimination.

Of interest to employers, attorneys, policymakers, and HIV-infected
persons.

6. WORKPLACE ISSUES

a. Books

596.   AMERICAN Management Association. *AIDS: The Workplace
       Issues.*   New   York: American   Management   Association
       Membership Publications Division, 1985.

Identifies and responds to questions raised by the incidence of AIDS
in the workplace.

Monograph

The four chapters deal with responding to AIDS in the workplace, the
legal issues, how insurance companies are responding, and medical
answers about AIDS. Three appendices demonstrate how to find resources in your area, how an employee assistance program (EAP) can
help, and the Bank of America Policy.

Of particular interest to managers and administrators.

597.   BOHL, Don L. (Ed.). *AIDS: The New Workplace Issues.* New
       York: American   Management   Association   Membership
       Publications Division, 1988.

Intended as a tool to help corporate decision makers establish policy regarding AIDS in the workplace and work through the specifics of workplace education.

Text

The six chapters address: how companies have responded to AIDS-related issues; questions and answers regarding dealing with workplace problems; the role of corporate policy; planning an effective workforce education program; case management; and the legal issues: what every manager should know. Three appendices address workplace testing for HIV infection; how public perceptions impact business patronage; and how to run an effective educational program. The authors advise readers not to rely solely upon any publication, but to consult, as appropriate, with knowledgeable individuals in the legal, medical, and adult education fields.

Of particular interest to employers, managers, and administrators.

598. COMMERCE Clearing House Editorial Staff. *AIDS: Employer Rights and Responsibilities.* Chicago: Commerce Clearing House, 1985.

Presents information on how management should view AIDS as a public issue and a workplace issue.

Report

The two parts of this report about AIDS in the workplace discuss 1) the practical employment relations problems that management will face when AIDS becomes a workplace issue, and 2) the legal issues that influence any personnel action taken with respect to AIDS.

Of interest to employers in general.

599. PUCKETT, Sam B., and Alan R. Emery. *Managing AIDS in the Workplace.* Reading, MA: Addison-Wesley, 1988.

Shares with readers what managers in organizations of all types, sizes, and locations have learned about managing the AIDS epidemic.

Text

The seven chapters cover: the AIDS epidemic and the workplace; understanding AIDS: the epidemic, the virus, and the disease; managing the fear of managing AIDS in the workplace; step by step management of AIDS in the workplace; designing and implementing AIDS education programs; a primer on prevention; and the future of corporate responsibility and employee health.

Of interest to all employers and to the general public.

600. SANKS, David. *Managing AIDS in the Workplace: A Managerial Guide to the Practicalities and Economics.* Fullerton, CA: DaSak Associates, 1988.

Provides a legal background as well as a practical and analytical framework for dealing with AIDS-related issues in the workplace.

Guidebook

An informative, practical book filled with factual, useful information to help the reader deal effectively with AIDS-related issues. The book provides: a detailed discussion of the legal options facing employers; guidelines for formulating AIDS policies; guidelines for educating the workforce; a discussion of the economic impact of AIDS in the workplace; guidelines for employment practices to minimize discriminatory problems; a glossary of AIDS-related terms; and a source list for obtaining additional educational materials and assistance for employees with AIDS.

Of interest to employers and managers.

601. SCHACHTER, Victor, and Susan von Seeburg. *AIDS: A Manager's Guide*. New York: Executive Enterprises, 1986.

Identifies key legal issues and answers practical questions to help managers make knowledgeable, lawful, humane responses to AIDS issues in the workplace.

Resource Book

Six chapters outline the basic medical facts about AIDS; address the issue of whether it can be considered a "physical handicap," identify state tort claims that might provide the basis of a lawsuit by an applicant or employee with AIDS, and summarize the statutory claims available to an employee or applicant who has AIDS; outline practical strategies for company managers to use in an effective response to AIDS issues; and identify specific workplace concerns and employment practices which can be implemented to avoid liability. The appendix includes a sample AIDS policy, the most recent CDC Guidelines, relevant laws, and a key agency decision defining AIDS as a physical handicap.

Of particular interest to employers, managers, and administrators.

602. WEXLER, Richard H. *Focus, AIDS in the Workplace*. Paramus, NJ: Prentice-Hall, 1986.

Proposes that organizations must be aware of the problems and dilemmas AIDS can bring to the workplace, and suggests guidelines to be used in determining how to respond to such problems.

Guidebook

Addresses what organizations must consider, some courses of action and their consequences with respect to discrimination; describes what some organizations are doing; details how organizations can protect themselves; and presents relevant excerpts from *Morbidity and Mortality Weekly Report* regarding AIDS in the workplace.

Of special interest to personnel managers, and to CEO's and management level employees in all sizes and types of organizations.

b. Articles

603. ABERTH, John. "AIDS in the workplace." *Management Review* 74, no. 12 (1985): 49-51.

Discusses the legal, insurance, and human relations issues of AIDS in the workplace.

Descriptive

Legal questions generally arise in the workplace when employers discriminate against PWAs, who are protected in most states from firing or mandatory testing by fair employment laws forbidding discrimination based on a handicap or physical disability. Many insurance companies claim that a preexisting condition or an undisclosed history of sexually transmitted diseases warrants non-payment of insurance claims. A notable exception is Equitable Assurance Society, which has reduced insurance costs by covering outpatient and home care. Aggressive AIDS education for managers and employees minimizes human relations problems in the worksite.

Of interest to employers and insurance officials.

604. BAKER, Constance H. and Megan W. Arthur. "AIDS in the hospital workplace: Theories of hospital liability." *Tort and Insurance Law Journal* 24 (1988): 1-17.

Addresses several areas of potential hospital liability.

Descriptive

As health care providers and employers, hospitals will probably experience the greatest impact from the AIDS epidemic. Patient care obligations may often conflict with the safety and welfare of health care workers and third parties. The situation is further complicated by the major financial problems stemming from inadequate reimbursement of medical costs. As the crisis continues, changes are slowly occurring. Medical and legal authorities are providing guidelines and recommendations that hospitals can use to carefully balance the rights of patients and employees. Changes in reimbursement programs designed to meet the special needs of AIDS patients may relieve some of the financial strain on the entire health care delivery system. As these changes continue, hospitals must carefully monitor the myriad of laws, regulations, and court decisions relating to AIDS to guide their policies and actions affecting patients and employees.

Of particular interest to hospital administrators.

605. BAYER, Ronald, and Gerald Oppenheimer. "AIDS in the workplace: The ethical ramifications." *Business and Health* 3, no. 3 (1986): 30-34.

Discusses the need to provide guidance and limitations for employers and insurers regarding persons with AIDS.

Discussion

AIDS poses a social and moral challenge to society. We can respond to its presence with compassion and reason, treating its victims with dignity, or we can succumb to hysteria and treat them as pariahs, robbing them of privacy and the right to function as members of the community. Among the most crucial issues facing the sick and infected are those involving employment, health insurance protection, and access to life insurance. While no greater justification for denial of employment exists for AIDS victims than for victims of any other illness, the cost of health care to the employer could be astronomical. The insurance industry, too, fears the potential effect of AIDS upon an industry that has not allocated reserves for such a purpose. There are no easy answers to this extremely complex problem, but these matters deserve broad public discussion in which the principle of equity ought to be given a central role.

Of interest to employers, insurers, lawyers, and legislators.

606. ———. "Living with AIDS in the workplace." *Across the Board* 23, no. 9 (September 1986): 56-61.

Discusses employment and insurance issues associated with AIDS.

Descriptive

Among the most crucial social and moral issues of the AIDS epidemic is the degree to which those who are sick or infected with HIV will find themselves excluded from employment, health insurance protection, and life insurance. Casual contact with persons with HIV infection or AIDS poses no risk to the public, and most restrictions on those who are ill or are carriers are inappropriate. The refusal to hire or the decision to fire someone with a medical condition, if he is capable of performing a job, generally is deemed a violation of the law. Employers who fear the potential health care costs of HIV infected employees and insurers who want to minimize their vulnerability wish to require antibody tests as screening devices. Preexisting condition clauses are being used by insurance companies to justify refusal to pay on life insurance policies. Pools have been created to cover people whose applications for health insurance are refused because of risk factors or health conditions, but the right to life insurance has no such support. Whether insurers should be permitted to deny coverage to persons at risk or whether life insurance should be socialized, are matters that require broad public discussion.

Of interest to employers, insurers, and legislators.

607. BROCKHOEFT, John E. "AIDS in the workplace: Legal limitations on employer actions." *American Business Law Journal* 26, no. 2 (1988): 225-304.

Discusses the nature of employment in the United States and its relevancy to AIDS, and identifies the major sources of legal liability for the employer with an HIV-infected employee.

Review

Employment at the will of the employer, giving employers the right to hire and fire whomever they wish, has been the accepted standard in the U.S. workplace since the 1880s. The courts, however, have ruled to protect employees' rights in the workplace, some of which are particularly pertinent to employees with AIDS. Federal legislation, notably the Federal Vocational Rehabilitation Act of 1973 and the Employee Retirement Income Security Act of 1974, provide protection for employees, as do state handicap laws, local ordinances, and protective bargaining. A recent ruling of the Supreme Court stated that persons with contagious diseases and persons regarded by others as impaired are protected by handicap legislation, and a state court of appeals ruled that employers cannot reassign infected persons to "distasteful" positions if there is no occupational risk of transmission.

Of interest to employers, managers, lawyers, and persons with AIDS.

608. COLOSI, Marco Leo. "AIDS: Human rights versus the duty to provide a safe workplace." *Labor Law Journal* 39 (1988): 677-687.

Discusses various legal issues and principles as those pertain to AIDS in the workplace.

Review

To address the issues and problems discussed in an AIDS-employment context, there are few court decisions, and, therefore, creative human resource and legal posturing, research, and analysis are required. These include consideration of legal principles, human resource concepts, and labor relations to develop a "decisional and probability of liability model" in determining policy. The model must consider current medical opinions and effect a marriage of those opinions with corporate policy and communications.

Of interest to employers, public health officials, and lawyers.

609. COOPERMAN, Harriet E. "AIDS and pregnancy discrimination: Balancing competing interests." *Trial* 24, no. 6 (1988): 14-17.

Addresses two areas in which employers must reconcile competing interests--AIDS and pregnancy discrimination.

Discussion

Discrimination laws have been enacted to ensure that individuals are treated fairly and given equal opportunities as long as their differences are unrelated to their ability to perform a job. However, in accommodating to the interests and needs of one employee, the employer sometimes spurs others to protest that their rights are being ignored and impaired. In other cases, the employer may find that important business considerations require taking actions against employees on a basis protected by discrimination laws. AIDS and pregnancy are two areas in which a balancing act develops in the attempt to reconcile competing interests. Specific examples are given and legal decisions cited. Employers are cautioned against such practices as requiring AIDS testing, disclosing information about an employee's or applicant's medical status, denying employment to an individual because of increased insurance costs, or treating a person differently from other employees because of that individual's physical status, and are given advice as to how they may successfully defend against a discrimination suit.

Of interest to employers, managers, and lawyers.

610. COX, Tom. "AIDS and stress." *Work and Stress* 2 (1988): 109-112.

A discussion of stress and AIDS, particularly the effect of stress on the AIDS patient's work.

Editorial

AIDS patients should not be exposed to working conditions or agents that further challenge the immune system. The AIDS sufferers' emotional reactions to their diagnoses are also important. If their reactions impair the sufferers' ability to work, they will undoubtedly be less attractive to an organization, and this will influence both management and peer behavior.

Of interest to employers, occupational health professionals, and rehabilitation counselors.

611. FAGOT-DIAZ, José G. "Employment discrimination against AIDS victims: Rights and remedies available under the Federal Rehabilitation Act of 1973." *Labor Law Journal* 39, no. 3 (1988): 148-166.

Presents a brief overview of AIDS, shows how it relates to employment discrimination litigation, demonstrates how existing laws forbidding handicap discrimination can be applied to the protection of AIDS carriers and victims in the workforce, and offers some guidelines and recommendations for employers.

Review

The disease known as AIDS will be protected as a "handicap" under the Rehabilitation Act of 1973. Employers, together with management personnel, should establish a well-defined AIDS in the workplace policy. Any allegation that an employer cannot accommodate the AIDS victim or carrier should be well documented and include all types of costs. Management and union representatives might consider the implementation of carefully scrutinized health benefit plans protecting AIDS afflicted employees, taking into consideration the medical costs surrounding the epidemic. Specific legislation relating to employee discrimination should be carried out statewide. Of paramount importance to the employer, is work force education relating to the AIDS issue.

Of particular interest to employers and management personnel.

612. GERBERT, Barbara, Bryan Maguire, Victor Badner, David Altman, George Stone. "Why fear persists: Health care professionals and AIDS." *Journal of the American Medical Association* 260 (1988): 3481-3483.

Discusses fear of AIDS in the workplace on the part of health care professionals.

Commentary

Recent studies have shown that fear is a basic and continued reaction to the HIV epidemic among health care professionals. Three reasons for this continuing fear have been identified: health care authorities have tended to downplay the real risk of occupational exposure; use of infection control procedures does not guarantee against HIV transmission; and communication between authorities and health care professionals is hindered by differences in the values and goals of the two groups. As long as the risk of HIV transmission in the workplace continues to exist, health professionals' fear of getting AIDS will persist. The authors make five suggestions for addressing that fear without denying the problem. The goal is not to eradicate the fear, but to prevent it from compromising the quality of patient care or threatening the health professionals' own well-being.

Of particular interest to hospital administrators and health educators.

613. JOHNSTON, George W. "Coping with AIDS: Today's major workplace issue." *Labor Law Journal* 40 (1989): 302-306.

Discusses the challenges AIDS presents for employers.

Discussion

Management can best prepare to confront AIDS and the conflicting legal issues it raises by formulating a detailed plan of action for dealing with the disease. Through such a plan, fair decisions can be made and the rights of everyone be recognized.

Of interest to employers and managers.

614. KANDEL, William L. "AIDS in the workplace." *Employee Relations Law Journal* 11 (1986): 678-690.

Surveys some of the new issues regarding AIDS in the workplace, which employers will have to confront.

Review

The employer and legal communities should now be taking affirmative steps to eliminate employment discrimination against persons with AIDS. Recent data indicate that workplace risks are negligible. Employers have the responsibility to educate themselves and then to ensure that their employees are made aware of the current facts. Although AIDS remains a medical crisis, it need no longer create a crisis of misunderstanding in the workplace.

Of interest to employers, managers, and corporation lawyers.

615. KIRP, David L. "Uncommon decency: Pacific Bell responds to AIDS." *Harvard Business Review* 67, no. 3 (1989): 140-151.

Describes the enlightened policies and programs established by Pacific Bell Telephone in response to AIDS.

Descriptive

The fears expressed by some Pacific Bell employees about encountering AIDS while serving customers led to an investigation of the company's 1984 records regarding AIDS deaths among employees, followed by the establishment of non-discriminatory policies, the expansion of employee health benefits to cover home and hospice care, and the establishment of an AIDS education program for employees. Pacific Bell co-sponsored the first conference on "AIDS in the Workplace" as well as production of the videotape, "The Epidemic of Fear". In 1986, the corporation publicly opposed a proposition to bar persons with AIDS from workplaces and school, and in 1988 opposed another proposition, which would have banned anonymous HIV testing. Bell also initiated AIDS support groups and programs about safer sex for employees. The corporation has received recognition from the media as well as a presidential citation for its enlightened policies.

Of interest to employers and managers, health educators, public policymakers, and members of the general public.

616. KRAPFL, Mike. "As AIDS hysteria spreads, so does the need for cool-headed education." *Occupational Health and Safety* 55, no. 3 (1986): 20-26.

Emphasizes the need for AIDS education in the workplace.

Descriptive

Fear and ignorance about AIDS have pervaded the workplace, and debate rages as to whether workers should be screened for the virus, how the disease is spread, and when and if it can be confronted and controlled. In March of 1986, California and Wisconsin were the only states to have laws forbidding testing for AIDS in the workplace to determine employability and insurability. Nevertheless, employers in both states continued to try to screen employees. One employer who screens for exposure to HIV is the Ensearch Corporation of Dallas, which screens its food service employees and has yet to be challenged. The military screens all recruits to avoid potential problems arising from placing a person with an immune deficiency in a situation threatening his/her health or the health of other service persons. Although the military can screen for HIV, it is a matter of debate whether private employers can legally do so. AIDS education in the workplace can benefit employers and employees. Occupational health nurses can play key roles in AIDS education.

Of interest to employers, managers, employees, health educators, and occupational health nurses.

617. LUCEY, Gerald R., and Gabriela B. Georgi. "Privacy in the workplace: Health and liability." *Human Rights* 14, no. 3 (1987): 45-47.

Discusses the conflict between the patient's right to privacy and the need to protect hospital employees from AIDS.

Commentary

Patient privacy laws sometimes make it illegal for a hospital to inform the staff that a patient has AIDS, and the law requires that the results of HIV antibody tests be confidential. Added to this, a hospital has the responsibility to accommodate any employee with AIDS. This issue is particularly problematic in the context of workers' compensation claims when an employee thinks he contracted AIDS on the job. Hospitals must maintain a delicate balance between their obligation to ensure worker safety and their obligation to protect the privacy of their patients and staff.

Of particular interest to hospital administrators and hospital staff.

618. LUTGEN, Lorraine. "AIDS in the workplace: Fighting fear with facts and policy." *Personnel* 64, no. 11 (November 1987): 53-57.

Provides guidelines for employers and human resources managers who wish to provide a safe work environment while maintaining a setting that is free from discrimination.

Guide

An organization should start with a clear policy statement, which is communicated to all employees. Specific policies on testing for AIDS among prospective and current employees should be set down along with clear guidelines on work-unit accommodations and work assignments of employees with AIDS. The organization should also define its position on providing inclusive health benefits to employees with AIDS and clarify the effect of its policy on the total work group. Finally, it is essential that a comprehensive mandatory training program, which dispels misinformation about the AIDS virus and reassures employees about their risk of contracting AIDS in the workplace, be provided for all employees.

Of interest to employers, managers, administrators, and human resource directors.

619. MASI, Dale A.   "AIDS in the workplace: What can be done?"
     Personnel 64, no. 7 (1987): 57-60.

Discusses AIDS in the workplace and possible strategies for employers to use in dealing with it.

Essay

A majority of companies have no program for dealing with AIDS despite the fact that an estimated 1.5 million Americans are infected with it.   Companies need to formulate non-discriminatory AIDS policies regarding hiring, testing, health benefits, and changes in job category.   Pressure should be placed on insurers to offer case management for employees with catastrophic illness.   Employee assistant programs should be involved in training and educating personnel and establishing procedures.   Managers must be trained to overcome personal prejudices and educate employees about the truths regarding AIDS, and employees going overseas should be given guidelines for protecting themselves against HIV infection.   Knowledge is the best weapon currently available to combat this disease.

Should interest all managers and administrators.

620. MYERS, Donald W., and Phyllis S. Myers.   "Arguments
     involving AIDS testing in the workplace." *Labor Law Journal*
     Journal 38, no. 9 (1987): 582-590.

A broad overview of current public health statistics, clinical manifestations of AIDS, and arguments for testing in the workplace.

Review

The question response format of this article provides excellent point counterpoint on reasons for testing, including such issues as legal protection of the employer, limitations of liability in services to the public, and limitations of benefit extensions to employees ill with AIDS or ARC.

Useful to labor law specialists, personnel managers, policymakers, and others concerned with the legal and ethical issues of HIV infection.

621. POSTOL, Lawrence P.   "Handicap discrimination considerations
     in treating the impaired worker: Drugs, alcohol, pregnancy,
     and AIDS in the workplace." *Journal of Occupational Medi-*
     cine 30 (1988): 321-327.

Discusses problems faced by employers regarding applicants and employees who are disabled by drugs, alcohol, pregnancy, or AIDS, and makes recommendations for dealing with these problems.

Guidelines

Administrators must comply with handicap and pregnancy discrimination statutes, any union collective bargaining agreement, and any state or local statutes specifically directed at protecting certain classes of handicapped persons when dealing with applicants and employees. Reasonable accommodations, which allow a disabled worker to perform the job, must be made, although accommodations which provide an undue hardship need not be implemented. An employee who cannot safely perform the essential functions of the job need not be hired or retained. However, current employees who are impaired should be treated with tolerance and patience. Employers must recognize their responsibilities and liability under their health benefit plans and other liability statutes, and attempt to minimize their exposure.

Of interest to managers and administrators.

622. ROWE, Mary P., Malcolm Russell-Einhorn, Michael A. Baker. "The fear of AIDS." *Harvard Business Review* 64, no. 4 (July-August 1986): 28-36.

Discusses fear of AIDS in the workplace as a problem for management.

Theoretical

When a worker has, or is rumored to have AIDS, fear among his co-workers can cause extraordinary tension and stress in the workplace. Managers need to initiate and support task forces and training programs inside their own companies, and executives need to face their own fears about AIDS to deal effectively with fear of AIDS at work. Education, compassion, and rational discussion are among the most valuable tools for dealing with fear of AIDS, and education in the workplace can sharply reduce fear and stress.

Of particular interest to managers, administrators, and health educators.

623. RYAN, Caitlan. "AIDS in the workplace: How to reach out to those among us." *Public Welfare* 44, no. 3 (1988): 29-33.

Discusses how employers and managers can prepare to cope with eventual cases of AIDS within the workplace.

Commentary

By the end of this century, everyone will be affected in some way by AIDS. The workplace has a critical role to play in dispelling the myths and fears surrounding the disease and encouraging an appropriate response to those affected by it. Management can help to ensure a compassionate, supportive, and understanding response to persons affected by AIDS by working with communities to develop essential support services, by educating employees, and by assisting employees with AIDS in a sensitive, responsive manner.

Of interest to employers, managers, and personnel directors.

624. STEIN, Robert E.   "Strategies for dealing with AIDS disputes
     in the workplace." *Arbitration Journal* 42, no. 3 (1987):
     21-29.

Focuses on the legal aspects of the AIDS crisis that impact on the
workplace.

Theoretical

Discusses how the law describes the rights and duties of employers and
employees, including coworkers of a person who has AIDS, ARC, or is
HIV antibody positive; what is really happening in the employment
world; and what strategies can help both employers and employees deal
more effectively with AIDS-related disputes.

Should interest managers and administrators, specialists in labor
relations, lawyers, public policymakers, persons with HIV infection,
and members of the general public.

625. TREBILCOCK, Anne M.   "AIDS and the workplace: Some policy
     pointers from international labour standards." *International
     Labour Review* 128 (1989): 29-45.

The principles drawn up by the World Health Organization and the ILO
are discussed with respect to the formulation of policies protecting
the rights of workers and the interests of public health.

Descriptive

Reference to internationally agreed standards can ensure that the
adoption of a consistent approach to the formulation of policies on
HIV/AIDS that combine public health concerns with respect for
individual rights.   Public policymakers need to take the lead, with
consultations and collective bargaining also playing an important
role.   This brief communication of selected ILO standards is a
starting point.   ILO instruments can serve as useful guideposts in the
search for policies that are both reasonable and humane.

Of interest to public policymakers, lawyers, employers, and public
health officials.

626. TURK, Harry N.   "AIDS: The first decade."   *Employee
     Relations Law Journal* 14 (1989): 531-548.

Chronicles the evolution of federal, state, and local law concerning
AIDS and the workplace.

Descriptive

Although some clear-cut answers and guidelines address the relationship of employer and employee to the AIDS epidemic, current legislation and enforcement of those laws does not adequately address the
person with AIDS as a handicapped individual.   The author emphasizes

the problems peculiar to the health care industry, the constitutionality of present legislation, and the AIDS victim's right to privacy versus the employer's need to know. Some practical solutions and guidelines are presented to help employers deal with a person with AIDS and his or her co-worker.

Of interest to employers, attorneys, educators, and counselors.

627. WAGEL, William S. "AIDS: Setting policy, educating employees at Bank of America." *Personnel* 65, no. 8 (1988): 4-8.

Describes the method Bank of America used in developing an AIDS policy and providing education and support for all employees.

Descriptive

A Bank of America interdepartmental task force made up of representatives from the equal opportunity, personnel, benefits, medical, and legal departments developed a corporate policy, which addresses all life-threatening illnesses of employees, and a comprehensive AIDS educational/support program. The education component makes use of pamphlets, videotapes, programs, and counseling. Health care costs for a person with AIDS are less than the California average since the Bank of America is self-insured and utilizes home and hospice care.

Of interest to corporate executives, personnel and benefits officers, and workplace educators.

628. WALDO, William S. "The work environment: A practical guide for dealing with AIDS at work." *Personnel Journal* 64, no. 8 (1987): 135-138.

Discusses the legal rights of AIDS victims in the workplace and the legal obligations of the employer.

Guide

Discusses employment and labor laws that apply to workers who are afflicted with AIDS and their employers, and, by employing a set of hypothetical situations, offers practical guidelines for employers who may have to deal with difficult situations created by the presence of AIDS in the workplace.

Of interest to all managers, administrators, and employers.

629. WORLD Health Organization. "AIDS and the workplace." *Lancet* 2, no. 8615 (1988): 841-842.

Participants from 18 countries examined the topic of AIDS and the workplace from three aspects: risk factors associated with HIV infection in the workplace; responses by business and workers to HIV/AIDS; and the use of the workplace for health education activities.

Commentary

Workers with HIV infection who are healthy should be treated just like
any other worker. Consistent policies and procedures should be
developed at national levels through consultations between workers,
employers, and their organizations. HIV/AIDS workplace policies
should be communicated to all concerned, continually reviewed,
monitored for their successful implementation, and evaluated for their
effectiveness. Preemployment HIV/AIDS screening as part of the
assessment of fitness to work is unnecessary and should not be
required. For persons in employment, HIV/AIDS screening should not be
required. Employees and their families should have access to
information and educational programs on HIV/AIDS as well as to
relevant counseling and referral.

Of interest to health professionals, public health officials, and
laymen.

Chapter 4

EDUCATION AND PREVENTION

1. THEORY AND PROCESS

a. Articles

630. ARCHER, Victor E. "Psychological defenses and control of AIDS." *American Journal of Public Health* 79 (1989): 876-878.

The well-known psychological defenses of avoidance, repression, and denial against the knowledge that one has, or might have, a fatal disease must be considered in control programs for HIV.

Commentary

Current programs of education, voluntary testing, and counseling do not consider defense mechanisms and may, therefore, provide inadequate control. Compulsory HIV testing programs and the development of an "HIV parole" system may be needed if the HIV epidemic worsens.

Of interest to health educators, counselors, and public health officials.

631. CATES, Willard, Jr., and G. Stephen Bowen. "Education for AIDS prevention: Not our only voluntary weapon." *American Journal of Public Health* 79 (1989): 871-874.

The authors suggest that education, while critically important to our efforts to stop transmission of HIV, needs to be bolstered by additional voluntary approaches.

Commentary

Control of parenteral drug use, prevention of ulcerative sexually transmitted diseases, provision of expanded contraceptive services to seropositive reproductive age women, and reinforcement of risk-reduction behaviors through extended follow-up interventions, as well as education, are required to put a stop to the transmission of HIV.

Of interest to health educators and public health officials.

632. FELDBLUM, Paul J., and Judith A. Fortney. "Condoms, spermicides, and the transmission of human immunodeficiency virus: A review of the literature." *American Journal of Public Health* 78 (1988): 52-54.

Reviews studies on the effectiveness of condoms and spermicides in preventing the transmission of HIV.

Literature Review

Barrier methods of contraception appear to be the only method apart from abstinence, monogamy, and curtailment of sexual activities of preventing sexual transmission of AIDS. However, evidence for the widespread assumption that condoms, and possibly spermicides, can effectively prevent the transmission of HIV is not strong. Suggestions are offered for future research.

Of interest to public health professionals and epidemiologic researchers.

633. GOCHROS, Harvey L. "Risks of abstinence: Sexual decision making in the AIDS era." *Social Work* 33 (1988): 254-256.

Explores efforts to reduce the sexual transmission of AIDS, and responds to those who suggest sexual abstinence as the primary solution to the AIDS crisis.

Descriptive

One sexual standard cannot be adopted for all people. Each person must think through his or her own responsible sexual choices. Social workers can help the process by sharing the facts of HIV infection. Social workers cannot support the thesis that the only alternatives to abstinence are amorality, permissiveness, and sure death.

Of interest to counselors, social workers, mental health professionals, and health educators.

634. GOLDSTEIN, Mel L., and Frank M. Yuen. "Coping with AIDS: An approach to training and education in a therapeutic community--the Samaritan Village Program." *Journal of Substance Abuse Treatment* 5 (1988): 45-50.

Focuses on one research approach using risk reduction strategies to prevent AIDS in a residential therapeutic environment.

Descriptive

The authors offer a practical working model that might be applicable in a variety of settings. It should be emphasized that this is not a one-step presentation of AIDS information, but rather that it is an ongoing program of AIDS education.

Of interest to health educators and substance abuse counselors.

635. GORDON, Richard. "A critical review of the physics and statistics of condoms in individual versus societal survival of the AIDS epidemic." *Journal of Sex & Marital Therapy* 15 (1989): 5-30.

Examines the odds of condom failure during a lifetime of sexual activity and questions the confidence placed in them as protection against HIV transmission.

Commentary

Condom failure rates for HIV are substantially greater than for pregnancy, even when comdoms are used by highly motivated people. Although they provide ineffective lifelong protection against HIV infection, thereby providing inadequate risk reduction for the individual, they are sufficiently effective that if everyone used them, the AIDS epidemic would be stopped. Quantitative public health goals are needed to reduce the estimated HIV infection rate of 4-12 people per carrier to less than one. Government and scientific testing of condoms can be improved statistically and by using relevant physics.

Of special interest to health educators and public health officials.

636. GOTZCHE, Peter C., and Meéte Hording. "Condoms to prevent transmission do not imply truly safe sex." *Scandinavian Journal of Infectious Diseases* 20 (1988): 233-234.

Thirty female prostitutes and 16 persons from the hospital staff each tested 10 latex condoms by vaginal intercourse.

Short Communication

Although encouragement to condom use is prudent in an epidemiological scale, truly safe sex, using condoms with an HIV positive partner, is a dangerous illusion.

Of interest to health educators and public health officials.

637. GREGORIO, David I., and Jeanne V. Linden. "Screening prospective blood donors for AIDS risk factors: Will sufficient donors be found?" *American Journal of Public Health* 78 (1988): 1468-1471.

252   Education and Prevention

Estimates the proportion of the U.S. population that should be deferred as blood donors because of personal histories of high risk behaviors for AIDS.

Discussion

It is estimated that 14-19% of American males and two percent of females, aged 17-75, have personal histories of behaviors that place them at high risk for HIV transmission, and many of these persons are unsuitable as blood donors for other reasons. Therefore, about 10-14% of adult males and one percent of females should be deferred from giving blood. Eliminating these people from the blood donor pool would not endanger the blood supply; there are about 100 million persons in the U.S. who are suitable blood donors.

Of interest to blood banking specialists, public health professionals, and public policymakers.

638. HEARST, Norman, and Stephen B. Hulley.   "Preventing the heterosexual spread of AIDS: Are we giving our patients the best advice?" *Journal of the American Medical Association* 259 (1988): 2428-2432.

Considers strategies for controlling the spread of AIDS through sexual contact.

Report

Current recommendations for controlling the spread of HIV through sexual contact include educating the public to: reduce the number of sexual partners, eliminate such high risk practices as anal intercourse, use condoms, practice abstinence or lifelong monogamy, or avoid sex with anyone who has not been tested and shown to be uninfected by HIV.   These strategies are imperfect as pragmatic guidelines for the public, and are difficult to follow. The authors use quantitative estimates of the risk of HIV infection in various circumstances to demonstrate that, at the present time, the single most important recommendation for physicians to give their patients is to avoid choosing a sexual partner who may be at high risk of carrying HIV.

Of interest to all health professionals.

639. KAPLAN, Edward N., and Paul R. Abramson.   "So what if the program ain't perfect?   A mathematical model of AIDS education." *Evaluation Review* 13 (1989): 107-122.

Proposes a simple mathematical model of withdrawal from risky behavior and recidivism to risky behavior within the context of the HIV epidemic, and discusses the policy implications of the results obtained.

Descriptive

The authors demonstrated that an imperfect intervention program can result in a large reduction in new HIV infections. This finding is important for policy considerations. AIDS educational programs that initially appear ineffectual, in the long run, have significant impacts on future AIDS outcome measures. The results of the present model suggest a more optimistic appraisal of AIDS education because the prospects for prevention seem reasonable, despite the inevitability of only partially effective interventions.

Of interest to researchers and health educators working in AIDS education.

640. KELLY, Jeffrey A., and Janet S. St. Lawrence. "AIDS prevention and treatment: Psychology's role in the health crisis." *Clinical Psychology Review* 8 (1988): 255-284.

Briefly reviews medical, epidemiological, and risk behavior findings concerning AIDS that are relevant to psychological interventions.

Review

The status of AIDS prevention efforts is reviewed with particular attention to behavioral factors that influence risk conduct among such populations as gay or bisexual men, IV drug users, heterosexuals, and adolescents. Research on the psychological needs of persons with HIV infection and AIDS is reviewed, and relevant therapy interventions are considered. Concludes with a discussion of several areas where further research attention is needed.

Of interest to psychologists and behavioral scientists.

641. ———. "Behavioral intervention and AIDS." *Behavior Therapist* 6 (1986): 121-125.

A review and critique of behavioral intervention at the level of individual clients, groups, and communities to reduce the risk of AIDS, prevent its transmission, and assist its victims.

Descriptive

Summarizes currently understood characteristics of AIDS; outlines areas to which clinical intervention and behavioral research might usefully be directed; considers issues relevant to behavioral intervention for persons with AIDS; and discusses special sensitivities needed by clinicians and investigators who work with populations at risk for AIDS.

Of interest to social and behavioral scientists.

642. ———. "The prevention of AIDS: Roles for behavioral intervention." *Scandinavian Journal of Behavior Therapy* 16 (1987): 5-19.

Summarizes research on AIDS risk behavior and discusses large scale behavioral community level intervention.

Summary and Discussion

Prevention messages and strategies are presented. Other potentially useful topics for applied behavioral community research include evaluating methods to better prompt risk group members, following AIDS risk education, to adopt lower risk practices; develop and employ audiovisual presentations, such as risk reduction educational videos, in settings such as bars or clubs frequented by risk group members; develop methods to better educate and train public health personnel, including physicians and nurses, in ways to interview and behaviorally counsel their patients on risk reduction; and explore intervention strategies to promote wide-scale risk behavior change.

Of interest to health educators and public health professionals.

643.   MOATTI, J.P., W. Dab, L. Abenhaïm, S. Bastide. "Modifi-
       cations of sexual behavior related to AIDS: A survey in
       Paris region." *Health Policy* 11 (1989): 227-231.

A survey of 900 persons, 18 years of age and older, in the region of Paris, France, was conducted to determine the effects of AIDS upon sexual behavior.

Research

Among those who identified themselves as sexually active, about 14% had been tested for HIV at least once in 1987; 11% had refused sex at least once in the preceding six months because of fear of AIDS, and 12% said they used condoms regularly. About half of those who used condoms were motivated to do so by fear of AIDS. Multivariate analysis showed that being single, declaring multiple sexual partners, and having been tested for HIV were the main predictors for use of condoms.

Of interest to health educators.

644.   NIGHTINGALE, Stuart L. "AIDS and condoms." *American
       Family Physician* 36, no. 6 (1987): 235-236.

A report from the FDA on the use of condoms for AIDS prevention.

Review

Intact, latex condoms offer the best protection from AIDS besides abstinence or mutually monogamous relationships. Labeling instructions for the use of condoms are described.

For a general audience.

645.   SIEGEL, Karolynn.   "Public education to prevent the spread
       of HIV infection." *New York State Journal of Medicine* 88
       (1988): 626-646.

Draws upon the knowledge and insights accumulated in other public health education programs to deal with public education to prevent HIV infection.

Review

Discusses who should be educated, what messages should be communicated, and who should do the educating.

Of interest to health educators and public health officials.

646. ———, Phyllis B. Grodsky, Alan Herman. "AIDS risk-reduction guidelines: A review and analysis." *Journal of Community Health* 11 (1986): 223-243.

A content analysis of 22 brochures obtained from public and private health organizations, nationwide, focused on the extent to which they incorporated the elements of a standard model of health communication.

Discussion

Until an effective treatment of vaccine for AIDS is discovered, the principal strategy for controlling its spread will remain persuading at-risk and diseased populations to modify behaviors implicated in the disease transmission. For homosexuals/bisexuals the risk-reduction or safe-sex brochure has emerged as the most widely used public health intervention modality.

Of interest to health educators and social and behavioral scientists.

647. SISK, Jane E., Maria Hewitt, Kelly L. Metcalf. "The effectiveness of AIDS education." *Health Affairs* 7 (Winter 1988): 37-51.

Summarizes the major findings and recommendations of the Office of Technology Assessment on the effectiveness of AIDS education.

Descriptive

Although the public's knowledge about AIDS has increased and the public's fears have declined, it is not clear whether these changes are a result of organized education or of general media coverage. Problems in evaluating program effectiveness range from poor study designs to a lack of basic information on sexual practices. Educational interventions in the homosexual community in San Francisco have been effective in reducing risky sexual behaviors, and projects to assess the effectiveness of educational interventions among IV drug users are presently being sponsored by the NIDA, NIMH, and CDC. For education to be effective, the content of a program and the dissemination of its messages must be tailored to reach people at high risk. Since AIDS has affected large numbers of blacks and Hispanics, educational approaches should be designed to target people in these and other social and cultural groups. Current educational programs should be evaluated for their effectiveness and the findings incorporated into future educational programs.

Of interest to health educators and program evaluators, public health professionals, and funding agencies.

648.   SOLOMON, Mildred Zeldes, and William De Jong.   "Recent sexually transmitted disease prevention efforts and their implications for AIDS health education."   *Health Education Quarterly* 13 (1986): 301-316.

An analysis of three recent studies to determine whether education efforts can successfully motivate the adoption of key behaviors relevant to the control of a variety of sexually transmitted diseases.

Research/Analysis

Analysis of two studies, which are completed, and prelimary data from a third study, have documented dramatic changes in behavior, knowledge, and attitudes among clients in inner-city public health clinics.   There is a consensus about what AIDS risk reduction messages should be, and there is a growing body of knowledge about how best to shape, package, and deliver those messages.   There now need to be concerted efforts to develop and implement innovative programs.

Of particular interest to health educators.

649.   SY, Francisco S., Donna L. Richter, Gene Copello. "Innovative educational strategies and recommendations for AIDS prevention and control."   *AIDS Education and Prevention* 1, no. 1 (1989): 53-56.

A list of recommendations from the First International Conference on AIDS Education, held in Columbia, South Carolina, July 31 to August 1, 1987.

Descriptive

Ten sets of recommendations were offered in the following categories: educational strategies for sexually active individuals; outreach programs for IV drug abusers; prevention programs for women and newborns; education and prevention programs in schools; educational training programs for health care workers; educating the general public; education outreach programs for minorities; worksite prevention and education programs; education and prevention programs in correctional systems; and education and prevention programs in developing countries.

Of interest to health educators, social and behavioral scientists, and public health officials.

650.   TRICE, Ashton D., and Judith Price-Greathouse.   "Locus of control and AIDS information-seeking in college women."   *Psychological Reports* 60 (1987): 665-666.

Describes a study to determine personality factors which influence women at low risk to seek information about AIDS.

Research

One hundred and twenty-four women at a liberal arts college, who completed the Chance subscale of the Multidimensional Health Locus of Control Scale, the Academic Locus of Control scale, and a 20-item pretest on AIDS information, were offered college credit for attending an informational seminar on AIDS. Scores on the two locus of control measures were not related, but both measures were significantly predictive of seminar attendance. Those scoring in the internal direction on the Academic Locus of Control attended at a higher rate than those scoring externally, and those with low chance scores on the health measure attended at a higher rate than those with high chance scores. Those who attended the sessions also knew more about AIDS before the sessions, as shown by the 20-item test, than those who did not attend. The findings suggest that not only are health attitudes and beliefs important in determining whether individuals will obtain information about AIDS; attitudes about the delivery systems may also influence information seeking.

Of interest to health educators.

651. TURNER, Norma Haston, Judith McLaughlin, Jacque Crist Shrum. "AIDS education: Process, content, and strategies." *Health Values* 12, no. 3 (1988): 6-12.

Presents a planning process, program content, and teaching strategies to be used for AIDS education in schools, worksites, and communities.

Descriptive

Education presently represents the best available method for slowing the spread of the AIDS epidemic. To be effective, educational programs must be well planned, timely, and appropriate to the needs of the learner.

Of interest to health educators and public health officials.

652. VALDISERRI, R.O. "Cum hastis sic Clypeatis: The turbulent history of the condom." *Bulletin of the New York Academy of Medicine* 64 (1988): 237-245.

A historical analysis of condom use as a means of preventing sexually transmitted infections.

Descriptive

With no effective treatment yet available for HIV infection, the ongoing epidemic of AIDS demands an aggressive approach to prevention. This will undoubtedly include the recommendation that condoms be used to prevent viral transmission. We can expect to encounter negative reactions to this recommendation based, in part, on historical precedent. Condoms are not the solution to AIDS. However, it is important to recognize the contribution they can make and to divorce their ability to prevent disease from their turbulent past.

Of interest to historians and social and behavioral scientists.

653. WEDDINGTON, William W., and Barry S. Brown. "Counseling regarding human immunodeficiency virus-antibody testing: An interactional method of knowledge and risk assessment." *Journal of Substance Abuse Treatment* 6 (1989): 77-82.

Summarizes issues regarding the administration of HIV-antibody testing and presents an interactional model of communicating information to patients regarding AIDS, transmission of HIV, and the meaning of HIV-antibody test results.

Descriptive

HIV-antibody testing, when associated with pretest and posttest counseling, can be used to educate individuals at risk for HIV infection and AIDS and can serve as an intervention to prevent the spread of HIV. The authors describe the interactional method that they have used with over 250 outpatients who sought treatment for cocaine dependency. The method is easily administered by medical and non-medical staff and well accepted by patients.

Of interest to substance abuse counselors.

654. WYKOFF, Randolph F., Clark W. Heath, Jr., Shirley L. Hollis, Sharon T. Leonard, Clarence B. Quiller, Jeffrey L. Jones, Marc Artzrouni, Richard L. Parker. "Contact tracing to identify human immunodeficiency virus in a rural community." *Journal of the American Medical Association* 259 (1988): 3563-3566.

Describes a contact investigation conducted in rural South Carolina to identify, counsel, and educate persons infected with or exposed to HIV.

Descriptive

Contact tracing succeeded, in this investigation, in identifying specific individuals infected with HIV or exposed to the virus and in providing opportunities for highly directed and personal counseling to these high-risk persons. This constitutes an efficient use of HIV testing (18% case detection) and targeted application of educational efforts.

Of special interest to public health professionals.

b. Chapter

655. COUGHLIN, Thomas A., III. "AIDS in prisons: Recommended policies and procedures." *In* Richard Rosner, and Ronnie B. Harmon (Eds.). *Correctional Psychiatry*. (Critical Issues in American Psychiatry and the Law, Volume 6). New York: Plenum, 1989.

Focuses on documenting the steps that are necessary to meet the AIDS crisis in the correctional setting and demonstrating the importance of developing an integrated approach to AIDS policies and procedures.

Discussion

Discusses policy and protocol development, identification and movement of inmates, placement and programming, education efforts, testing, condoms, needles, legal and confidentiality issues, case review, and budgets.

Of interest to prison administrators and health professionals in correctional institutions.

c. Dissertations

656. CARDON, Marie-Claude. "Effects of different presentation modes and personality variables on recall of information about AIDS and sexually transmitted diseases." Ph.D. dissertation, University of Miami, 1988.

A study to determine whether method of presentation of information about sexually relevant topics and subjects' levels of sex guilt affect recall of information.

Research

A sample of 114 undergraduates, divided into two groups—LSGs (low sex guilt), and HSGs (high sex guilt)—according to sex guilt scores on the Revised Mosher Guilt Inventory, were shown videotapes presenting information about AIDS and STDs, either in a "personalized format" or in an impersonal, lecture-type format. No interaction between conditions and levels of sex guilt emerged as significant. LSGs did not remember more information overall than HSGs, but there was a significant difference between the two groups in the personalized condition. More LSGs reported being sexually active, and more frequently, than HSGs. LSGs were more likely to report being concerned about contracting AIDS and STDs than HSGs. There was no difference among subjects in their reported intention to use protective measures against AIDS and STD, but LSGs reported using condoms as a precaution at a three-week posttest. Implications for sex educators and suggestions for future studies were discussed.

Of interest to sex educators and mental health professionals.

657. WILKINSON, Mary Ann. "The impact of neurolinguistic programming rapport skills training for registered nurses on one-on-one teaching of acquired immune deficiency syndrome prevention." Ed.D. dissertation, Virginia Polytechnic Institute and State University, 1988.

Investigates the effect of neurolinguistic programming (NLP) as a rapport builder and teaching technique in one-on-one nurse-client teaching transactions including client satisfaction with the relationship and retention of knowledge of AIDS prevention information.

Research

A quasi-experimental design was used. Volunteer nurses were trained to teach AIDS prevention, using adult volunteer clients as the treatment group. The control group were taught by the nurses using the basic AIDS prevention curriculum. The two groups were then compared according to the results of pre- and post-test knowledge scores and satisfaction ratings for the nurse teacher. Data were analyzed using analysis of covariance and analysis of variance. There were no significant differences between the two groups. Qualitative data, collected after the completion of the teaching, supported usefulness of the techniques for teaching. Further studies were recommended.

Of interest to health educators and nursing educators.

2. INTERNATIONAL

a. Books

658. SCHINAZI, Raymond F., and André J. Nahmias (Eds.). *AIDS in Children, Adolescents & Heterosexual Adults: An Interdisciplinary Approach to Prevention.* New York: Elsevier, 1988.

Based on an international conference, held in 1987, to discuss AIDS in children, adolescents, and heterosexual adults.

Book of Readings

Contains papers related to public health issues; legal, social, ethical, and religious issues; economic considerations; community resources; the role of the media; epidemiological issues; infection control; psychosocial aspects of the pregnant woman; the dilemmas of adoption; foster care and day care; medical and nursing management issues; education and behavior change; AIDS in schools, colleges, and universities; and the sexually active adolescent.

Of interest to health professionals, public health professionals, and health educators.

659. WORLD Health Organization. *AIDS Prevention and Control.* Oxford: Pergamon Press, 1988.

A jointly organized meeting by the Government of the United Kingdom and the World Health Organization, held in London on January 26-28, 1988 to exchange views on the role of education and information programs in the fight against AIDS.

Monograph

The five sections of this document, consisting of invited presentations and papers, are: AIDS: A global challenge; AIDS prevention through health promotion; health promotion programs for specific groups; the critical role of counseling; arming health workers for the AIDS challenge; and closing addresses.

Of interest to all health professionals, public health officials, policymakers, social and behavioral scientists, and laymen.

660. ————. *Guidelines for the Development of a National AIDS Prevention Control Programme.* Geneva: World Health Organization, 1988.

The first in a series of publications to be produced by the World Health Organization with the aim of helping national authorities meet the challenge of AIDS.

Monograph

Provides information on the establishment and organization of a national program for the prevention and control of AIDS, covering definition of program objectives, development of strategies, identification of appropriate activities, and evaluation of achievements and disease trends.

Of interest to public health officials and government officials in health services.

661. ————. *Report of Meeting on Educational Strategies for the Prevention and Control of AIDS.* Geneva: World Health Organization, June 17-19, 1986.

Reports on a meeting convened to assist the Central Programme on AIDS in exploring the complex educational issues involved with AIDS prevention.

Report

Reviews the context for educational strategies for the prevention and control of AIDS; formulates recommendations for a WHO global communication program on AIDS and national programs for the prevention and control of AIDS; and outlines the methodology with which WHO can assist its member states in the implementation of AIDS prevention strategies.

Of interest to public health professionals and health educators.

b. Articles

662. "AIDS--An international perspective." *Health Education Journal* 46, no. 2 (1987): Entire Issue.

A collection of articles about AIDS education and prevention efforts around the world.

Special Journal Issue

The articles cover: AIDS as a global challenge; AIDS experience in seven European countries; the British context; AIDS, Africa, and education; AIDS and intravenous drug users; the development of AIDS publicity; the work of the National Advisory Service on AIDS; people's perception of the risk of AIDS and the role of the mass media; teaching about AIDS in schools; HIV antibody testing and counseling; AIDS and female prostitution; training about AIDS; AIDS education in black America; a guide to books on AIDS; the professional response to AIDS; and the view from a GP's surgery.

Of general interest.

663. AIRHIHENBUWA, Collins O. "Perspectives on AIDS in Africa: Strategies for prevention and control." *AIDS Education and Prevention* 1, no. 1 (1989): 57-69.

Presented here is the incidence of HIV and AIDS in Africa, patterns of HIV transmission, a conceptual model for health education strategies, barriers to progress in primary health care, and the need and utility of AIDS research.

Analytical

While the incubation period for measles, diarrhea, malaria, and syphilis are hours and days, the incubation period for AIDS appears to be five to ten years. The duration of illness ranges from three weeks for smallpox to two to four years for syphilis, while it is life-long for AIDS. The carriers of the HIV infection can infect others even before developing any symptoms themselves. Whereas there are available drugs and/or vaccines for the other diseases mentioned, there is presently no AIDS vaccine and none is expected for the next five to ten yers. Additionally, there is no currently effective treatment or cure. Given the facts, it is clear that the only weapon against the spread of HIV infection is health education.

Of interest to public health officials and epidemiologists.

664. ASSAAD, Fakhry, and Jonathan M. Mann. "AIDS--an international perspective." *Journal of the Royal Society of Health* 107, no. 3 (1987): 77-78.

Discusses the international health problem created by AIDS, and summarizes the perspective and plans for global HIV prevention and control of the World Health Organization.

Editorial

Prevention of HIV infection presents a serious challenge to medical and public health practice. It will require long-term changes in sexual behavior, modifications in blood services and other medical and paramedical practices, and aggressive approaches to the control of perinatal transmission. Member states of the WHO need to unite their material and intellectual resources to confront this major challenge.

The WHO AIDS control strategy, which involves coordinated and complementary actions at international and national levels, is outlined.

Of interest to epidemiologists, public health professionals, and public policymakers and planners.

665. BOYD, Neil T., and Margaret A. Jackson. "Reducing the risks of pleasure: Responding to AIDS in Canada." *Canadian Public Policy* 14 (1988): 347-360.

Points out the high risk behaviors that lead to transmission of AIDS and suggests strategies for risk reduction.

Descriptive

The behaviors that place people at the highest risk for acquiring AIDS are identified as multiple partner anal intercourse, a multiple partner sexual lifestyle, and intravenous drug use. From a public policy standpoint, it is contended that these behaviors should be the focus of the greatest consideration. The well-known risk reduction techniques, the use of condoms and the solitary use of sterilized needles, should be encouraged, although at risk groups can be particularly difficult to reach and persuade. In the face of continuing state discrimination against homosexual men and women, there has been understandable reluctance to listen to the message of government. Members of some groups must still be convinced of their vulnerability to infection. A review of the social psychological literature on attitude and behavior change suggests several policy initiatives.

Of interest to public policymakers, public health officials, and health professionals.

666. BRORSSON, Bengt, and Claes Herlitz. "The AIDS epidemic in Sweden: Changes in awareness, attitudes and behavior." *Scandinavian Journal of Social Medicine* 16 (1988): 67-71.

Questionnaire surveys concerning awareness, attitudes, and beliefs about HIV and AIDS in Sweden were conducted in March/April of 1986, February/March of 1987, and May 1987.

Research

The number of individuals compared in the three surveys were 2622, 1805, and 707 respectively. The surveys indicate that the general public views the AIDS epidemic with growing concern and believes that researchers and public officials cannot effectively combat the problem. To a growing extent, they believe that it is up to individuals to appropriately adapt their behavior if the spread of the disease is to be slowed, and, to a certain extent, changes in sexual practices seem to have occurred. Changes in awareness, attitudes, and beliefs have accelerated since March 1987, the start of the Swedish AIDS Information Campaign.

Of interest to health educators and public health officials.

667. CHEN, Lincoln C. "The AIDS pandemic: An internationalist approach to disease control." *Daedalus* 116 (1987): 181-195.

Although the U.S. has 75% of all AIDS cases, 98 other countries also have AIDS. The author appeals for an international perspective in combatting the disease.

Discussion

The AIDS pandemic is distinguished from those of history by lifelong infection, long latency, and asymptomatic transmission, and also by a rapid transmission throughout the world. Three approaches to AIDS control are possible--prevention and treatment, interruption of transmission, and slowing the spread between populations--and each requires international cooperation to be effective.

Of interest to social and political scientists.

668. CLARKE, Janette, Michael A. Waugh, Charles J.N. Lacey, Milton H. Hambling. "HIV antibody testing: Experience in a provincial sexually transmitted disease clinic." *Public Health* 102 (1988): 251-255.

HIV antibody test requests from April 1984 to May 1987 at a clinic in Leeds were reviewed to assess the effects of late 1986 and early 1987 health education campaigns to inform the public about AIDS.

Research

There were large increases in the number of tests performed following the campaigns, but numbers returned to pre-campaign levels by May 1987. A majority of the women requesting tests were from high risk groups. Compared to reports from clinics in London, a very high percentage of the homosexual men attending the clinic in Leeds requested HIV antibody testing in 1986. Future plans for HIV health education should take into consideration the considerable regional variations in the behavior of target groups.

Of interest to health educators and public health officials.

669. COHEN, Erik. "Tourism and AIDS in Thailand." *Annals of Tourism Research* 15 (1988): 467-486.

Considers the complex problems that the appearance and worldwide dissemination of AIDS have created for the tourist industry in Thailand.

Case Study

The tourist industry and tourism policymakers are just beginning to grapple with AIDS-related problems, which are especially acute in countries such as Thailand, where sexual attractions have been an important determinant of the tourist flow. The author examines the dilemma facing authorities of protecting tourism by downplaying the threat of AIDS versus protecting public health by acknowledging it; traces the changes in policies toward AIDS, and in public attitudes to foreigners and tourists, in the wake of an AIDS scare; and discusses the problems of protecting sex workers from infection. Changes in national tourism policies are indicated, and some general conclusions regarding the interface of tourism and AIDS are proposed.

Of interest to social scientists, public health professionals, tourism policymakers, and tourist industry personnel.

670. COHEN, Lynne. "The Federal Centre for AIDS: Working against a plague mentality." *Canadian Medical Association Journal* 138 (1988): 839-840.

Describes the role of the Canadian government's Federal Centre for AIDS.

Descriptive

The Federal Centre for AIDS (FCA), located in Ottawa, is Canada's first one-disease directorate and has the same status as the Laboratory Centre for Disease Control. It was created by the National Advisory Council on AIDS (NACAIDS), which was established to advise the Health Minister on all aspects of the problem of AIDS in Canada. The FCA provides the secretariat for NACAIDS and administers the National AIDS Program, which functions to provide research support, to educate the public and health care professionals, to provide advisory committees at the national and interprovincial levels, to provide financial and informational support for community-based private AIDS groups, to fund and enhance diagnostic centers throughout Canada, and to organize and host the Fifth International Conference on AIDS, which will be held in Montreal in 1989.

Of general interest.

671. DiCLEMENTE, Ralph J., Cherrie B. Boyer, Stephen J. Mills, Michael Helquist (Eds.). "AIDS." *Health Education Research* 3, no. 1 (1988): Entire issue.

The purposes of this special issue are two-fold: to increase awareness of relevant AIDS prevention activities occurring in other countries, and to provide in-depth analyses of various research and relevant theoretical issues which may impact on the development and implementation of AIDS health education/prevention programs.

Special Journal Issue

The global nature of the AIDS epidemic creates the need for cross-cultural collaboration. The 14 papers in this issue address a broad spectrum of important health education issues for controlling the spread of HIV infection, focusing on the breadth of AIDS-prevention programs from around the world to provide cross-cultural perspectives on the development of risk reduction programs.

Of interest to health educators, health education researchers, and public health officials.

672. DRUMMOND, C., G. Edwards, A. Glanz, I. Glass, P. Jackson, E. Oppenheimer, M. Sheehan, C. Taylor, B. Thom. "Rethinking drug policies in the context of the acquired immunodeficiency syndrome." *Bulletin on Narcotics* 39, no. 2 (1988): 29-35.

A policy analysis of the needed responses to the problems associated with AIDS and drug misuse that are now being experienced in the United Kingdom and Northern Ireland.

Descriptive

International communication must be strengthened. The AIDS epidemic requires a reexamination of the penal handling of drug misusers. Treating some patients earlier may contribute significantly to prevention strategies, and methods of "harm reduction" deserve attention. Compulsory treatment or testing for HIV infection is not favored. The importance of professional training and of research is stressed.

Of interest to public policy analysts, political scientists, and public health officials.

673. EISENBERG, Leon. "Health education and the AIDS epidemic." *British Journal of Psychiatry* 154 (1989): 754-767.

Discusses the need for effective health education, the focus of which should vary from country to country to accommodate local differences in prevalence and predominant modes of transmission.

Review

What is known about the biology of AIDS is reviewed. Social factors, which influence disease transmission and public attitudes, are considered. The methods available to control the epidemic are evaluated, and the reasons why public health measures undertaken, to date, have had limited success are considered. The ethical debate on public health policy is analyzed, and the need for a nationwide educational program on AIDS, which is responsive to the rights and obligations of citizens in a democratic society, is emphasized.

Of interest to health educators and public health officials.

674. FELDMAN, Douglas A., Samuel R. Friedman, Don C. Des Jarlais. "Public awareness of AIDS in Rwanda." *Social Science and Medicine* 24 (1987): 97-100.

Because AIDS is a rapidly growing epidemic in Kigali, Rwanda, 33 informants (15 men and 18 women) in that city were interviewed, in September 1985, to determine the level of public awareness of AIDS.

Research

Most of the informants (66.7%) said they first heard of the disease within the previous eight months. About half (46.9%) could not mention one or more symptoms of AIDS; younger informants and women reported less knowledge of AIDS symptoms. Most knew the disease was stigmatized, but did not know why. Only 34.4% could correctly state the mode of AIDS transmission; people at greatest risk for the disease (unmarried men and women) were least likely to know how it is transmitted. Half of those who responded to the question about the origins of AIDS thought that it began in America. Although many informants were frightened of the disease, no one had, as yet, changed his/her sexual behavior in response to the epidemic. All agreed that more information about AIDS should be made available in Rwanda. The authors conclude that preventive measures against AIDS are urgently needed in central Africa.

Of interest to health educators and public health officials.

675. FORTIN, Alfred J. "The politics of AIDS in Kenya." *Third World Quarterly* 9 (1987): 906-919.

A discussion of the politics and etiology of AIDS in Kenya.

Editorial/Commentary

The author advocates more attention be given to the needs of persons with AIDS. The basic preventive strategy should involve those who suffer from the disease. An AIDS prevention program should address the social, political, and cultural views of those most directly affected. This kind of strategy cannot be adequately represented in the current monopoly of AIDS research by Western medicine.

Of particular interest to health policy analysts and epidemiologists.

676. HASTINGS, G.B., D.S. Leathar, A.C. Scott. "AIDS publicity, some experiences from Scotland." *British Medical Journal* 294 (1987): 48-49.

Discusses and provides a model for the evaluation of mass media publicity before its release.

Descriptive

It is important that mass media publicity be evaluated before it is widely released to determine whether it is saying the right thing to the right people in the right way. In 1986, the Scottish Health Education Group decided to produce a leaflet pointing out the implications of AIDS to heterosexuals as well as homosexuals and drug addicts. A rough draft of the pamphlet was produced and, in order to obtain responses to the pamphlet and explore general knowledge and attitudes on AIDS, groups of six to eight respondents were carefully selected, in social demographic terms, and brought together in

informal settings to discuss the subject in depth under the direction
of a psychologist or group moderator. The document was then revised
and tested a second time and is now undergoing another revision to
correct the specific weaknesses of the second draft. The advantages
of the described method, the lessons learned regarding the problems of
communication, and the need for consumer research in developing
effective mass media material are discussed.

Of special interest to health educators.

677. ⸺⸺. "Scottish attitudes to AIDS." *British Medical Journal*
      296, no. 6627 (1988): 991-992.

A representative sample of 988 persons, aged 15 and over, was surveyed
in Scotland in July 1986 and again one year later to measure the
cumulative impact of various education campaigns and interventions on
the general public's awareness of and attitudes towards HIV and AIDS.

Research

There is evidence of increasing awareness about the risk from AIDS to
the general public as well as to high risk groups. Fewer people
associate AIDS with specific groups only. There is great concern
about AIDS, with increasing proportions of the population seeing it as
a serious social problem. Anxiety is increasing, especially among
young people, and there is a growing demand for more information about
AIDS. Almost everyone is aware that such behavior as sharing needles
by IV drug abusers can spread AIDS. The survey findings suggest a
need to help relieve anxiety by providing information about how to
reduce the risk from AIDS, using materials designed to meet specific
needs. An increase in public awareness of the connection between drug
abuse and AIDS is unnecessary, and little is to be gained by trying to
induce fear or anxiety to reinforce existing knowledge, but there is a
need to address knowledge-behavioral inconsistency.

Of interest to health educators and public health officials.

678. HENDRICKS, M. "Underestimation of AIDS--there's nothing to
      be optimistic about." *South African Medical Journal* 73 (1988):
      573-574.

Expresses concern about the cautious optimism of the Third International Congress on AIDS.

Opinion

The future for containing the AIDS epidemic is bleak. AIDS will
spread among heterosexuals because of the permissiveness in society.
Monogamy and a return to morality must be emphasized by the media and
AIDS educators.

Of interest to educators, representatives of the media, public health
officials, and clergy.

679. IGLEHART, John K., L. Leighton Read, James A. Wells. "The socioeconomic impact of AIDS on health care systems." *Health Affairs* 6 (1987): 137-147.

A summary of a Project Hope conference on AIDS and its socioeconomic impact on health systems worldwide.

Conference Report

At this time, the best defense that nations can muster to protect their populations against the spread of AIDS is to educate people about how to guard against contracting the disease. The attack must be engaged on a global basis and must involve governments at all levels and the private sector.

Of interest to health professionals and laymen.

680. IJSSELMUIDEN, C.B., M.H. Steinberg, G.N. Padayachee, *et al.* "AIDS and South Africa: Towards a comprehensive strategy." *South African Medical Journal* 73 (1988): 455-467.

A series of three articles highlights the problems and controversial issues pertinent to strategies for the control of HIV infection and AIDS in South Africa and makes recommendations regarding these problems.

Review/Commentary

Part I considers the world-wide experience with the AIDS epidemic. It focuses on problems of case definition; differences between "African" and "Western" AIDS and the implications for South Africa; and problems with sensitivity and specificity of tests used at present; considers some of the ethical issues; and emphasizes differences between "notification" and "reporting." Part II considers controversies related to screening for HIV, the indications for and desirability of mandatory testing of certain groups at risk, and the place of voluntary testing in the control of HIV transmission and infection, and makes recommendations relating to these issues. Part III emphasizes the urgent need for a comprehensive strategy for the control of HIV infection and proposes steps for such a strategy, highlighting the fundamental importance of an education campaign and three critical essentials for its success. A plea is made for more psychosocial research.

Of particular interest to public health officials and health educators.

681. KRASNIK, Allan, Jacob Bjoerner, Birgit Westphal Christensen. "Community and individual considerations in legislation and test policy regarding HIV infection in the Nordic countries--a cross national comparative study." *Social Science and Medicine* 29 (1989): 577-584.

Compares the legislative and policy stances taken in five Nordic countries toward AIDS.

Research

Policies and legislation in Denmark generally are concerned with the protection of individual rights, while those in Sweden and Iceland focus more on the rights of the public. Policies in Finland and Norway more nearly balance competing issues. Reporting of infection is taking place in all the Nordic countries, and every country is attempting to secure some anonymity. AIDS issues are often publicly and emotionally debated, but the publication of program descriptions and evaluations is rare.

Of interest to international health professionals and public health policymakers.

682. LEHMANN, Philippe, Dominique Hausser, Bertino Somaini, Felix Gutzwiller. "Campaign against AIDS in Switzerland: Evaluation of a nationwide educational programme." *British Medical Journal* 295 (1987): 1118-1119.

An evaluation of the impact of a program in which a booklet about AIDS was mailed to every Swiss household in March 1986 and followed by a mass media campaign promoting the use of condoms.

Research

Of the population, aged 20-69, to whom the booklet was sent, 56% read the booklet. The results showed that those who read the booklet, compared to those who did not, displayed a greater improvement in knowledge and a better understanding of the risks of specific behaviors. The mean indices of knowledge and beliefs were significantly different. Having better information does not imply that people will change their behavior, but both the high reading rate and the increase in knowledge suggest that the educational program reached its objectives.

Of interest to health educators, public health officials, and policymakers.

683. McTIGUE, James F. "The United States and the international control of AIDS." *Annals of the American Academy of Political and Social Science* 500 (November 1988): 91-104.

Reviews three distinct epidemiological patterns that have emerged throughout the world with respect to AIDS.

Descriptive

AIDS cases will increase in number dramatically over the next three years, with devastating social and economic consequences. Health-care systems and economic resources in large cities in the U.S. will be severely strained. African countries will lose many educated and

economic leaders. Many Third World countries will have lower produc-
tivity and economic output. A global strategy is emerging to
understand and control the spread of AIDS. To provide the commitment
and leadership necessary to control AIDS in the rest of the world, the
U.S. must first demonstrate a stronger moral conviction and societal
will to control the disease in this country.

Of interest to health professionals, social scientists, and political
analysts.

684. MANN, Jonathan M. "AIDS: A global strategy for a global
    challenge." *Impact of Science on Society* 150 (1988): 159-167.

The author discusses the need for an orchestrated international
response to the AIDS epidemic.

Review

Specific prevention programs must be started to provide information
and education to prevent transmission of the disease; to prevent blood
transmission by making blood and blood products safe, curbing IV drug
abuse, educating and treating those who practice it, and insuring that
injection equipment and other instruments are sterile; and to prevent
mother-to-child spread. A comprehensive national AIDS program must
help people already infected with the AIDS virus, including persons
with AIDS, and help them to discharge their responsibility to protect
others.

Of interest to public health officials and international health
experts.

685. MASSARI, V., J.B. Brunet, E. Bouvet, A.J. Valleron.
    "Attitudes towards HIV-antibody testing among general
    practitioners and their patients." *European Journal of
    Epidemiology* 4 (1988): 435-438.

Reports on a study by the French Communicable Diseases Network to
identify the type of patient being tested for HIV and the reasons for
requesting the test.

Research

Data from two periods, November and December 1986 and March through
April 1987, were compared. Patients requesting testing during the
first period were predominantly males (82%) belonging to high risk
groups (66%). During the second period, the percentage of males
decreased to 47% and the percentage of high risk group members to 27%.
The number of persons with clinical symptoms requesting the test also
decreased, and more patients were tested because of present or past
STDs. Fewer seropositive patients were found during the second
period.

Of interest to physicians, epidemiologists, and public health
officials.

686. MOATTI, J.P., L. Manesse, C. Le Galés, J.P. Pagés, F. Fagnani. "Social perception of AIDS in the general public: A French study." *Health Policy* 9 (1988): 1-8.

Presents the results of the first national survey about social perception of AIDS in a representative sample of the French general public, carried out in June 1987.

Research

A large majority of the public (73.1% of respondents) supports mandatory screening for HIV, and a significant part (21.9%) favors isolation. False beliefs about transmission by casual contact are shown to be related to willingness to agree to measures that carry the danger of stigmatization for AIDS patients and HIV carriers, but, for a fraction of the public, attitudes about AIDS are determined by a priori ideological and ethical values rather than by risk perception. Results suggest that any ambiguity in scientific information about AIDS may increase social pressure, even among the educated, for unnecessary measures. Tentative conclusions are drawn for public policy on prevention and information about AIDS.

Of interest to health educators, public health professionals and public policymakers.

687. NGUGI, E.N., F.A. Plummer, J.N. Simonsen, D.W. Cameron, M. Bosire, P. Waiyaki, A.R. Ronald, J.O. Ndinya-Achola. "Prevention of transmission of human immunodeficiency virus in Africa: Effectiveness of condom promotion and health education among prostitutes." *Lancet* 2, no. 8616 (1988): 887-890.

Describes the effect of an AIDS education program and the distribution of free condoms on condom use among the prostitutes.

Description

The study provides evidence that public education programs on AIDS in Africa can effect important changes in sexual behavior that reduce the risk of transmission of HIV. It emphasizes the efficacy of health promotion offered through a primary health care structure in a high risk group. This program has prevented the transmission of a large number of HIV infections in men--approximately a one-third reduction in the number of HIV infections transmitted.

Of interest to public health officials and health educators.

688. PELA, A. Ona, and Jerome Platt. "AIDS in Africa: Emerging trends." *Social Science and Medicine* 28 (1989): 1-8.

Reviews the literature on AIDS in Africa.

Review

Raises a number of questions relating to heterosexual behaviors. Other issues addressed include drug use behavior, homosexuality, and high-risk sexual activities of Africans and foreigners in Africa. The impact of the political and socioeconomic climate in most of Africa during the 60's and early 70's is evaluated. Suggestions are made that include confirmatory testing of HIV positive samples, conducting epidemiology and social science-based research, and developing innovative educational programs that are culturally relevant.

Of interest to public health professionals, health educators, and political analysts.

689. PENINGTON, David G. "The AIDS epidemic--where are we going?" *Medical Journal of Australia* 147 (September 21, 1987): 265-266.

Suggests directions for AIDS research, education, and planning.

Editorial/Commentary

Proposes a national strategy to curb the sexual spread of the AIDS virus: education that is designed to convince people that they must not allow themselves to be placed at risk of infection; and an obligation on the part of those persons who are presently at high risk of HIV infection to determine if they are infected and, if so, never to place another person at risk without their knowledge and consent.

Of general interest to laymen and health professionals.

690. PIOT, Peter, Francis A. Plummer, Fred S. Mhalu, Jean-Louis Lamboray, James Chin, Jonathan M. Mann. "AIDS: An international perspective." *Science* 239 (1988): 573-579.

Describes the global patterns and prevalence of AIDS, the impact on health and society, and the global control and prevention of AIDS.

Descriptive

Although the prevention and control of AIDS are ultimately dependent on the decisions of individuals, those decisions are influenced by local, national, and international customs. Educational programs must take these factors into consideration, and it will be necessary for these programs to involve experts in the social and behavioral sciences. One urgent need in all countries affected by AIDS is to resolve the difficult issue of disclosure of information about HIV-infected individuals. The control and prevention of AIDS will require a sustained and long-term commitment.

Of interest to epidemiologists and public health officials.

691. POULSEN, Asmus, and Susanne Ullman. "AIDS-induced decline in the incidence of syphilis in Denmark." *Acta Dermato-Venereologica* 65 (1985): 567-569.

Discusses a decline in the incidence of syphilis in Denmark resulting from the fear of AIDS.

Report

The incidence rate of acquired syphilis per 100,000 total population in Denmark, which had increased by 70% from 1978 to 1982, decreased by 61.2% in 1984, with a 62.3% decrease in the incidence of syphilis among the male population in 1983 and 1984. The decreasing number of acquired syphilis cases during these two years are correlated to a lower number of sexual contacts among homosexual men because of fear of AIDS.

Of interest to health educators and public health officials.

692. SHERR, L. "An evaluation of the U.K. government health education campaign on AIDS." *Psychology and Health* 1 (1987): 61-72.

Investigates the effectiveness of a health education campaign conducted through the use of full page newspaper advertisements by the United Kingdom Department of Health and Social Security.

Research

Groups of subjects at higher and lower risk for human immunodeficiency virus were questioned before and after the campaign. The desire for information was high and most respondents named the medical profession as the desirable source of information. The campaign was noticed and read by 31.1% of the lower risk group and 50% of the higher risk group. Although information scores were slightly increased, the campaign had no effect on adjusting misconceptions or lowering anxiety. Attitudes and behavior were not altered. The results are discussed in the light of a content analysis of the campaign.

Of interest to health educators.

693. TINKER, Jon. "AIDS in the developing countries." *Issues in Science and Technology* 4, no. 2 (1988): 43-48.

Discusses how the AIDS crisis will become a dominating issue in Third World development.

Descriptive

The AIDS pandemic demands an international mobilization of the richer nations' scientific resources, experience, compassion, and money. So far, however, neither the U.S. administration, nor competent private groups are exercising effective international leadership on AIDS, and the scientific effort in the U.S. remains focused on tackling the domestic public health crisis.

Of interest to public health officials.

694. WILSON, D., and C Wilson. "Knowledge of AIDS among Zimbabwean teacher-trainees prior to the Public Awareness Campaign." *Central African Journal of Medicine* 33 (1987): 217-221.

Two open-ended questions and a 22-item true/false inventory were used to assess knowledge of AIDS among 630 Zimbabwean trainee school teachers in January-February 1987.

Research

Contact with prostitutes was identified as a risk factor by 73% of the sample. Few believed AIDS to be primarily a homosexual disease in Africa. On the other hand, few cited the sexual partners of other high risk groups as a high risk category, and only 58% knew that condoms used during coitus reduce the risk of HIV transmission. More than half the sample believed HIV infection could result from exposure to towels and toilet seats, from saliva, and from caring for AIDS victims. The majority of respondents were not offended by sex-related questions. Results of the study suggest that further education efforts might emphasize the high risk status of sex partners of members of high risk groups and the effectiveness of condoms as a precaution against serotransmission and reassure individuals of the unlikelihood of transmission through casual contact.

Of interest to health educators.

695. WINN, Sandra. "The developing geography of AIDS: A case study of the West Midlands." *Area* 20 (1988): 61-67.

Examines the geography of HIV infection in the U.K., the pattern of infection in the West Midlands, the characteristics of the people in the West Midlands who are tested for HIV, and the impact of the government's AIDS information campaign.

Review

The only means of limiting the spread of HIV infection is by changing sexual behavior throughout the population as a whole. Evidence from the HIV tests in the West Midlands indicates that the government's AIDS information campaign had a considerable effect in raising levels of public awareness about AIDS, but the extent of success in modifying sexual behavior is, as yet, unknown. Mathematical modelling indicates that without behavior changes, a level of 20,000 to 40,000 deaths from AIDS per year will eventually be reached in the U.K. The actual level of HIV infection and deaths from AIDS in the U.K., and the geographical distributions of HIV infection and AIDS cases, will depend upon the extent to which different segments of the population modify their sexual behavior. This, in turn, will depend on the effectiveness of health education.

Of interest to health educators and public health officials.

696. WOOLEY, P.D., and G.R. Kinghorn. "AIDS publicity campaigns." *Lancet* 2, no. 8553 (August 1, 1987): 284.

Reports on the results, in Sheffield, of a publicity campaign on the dangers of AIDS.

Letter

The campaign increased anxiety among low-risk individuals. Of 777
patients making primary requests for tests for HIV seropositivity in
the six-month period following the start of the campaign, 429 (55.2%)
were from low-risk groups. However, individuals of both sexes from
high-risk groups, particularly those who had not been tested before,
were also motivated to request testing for HIV seropositivity. HIV
seropositivity was confined exclusively to the high risk male group.

Of particular interest to public health professionals.

697. "WORLD population and HIV." *Public Health* 101 (1987):
397-398.

Discusses the possible effect of HIV on human ecology.

Editorial

Despite current intense research on AIDS, there is little hope of a
cure or eradication in the near future. The disease is likely to
continue to spread all over the world, taking a severe toll on those
populations in which promiscuous sexual activity is common. Unless
all governments, and particularly those of the developing nations of
Africa and South America, actively encourage and facilitate social and
sexual behavior change, AIDS may prove to be the natural factor that
will halt the uncontrolled increase of human population that has taken
place during the past 150 years, but at a very great cost in human
suffering.

Of particular interest to health educators, legislators, and
policymakers.

3. UNITED STATES

a. Articles

698. BANKS, Taunya Lovell. "AIDS and government: A plan of
action?" *Michigan Law Review* 87 (1989): 1321-1337.

Points out the weaknesses of the Presidential Commission's final
report on the HIV epidemic as a national plan of action.

Commentary

The commission's recommendations that states enact statutes to punish
HIV-infected individuals who engage in behaviors likely to transmit
the virus, and that they strictly enforce prostitution laws, are
inconsistent with their warnings against criminalizing HIV infection.
Although the report stresses the need for informed consent and
counseling for HIV testing, it does not address mandatory HIV testing

at the worksite. It fails to point out that physicians may, in some circumstances, be under a legal duty to provide non-emergency care to persons with HIV infection who have no health insurance. Financial recommendations are stopgap measures that do not squarely address the problems of an inadequately financed health care system incapable of caring for the chronically ill, uninsured working poor, and racial/ethnic minorities. Although the Presidential Commission's report is flawed, it can still serve as a starting point from which President Bush can address the problems of the AIDS epidemic.

Important to public health officials, politicians, and the public.

699. DAN, Bruce B. "The National AIDS Information Campaign: Once upon a time in America." *Journal of the American Medical Association* 258, no. 14 (1987): 1942.

An overview of the Center for Disease Control's (CDC) National AIDS Information Campaign.

Editorial

Describes a massive public information campaign regarding AIDS. Objectives concentrate on learning about the opinions held by specific target audiences about the disease and its impact.

Of interest to all health professionals and the lay public.

700. FINEBERG, Harvey V. "Education to prevent AIDS: Prospects and obstacles." *Science* 239 (1988): 592-596.

A discussion of the obstacles to effective AIDS education.

Descriptive

A number of obstacles thwart effective education to prevent AIDS in the U.S. These include the biological basis and social complexity of the behaviors that must be changed, disagreement about the propriety of educational messages to prevent AIDS, uncertainty about the degree of risk to the majority of Americans, and dual messages of reassurance and alarm from responsible officials. The U.S. has yet to mount a nationwide, comprehensive, intensive, and targeted education program to prevent AIDS.

Of interest to health educators, health professionals, and public health officials.

701. FRANCIS, Donald P., and James Chin. "The prevention of acquired immunodeficiency syndrome in the United States: An objective strategy for medicine, public health, business, and the community." *Journal of the American Medical Association* 257 (1987): 1357-1366.

Reviews the current knowledge regarding the pathogenesis and transmission of AIDS in the U.S., outlines a prevention plan based on that
knowledge, and describes the major problems confronting effective
prevention and control.

Descriptive

The eventual extent of HIV transmission and the resulting morbidity
and mortality will be determined by how well we, as a society, can
design and implement a concerted AIDS prevention effort, and how we,
as individuals, heed the messages of that prevention effort and take
personal responsibility to protect ourselves.

Of interest to health professionals, public officials, and public
health personnel.

702. GERBERT, Barbara, and Bryan Maguire. "Public acceptance of
      the Surgeon General's brochure on AIDS." *Public Health
      Reports* 104 (1989): 130-133.

A nationwide telephone survey was conducted to ascertain whether
recipients had read the brochure, whether they were glad to receive
it, and whether they believed that it was a worthwhile use of tax
dollars.

Research

Public acceptance of the Surgeon General's brochure on AIDS was
extremely positive. Almost everyone who received it was glad to
receive it, few were offended by it, and most thought it was a good
use of their tax dollars. This finding confirms early press reports
about the public's reaction.

Of general interest to laymen and health professionals.

703. HERBOLD, John R. "AIDS policy development within the
      Department of Defense." *Military Medicine* 151 (1986):
      623-627.

Discusses the HIV antibody screening program initiated by the
Department of Defense.

Descriptive.

The Defense Department's initiation of an HIV antibody screening
program for members of the military represented a proactive approach
to the early detection and prevention of problems associated with HIV
infection. The events preceding implementation of this program are
reviewed, and the military public health and operational issues are
discussed.

Of interest to military administrators and public health officials.

704. KIRBY, Diana Gonzalez, and Tony A. Harvell. "U.S.
      government information policy and the AIDS epidemic."
      Government Publications Review 16 (1989): 157-161.

Discusses the role of the U.S. government in disseminating information on AIDS to the general public.

Analytical

The authors look at the history of AIDS-related information, its
format, content, and scope. They assert that this information is
essential for targeting and evaluating control and prevention efforts
at all levels. It is concluded that libraries have been underutilized
in providing AIDS information to the public.

Of interest to health professionals, social and political scientists,
and health educators.

705   KOOP, C. Everett. "Physician participation needed in AIDS
      education." *Journal of the American Osteopathic Association*
      88 (1988): 92-93.

Encourages osteopathic physicians to educate patients about sexual
transmission of HIV.

Editorial

States the rationale for physician involvement in patient education
about sexual transmission of HIV. Suggests that physicians give
patients information on the selection and use of condoms, the need for
avoiding sex with potentially seropositive partners and shunning anal
intercourse, and the HIV antibody test.

Should interest physicians and health educators.

706. KOSTERLITZ, Julie. "Educating about AIDS." *National Journal*
      18 (1986): 2044-2049.

An overview of PHS efforts to educate the public about AIDS,
delineating some of the obstacles to AIDS education.

Review

According to the Public Health Service (PHS), education to reduce
AIDS-related risk behaviors is the only mechanism for preventing the
further spread of HIV. Because AIDS issues include economics,
politics, and moralism, there have been many obstacles to education
and prevention. Until 1984, when the PHS received $1.4 million, they
had been given no money for AIDS education and risk reduction. Early
efforts focused on educating private and public health officials.
Money for education was funneled through the U.S. Conference of
Mayors. Problems arose, however, when one grant was used for
producing a videotape that contained explicit information about

homosexual sex.   State spending has ranged from $6.6 million in California to nothing in 11 states.   The education of drug users has been bogged down in controversies over the issue of providing clean needles to IV users.   National polls have shown considerable misinformation about AIDS on the part of the public.   Blacks and sexually active adolescents have been identified as groups in particular need of AIDS education.

Of interest to health educators and public health professionals.

707. MacDONALD, Donald Ian.   "Coolfont Report: A PHS plan for prevention and control of AIDS and the AIDS virus." *Public Health Reports* 101 (1986): 341-348.

The Public Health Service convened a meeting at the Coolfont Conference Center in Berkeley Springs, WV, June 4-6 1986, to review and modify the PHS plan according to current information, needs, and demographic projections through 1991.

Conference Report

Recommendations of the conference focused on five areas: information base, information and education, prevention of IV drug abuse transmission, prevention of sexual transmission, and prevention of transmissibility by blood and blood products.

Of interest to health professionals, public health officials, and the general public.

708. MASON, James O.   "Public Health Service plan for the prevention and control of acquired immune deficiency syndrome (AIDS)." *Public Health Reports* 100 (1985): 453-455.

This document provides an outline of the key goals and objectives that must be met to achieve prevention and control of AIDS.

Guidelines

The plan calls for action by federal agencies, state and local departments, professional organizations, and volunteer groups. Many of the objectives cannot be expressed in measurable terms because of inadequate current information, but are included even though modifications will be made as more data are generated.

Of interest to health professionals and the public.

709. SCHAFFNER, W.   "The evolution of hospital infection control policies concerning AIDS: The current United States debate." *Journal of Hospital Infection* 11, Supplement A (1988): 223-226.

Discusses the stages through which hospital control policies in the United States have passed.

Hospital control policies in the U.S. have undergone three stages: a period of confusion, a period of consolidation, and a period of renewed concern. The first stage, which reflected the epidemic of fear regarding AIDS, compromised the function of hospitals as places to care for the sick, and threatened the ethical foundations of the healing professions. Increased knowledge about transmission, the discovery of the HIV, and the availability of serological testing brought about the second stage, in which well-established infection protocols and intensive education programs for health care workers were implemented. The third stage began when three health care workers were infected by skin and mucous membrane exposures, renewing the epidemic of fear. In light of the debate regarding issues of safety, most hospitals have adopted a variety of protocols for protecting personnel and screening for antibodies to HIV. However, equal concern must be shown for providing the best possible care for patients.

Should interest health care workers and hospital administrators.

710. SIEGEL, Karolynn (Ed.). "AIDS education: The public health challenge." *Health Education Quarterly* 13, no. 4 (1986): 285-432.

A collection of articles that reflect the perspectives and insights of diverse professionals involved in seeking solutions to the public health problems raised by the AIDS epidemic.

Special Journal Issue

Contains articles on AIDS, social sciences, and health education; sexually transmitted disease prevention efforts and their implications for AIDS; health education about AIDS among seropositive blood donors; psychosocial predictors of reported behavior change in homosexual men at risk for AIDS; AIDS risk reduction recommendations and sexual behavior patterns among gay men; alcohol and drug use during sexual activity and compliance with safe sex guidelines for AIDS; health education and knowledge assessment of HIV diseases among intravenous drug users; AIDS health education for intravenous drug users; helping companies respond to the AIDS crisis; and a community health education intervention for minority high risk group members.

Of interest to health educators, health professionals, public health professionals, and members of the gay community.

711. SKILLMAN, Donald R., and Charles Clark. "HIV infection and the acquired immunodeficiency syndrome: A strategy for public education." *Military Medicine* 152 (1987): 479-480.

A description of a stepwise educational scheme for AIDS is presented.

Editorial

Supreme Headquarters Allied Powers Europe (SHAPE) is the military
command center for NATO.   All branches of the American military at
SHAPE were involved in the educational plan.   The program resulted in
more   responsible   and   compassionate   behavior   towards   infected
individuals.   Whether the program will result in any change in sexual
behavior is yet unknown.   Historically, intense educational efforts to
reduce drunken driving, teenage pregnancy, and drug use have had
disappointing results among American audiences.

Of particular interest to health professionals and officials in the
U.S. military.

712.   STAMBOVSKY, Joyce M.   "Human immunodeficiency virus (HIV)
       antibody total force screening in a clinic environment."
       Aviation Space and Environmental Medicine 59 (1988): 575-578.

Describes the process of establishing a screening clinic for HIV for
9,600 active duty Air Force personnel.

Descriptive

HIV screenings of large populations have some characteristics in
common.   The author describes the steps taken to organize an effective HIV antibody screening program that can be duplicated elsewhere.

Of interest to public health officials.

713.   TASK Force on Pediatric AIDS, American Psychological Associa-
       tion.   "Pediatric AIDS and human immunodeficiency virus
       infection: Psychological Issues."   *American Psychologist* 44
       (1989): 258-264.

Briefly reviews what is known about AIDS in children; addresses three
areas of concern--the delivery of clinical services to infected and
ill children and their families, the development of effective AIDS
education and prevention programs, and research needs--and makes
recommendations for action.

Descriptive

The Task Force recommends funding and implementation of a flexible
national model that can be adapted to the special needs of each
region; supports the rights of children with AIDS/HIV infection to
attend school; recommends that school systems develop educational
programs that provide current information on AIDS and HIV transmission
for parents; suggests the development of broad, community-based education and information on pediatric AIDS/HIV infection; supports the
Surgeon General's recommendation that AIDS education begin in early
childhood and extend through high school; and recommends that drug
rehabilitation programs be expanded to ensure that services are
available to active drug users who are seeking to change their
behavior.   HIV antibody testing is recommended as an adjunct to
prevention education and counseling efforts rather than its primary
focus.

Of special interest to educators, pediatricians, and child development specialists.

714. TOLSMA, Dennis B. "Activities of the Centers for Disease Control in AIDS education." *Journal of School Health* 58 (1988): 133-141.

Outlines the national program to prevent the spread of HIV infection among young people.

Descriptive

CDC is working with each of 15 national agencies, as well as the 15 state and 12 city departments of education currently funded by CDC, to help them evaluate, and improve, the effectiveness of their programs. As part of the National Adolescent Student Health Survey, baseline information about the AIDS knowledge and beliefs of the nation's eighth and tenth grade students was gathered by IOX Associates. The national data will be used to plan educational strategies in AIDS school health education. State and local education agencies are establishing systems to obtain baseline information and monitor AIDS-related knowledge, beliefs, and behavior among youth to plan and assess the effectiveness of their educational strategies.

Of interest to the general public as well as health professionals.

b. Chapters

715. DOWDLE, Walter R. "Strategy for AIDS prevention and control." *In* Robert A. Smith (Ed.). *HIV and Other Highly Pathogenic Viruses.* San Diego: Academic Press, 1988.

Discusses the education/information program designed by the CDC for four major audiences: the public at large, school and college age young people, persons at increased risk or already infected, and health workers.

Descriptive

After six years, the AIDS epidemic in the U.S. is still growing. Research on vaccines and antiviral drugs may provide options for the long term, but our best current efforts at prevention must employ a strategy based on information and education. Any successful effort to change attitudes and behavior must involve multiple channels including the federal, state, and local governments, medical professionals, teachers, parents, religious leaders, voluntary organizations, state and local departments of health and education, businesses, commercial organizations, and highly esteemed public figures. It must reach all segments of American society and involve a spectrum of activities ranging from one-on-one teaching and counseling programs to national media programs. The CDC has developed a program based upon this philosophy to inform and educate the U.S. population about AIDS.

Of interest to public health officials and health educators.

716. WINETT, Richard A., Abby C. King, David G. Altman.
      "Concepts, principles, and strategies to effectively use media
      for health promotion: Altering the course of the AIDS
      epidemic." *In* Richard A. Winett, Abby C. King, David G.
      Altman. *Health Psychology and Public Health: An Integrative
      Approach.* New York: Pergamon Press, 1989.

Discusses the use of media in health promotion, focusing on the AIDS
epidemic.

Review

The objectives of this chapter are to develop an approach for
designing effective media; to delineate strategies pertinent to
addressing monetary and regulatory barriers to media access; and to
synthesize the conceptual and technical material and demonstrate how a
media approach, in conjunction with multilevel analyses for planning
multilevel interventions, may be used to alter the course of the AIDS
epidemic.

Of interest to health educators and public health officials.

c. Dissertation

717. LEVINE, Helen Dorothy. "The state of Florida's response to
      acquired immune deficiency syndrome: A policy analysis."
      Ph.D. dissertation. The Florida State University, 1987.

Examines the development of public policies on AIDS in the public
education delivery system of Florida.

Research

Three conceptual models of policy formation and decision-making were
used as analytical frameworks from which to study state and local
education policy initiatives on AIDS. It can be concluded from the
research that, of the three models, the bureaucratic-politics model
best explained the policy formation process on AIDS and public schools
in Florida. The strengths of the model included the recognition of
the influence of organizational patterns, as well as individual
interests, on the policy formation process.

Of interest to public policymakers and analysts.

4. TARGET POPULATIONS

A. GAY AND BISEXUAL MEN

a. Book

718. DELANEY, Martin, and Peter Goldblum, with Joe Brewer.
      *Strategies for Survival: A Gay Men's Health Manual for the
      Age of AIDS.* New York: St. Martin's Press, 1987.

Designed to help gay people cope with the AIDS crisis and do battle against it.

Manual

Addresses people currently ill with AIDS or ARC, people who are not ill, but are seropositive, and people who are neither ill nor sero-positive, but are concerned. Chapter one discusses the meaning of health, and how the gay community has been affected by the AIDS crisis, and presents a four-step planning process for establishing a personal health plan. Chapters two through six address major life-style issues: sexual practices, the role of stress, substance use and abuse, social support, and exercise and nutrition. The final chapter discusses medical, political, and psychological strategies for meeting the threat that AIDS poses to the community. An appendix entitled "resources" directs readers to AIDS-related support services, organizations, and references.

Intended for members of the gay community, but useful to anyone touched by the AIDS epidemic.

b. Articles

719. CARNE, C.A., A.M. Johnson, F. Pearce, A. Smith, R.S. Tedder, I.V.D. Weller, C. Loveday, A. Hawkins, P. Williams, M.W. Adler. "Prevalence of antibodies to human immunodeficiency virus, gonorrhoea rates, and changed sexual behavior in homosexual men in London." *Lancet* 1, no. 8534 (March 21, 1987): 656-658.

Two markers of sexually transmitted infection, the prevalence of antibodies to HIV and rates of gonorrhea, in men routinely attending a sexually transmitted disease clinic were examined to determine the possible effect of any changes in sexual practices in London's homosexual population.

Research

A reduction in the number of sexual partners and a change to safer sexual practices was documented among homosexual and bisexual men taking part in a prospective study of the natural history of HIV infection. Data support the value of continuing preventive efforts to control viral spread in the absence of an effective vaccine or therapy.

Of interest to virologists, health educators, and public health officials.

720. COATES, Thomas J., Leon McKusick, Richard Kuno, David P. Stites. "Stress reduction training changed number of sexual partners but not immune function in men with HIV." *American Journal of Public Health* 79 (1989): 885-887.

The authors tested the impact of stress management training on sexual behavior and immune function in 64 gay men infected with HIV.

Research

Treatment subjects, at post-test, reported significantly fewer sexual partners during the preceding month.   There were no differences between groups in lymphocyte numbers and function.

Of interest to health educators, mental health professionals, and health professionals caring for AIDS patients.

721.   EVANS, Brian A., Kenneth A. McLean, Stephen G. Dawson, Steven A. Teece, Robert A. Bond, Kenneth D. McRae, Robert W. Thorp. "Trends in sexual behaviour and risk factors for HIV infection among homosexual men, 1984-7." *British Medical Journal* 298 (1989): 215-218.

Sexual behavior among 1050 homosexual men tested for HIV infection at a genitourinary medicine clinic in west London from November 1984 to September 1987 was monitored to assess whether the spread of infection can be reduced by changes in behavior among groups most at risk because of their sexual practices.

Research

Sexual behavior among homosexual men changed during the period studied, with a considerable drop in the proportion reporting casual relationships and high risk activities such as anoreceptive intercourse with casual partners, and the incidence of HIV infection fell. Nevertheless, half of the men in the last cohort studied reported having casual partners.   Behavioral risk factors for HIV infection most closely resembled those for hepatitis B.   A history of syphilis ranked above anoreceptive intercourse as the strongest predictor of HIV infection.   Actively bisexual men showed a much lower prevalence of HIV infection (5%) than exclusively homosexual men (30%).   More education programs directed at homosexual men are needed to reemphasize the dangers of infection.

Of interest to health educators and public health officials.

722.   JOSEPH, Jill G., Susanne B. Montgomery, Carol-Ann Emmons, Ronald C. Kessler, David G. Ostrow, Camille B. Wortman, Kerth O'Brien, Michael Eller, Suzann Eshleman. "Magnitude and determinants of behavioral risk reduction: Longitudinal analysis of a cohort at risk for AIDS." *Psychology and Health* 1 (1987): 73-96.

Reports the magnitude and predictors of longitudinal behavior change in a cohort of homosexual men at risk for AIDS.

Research

Self-reports of sexual behavior, obtained at two points in time separated by an interval of approximately six months, were used to construct both dichotomous and continuous measures of changes in behavior consistent with reduction in the transmission of the AIDS virus. Despite considerable variability in behavior, mean changes were consistently in the desired direction. Of all the factors examined, only the availability of supportive peer norms was consistently, significantly, and positively related to multiple measures of outcome. These results suggest that policies regarding HIV antibody testing should take into account the failure of a sense of risk to predict subsequent behavioral change and emphasize the important role of gay organizations in developing social norms supportive of behavioral risk reduction.

Of interest to health educators, health professionals, and public policymakers.

723. KELLY, Jeffrey A., Janet S. St. Lawrence, Harold V. Hood, Ted L. Brasfield. "Behavioral intervention to reduce AIDS risk activities." *Journal of Consulting and Clinical Psychology* 57 (1989): 60-67.

In this study, 104 gay men with a history of frequent AIDS high-risk behavior completed self-report, self-monitoring, and behavioral measures related to AIDS risk.

Research

The experimental intervention provided risk education, cognitive-behavioral self-management training, sexual assertion training, and attention to the steady and self-affirming social supports. Experimental group participants greatly reduced their frequency of high-risk sexual practices and increased behavioral skills for refusing sexual coercions, AIDS risk knowledge, and adoption of "safer sex" practices. Change was maintained at eight month follow-up.

Of interest to health educators, social and behavioral scientists, and public health professionals.

724. KLEIN, Daniel E., Greer Sullivan, Deane L. Wolcott, John Landsverk, Sheila Namir, Fawzy I. Fawzy. "Changes in AIDS risk behavior among homosexual male physicians and university students." *American Journal of Psychiatry* 144 (1987): 742-747.

Two samples of homosexual men, 64 physicians and 58 university students, reported profound decreases in several sexual practices linked to transmission of AIDS.

Research

The physicians showed the greater reduction. When sociodemographic variables, health beliefs, feelings of control over outcome, mood, sexual interest before the AIDS epidemic, and medical care utilization were correlated with decrease and/or increase in AIDS risk behaviors, the clusters of variables most strongly correlated with changes in risk. Behaviors differed between the physicians and students. Interventions designed to change behaviors should be tailored to specific subgroups.

Of interest to health educators, mental health professionals, and social scientists.

725. LANDRUM, Susan, Consuelo Beck-Sague, Stephen Kraus. "Racial trends in syphilis among men with same-sex partners in Atlanta, Georgia." *American Journal of Public Health* 78 (1988): 66-67.

Reports a decrease in incidence of early syphilis among white men at risk of HIV infection.

Review / Theoretical

During the 1970s, the percentage of reported cases of early syphilis rose among white homosexual males who reported at least one partner. A nationwide decline in early syphilis cases attributable to homosexual transmission since 1981 is consistent with the hypothesis that fear of AIDS has brought about sexual behavior change among gay men. In Atlanta, Georgia, the city with the highest 1985 rates of primary and secondary syphilis in the country, a decline in syphilis was reported in only one county, DeKalb. Analysis of the data from DeKalb County shows a decline from 191 early cases in 1981 to 97 in 1985. However, the decline occurred only among white homosexual males; early syphilis has risen among black men with same sex partners.

Of interest to epidemiologists, health educators, and public health professionals.

726. McCUSKER, Jane M., Jane G. Zapka, Anne M. Stoddard, Kenneth H. Mayer. "Responses to the AIDS epidemic among homosexually active men: Factors associated with preventive behavior." *Patient Education and Counseling* 13 (1989): 15-30.

This study explored factors that are related to AIDS preventive behavior in 201 asymptomatic homosexual and bisexual men seen at a community health center.

Research

Results suggested that greater reported behavioral effect was associated with greater perceived susceptibility to and severity of AIDS, with involvement in informational activities, and with beliefs of friends and lovers. Fewer anogenital partners were significantly associated only with fewer lifetime partners and older age. Knowledge of high risk behavior was not associated with either the effort to reduce high risk behavior or the number of anogenital partners during the previous 6 months.

Of interest to counselors and mental health professionals.

727. McKUSICK, Leon, Marcus Conant, Thomas J. Coates. "The AIDS epidemic: A model for developing intervention strategies for reducing high-risk behavior in gay men." *Sexually Transmitted Diseases* 12 (1985): 229-234.

The authors conducted a conference at the University of California at San Francisco to provide a framework for developing health education programs to reduce high-risk sexual activity associated with AIDS.

Symposium Commentary

Operating on a consensus model, four groups of experts defined the sexual behaviors that place an individual at high risk for AIDS, the principles of health psychology that can be applied to health education programs for reducing high-risk sexual activity among gay men, the health education and media strategies that might be used, and the factors unique to gay men that need to be considered. It is hoped that these reports will provide a foundation for discussion of health education strategies for reducing the risk of AIDS and also prove useful to local, regional, and national organizations in developing such programs.

Of interest to health educators and public health officials.

728. McKUSICK, Leon, William Horstman, Thomas J. Coates. "AIDS and sexual behavior reported by gay men in San Francisco." *American Journal of Public Health* 75 (1985): 493-496.

In November 1983, 655 gay men in San Francisco were surveyed regarding their sexual practices during the previous month and the same month one year earlier.

Research

Among men who regularly frequented bathhouses and gay bars, there was little change in frequency of attendance or in number of sexual partners from those locations. However, substantial reductions in frequency of sexual contacts from bars, baths, T-rooms, and parks were shown by men who went to neither place and by those in primary relationships. Men in monogamous relationships showed little change in sexual behavior within their relationships, while men in non-monogamous relationships and men not in relationships reported substantial reductions in high-risk sexual activity, but no corresponding increase in low-risk sexual behavior. Although knowledge of health guidelines was high, it had no relation to sexual behavior. Frequency and type of sexual behavior were related to the use of sex to relieve tension, the use of sex to express gay identity, and the knowledge of persons with AIDS who were in the late stages of the disease.

Of interest to social and behavioral scientists, health educators, and public health officials.

729. McKUSICK, Leon, James A. Wiley, Thomas J. Coates, Ronald
     Stall, Glen Saika, Stephen Morin, Kenneth Charles, William
     Horstman, Marcus A. Conant. "Reported changes in the
     sexual behavior of men at risk for AIDS, San Francisco,
     1982-84--the AIDS Behavioral Research Project." *Public
     Health Reports* 100 (1985): 622-629.

In November 1983 and in May 1984, 454 men were surveyed regarding
their sexual practices during the month before the survey. In the
1983 survey, reports about sexual behavior during the same month one
year prior to the survey were requested.

Research

There were substantial changes found in reported sexual behavior with
persons other than a primary partner. The average number of male
partners declined from 6.3 in November 1982 to 3.9 in May 1984.
Receptive anal intercourse without a condom declined from 1.9 to 0.7,
oral-anal contact declined from 1.1 to 0.3, and swallowing semen
declined from 2.8 to 0.7 in terms of the number of times that the
respondent engaged in the act in the last month. These changes did
not occur in relation to sex with a primary partner. Only increased
length of time since the first homosexual experience distinguished
persons maintaining few sexual partners from those increasing the
number of partners, while four variables were found to distinguish
those retaining high numbers of partners from those lowering the
number of partners.

Of interest to physicians, health educators, and public health
officials.

730. MARTIN, John L. "The impact of AIDS on gay male sexual
     behavior patterns in New York City." *American Journal of
     Public Health* 77 (1987): 578-581.

In 1985, a sample of 745 gay men between the ages of 20 and 65 were
interviewed to determine the impact of the AIDS epidemic on the non-
ill but at-risk population.

Research

Sexual activity since learning about AIDS, measured by the number of
different sexual partners, was reported to have declined by 78
percent. The frequency of sexual encounters involving the exchange of
body fluids and mucous membrane contact declined by 70 percent. Use of
condoms during anal intercourse increased from 1.5 to 20 percent.
There was no change over time in abstinence from gay sex.

Should interest health educators, public health professionals, and
social and behavioral scientists.

731. PRICE-GREATHOUSE, Judith, and Ashton D. Trice. "Chance
     health-orientation and AIDS information seeking."
     Psychological Reports 59 (1986): 10.

Investigated attendance at education sessions on AIDS by at-risk individuals living in an area with a low incidence of AIDS.

Research

Sixty-six sexually active male homosexuals who reported more than one partner were administered Form A of the Multidimensional Health Locus of Control Scales. Only the Chance subscale, which has items on the importance of chance factors in health, predicted subsequent behavior. Half scored above the mean (external), while half scored below (internal). Fifteen (45%) of the external subjects attended one or more of three informational meetings, while 23 (70%) of the internal subjects attended; more internal scorers attended two or more sessions than did external scorers. At the beginning of the program, a 25-item objective test indicated that the 33 external scorers (58%) knew less about the disease than the 33 internal scorers (65%). While these differences were nonsignificant, by the end of the program, they were significant (69% vs. 87%). The findings suggest that a chance-health orientation may identify a group that is less informed and may acquire less information, which, considering the nature of AIDS, places them at considerable risk.

Of interest to psychologists and health educators.

732. REAGAN, Patricia, Jeffrey Dykes, George White. "An AIDS intervention curriculum for gay and bisexual men." *Health Values* 11, no. 3 (1987): 16-21.

Discusses the merits and weaknesses of the Health Belief Model in promoting behavior change among gay and bisexual men, and outlines a possible behavior change intervention for health educators for those particular high-risk groups.

Theoretical/Descriptive

The Cognitive Behavioral Curriculum, based on the Health Belief Model and Personal Choice Models of behavior change, is a risk reduction intervention, developed by the New York City AIDS Project, that provides "positive reinforcement for healthy behaviors, enhancing self-esteem, and promoting gay identity and sexuality." It takes into account the problems associated with changing behaviors and promoting health in high risk groups. Non-sexual outlets for meeting human intimacy needs are stressed, and role modeling, desensitization, and stress management skills are taught. Modifications in the curriculum should be made to fit individual communities.

Of interest to health educators and concerned members of the gay community.

733. RICHWALD, Gary A., Donald E. Morisky, Garland R. Kyle, Alan R. Kristal, Michele M. Gerber, Joan M. Friedland. "Sexual activities in bathhouses in Los Angeles County: Implications for AIDS prevention education." *Journal of Sex Research* 25 (1988): 169-180.

Describes the sociodemographic and behavioral characteristics of men attending bathhouses.

Research

The data suggest that the majority of sexually active men attending bathhouses in Los Angeles County practice low risk sexual behaviors. However, an identified minority, who are more likely to be young, less educated, and of lower income, were found to practice sexual behaviors that would place them at increased risk of HIV transmission. Consequently, AIDS educational interventions tailored for this high risk group are an immediate priority.

Of interest to health educators and public health officials.

734.   ROSS, Michael W.   "Personality factors that differentiate homosexual men with positive and negative attitudes toward condom use."   *New York State Journal of Medicine* 88 (1988): 625-628.

The Attitudes Toward Condoms scale together with two personality and mood inventories, The Adjective Check List and the Profile of Mood States, were administered to 148 homosexually active men.

Research

Attitudes toward condom use were consistently positive among those who scored high on the dominance and aggression scales and negative among those who scored high on the abasement, deference, and tension-anxiety scales.   It appears that education should be directed toward assertiveness training in sexual encounters rather than the provision of information on condom efficacy.

Of interest to health educators, public health officials, and sexuality counselors.

735.   ———.   "Relationship of combinations of AIDS counselling and testing to safer sex and condom use in homosexual men."   *Community Health Studies* 12 (1988): 322-327.

This study investigated the distribution of sexual risk behaviors and condom use, and the relative effects of testing, counseling, both, or neither on risk behaviors and condom use, and determined what variables are associated with increased condom use in homosexually active men.

Research

Findings suggest that provision of free condoms in a context of professional and peer support may enhance condom usage during behaviors known to transmit HIV.

Of interest to physicians and health educators.

736. SCHECHTER, Martin T., Kevin J.P. Craib, Brian Willoughby, Bruce Douglas, W. Alastair McLeod, Michael Maynard, Peter Constance, Michael O'Shaughnessy. "Patterns of sexual behavior and condom use in a cohort of homosexual men." *American Journal of Public Health* 78 (1988): 1535-1538.

To measure the magnitude of risk reduction within a cohort of homosexual men, questionnaire responses in April 1984 - March 1985 were compared to those in October 1986 - September 1987.

Research

The annual number of sex partners declined significantly with no difference between the serologic groups. The number of subjects reporting no receptive anal intercourse increased, as did condom use during anal receptive intercourse. More seropositive subjects reported no condom use during receptive anal intercourse with regular partners and with casual partners. Among subjects with the most casual sexual contacts at the second visit, 33.3% of seronegatives and 29.2% of seropositives did not report usual condom use during receptive anal intercourse with casual partners. Safe sex practices are still not universal and a few individuals continue to put themselves at extremely high risk.

Of interest to public health officials and health educators.

737. VALDISERRI, Ronald O., David D. Lyter, Lawrence A. Kingsley, Laura C. Leviton, Janet W. Schofield, James Huggins, Monto Ho, Charles R. Rinaldo. "The effect of group education on improving attitudes about AIDS risk reduction." *New York State Journal of Medicine* 87 (1987): 272-278.

Four hundred and sixty-four homosexual and bisexual men, recruited from a cohort of 1700 men enrolled in a study of the natural history of AIDS, participated in a peer-led, small group educational session promoting AIDS risk reduction.

Research

Despite relatively high levels of knowledge about AIDS and HIV transmission, at least 60% of the men reported having engaged in receptive anal intercourse with more than one partner in the preceding six months. Prior to intervention, a substantial number of the men had mixed feelings or endorsed negative attitudes about AIDS risk reduction. In five of the six areas surveyed, attitudes improved significantly after the session. The success of the group educational session in positively influencing attitudes about AIDS risk suggests that this type of intervention might be effective in enabling homosexual and bisexual men to adopt low-risk sexual activities by influencing the nonhealth motives of sexual behavior, especially peer norms about safe sex. The authors stress the importance of incorporating existing health promotion research findings into the design and evaluation of AIDS risk reduction programs.

Of interest to health educators and counselors.

738. VALDISERRI, Ronald O., David W. Lyter, Laura C. Leviton, Catherine M. Callahan, Lawrence A. Kingsley, Charles R. Rinaldo. "Variables influencing condom use in a cohort of gay and bisexual men." *American Journal of Public Health* 78 (1988): 801-805.

Nine hundred fifty-five of 1,384 gay and bisexual men enrolled in a prospective study of the natural history of HIV infection, who reportedly engaged in anal intercourse in the past six months, were surveyed about condom use practices for both insertive and receptive anal intercourse.

Research

Multiple logistic regression analysis showed the following variables associated with both insertive and receptive condom use: condom acceptability, a history of multiple and/or anonymous partners in the past six months, and the number of partners with whom one is "high" during sex. Knowledge of positive HIV serostatus was more strongly associated with receptive than with insertive use. Condom use is a complex health-related behavior, and condom promotion programs should not limit themselves to stressing the dangers of unprotected intercourse.

Of interest to health educators and public health professionals.

739. VALDISERRI, Ronald O., David W. Lyter, Laura C. Leviton, Kerry Stoner, Anthony Silvestre. "Applying the criteria for the development of health promotion and education programs to AIDS risk reduction for gay men." *Journal of Community Health* 12 (1987): 199-212.

Describes the development and implementation of an AIDS risk reduction program for gay and bisexual men.

Descriptive

Five criteria were used for developing health promotion programs in the context of AIDS risk reduction.

Of interest to public health professionals, health educators, and community health workers.

740. VALLE, Sirkka-Liisa. "Sexually transmitted diseases and the use of condoms in a cohort of homosexual men followed since 1983 in Finland." *Scandinavian Journal of Infectious Disease* 20 (1988): 153-161.

Reports the change that was observed, both in the occurrence of STDs and the use of condoms, in a cohort of homosexual men who were repeatedly given practical advice and general risk reduction guidelines for avoidance of HIV infection.

Research

The study participants were repeatedly given detailed advice for avoiding HIV infection, and a tendency towards "safer" sexual practices resulting in a decrease in incidence of most STDs was noted during the course of the study. However, further spread of HIV is to be expected because 57% of the men still reported practicing anal sex at the end of the follow-up, 42% of them without condoms.

Of interest to health educators and public health officials.

741. van GRIENSVEN, Godfried J.P., Ernest M.M. de Vroome, Robert A.P. Tielman, Jaap Goudsmit, Jan van der Noordaa, Frank de Wolf, Roel A. Coutinho. "Impact of HIV antibody testing on changes in sexual behavior among homosexual men in the Netherlands." *American Journal of Public Health* **78** (1988): 1575-1577.

The relation between the disclosure of HIV antibody status and subsequent sexual behavior in 746 homosexual men was analyzed.

Research

Seropositives initially reported more sexual partners than seronegatives; they also showed a greater reduction in the number of sexual partners and the number of partners with whom all forms of sexual practices were performed than did seronegatives. In both groups, subjects were more likely to terminate orogenital intercourse than anogenital intercourse and masturbation.

Of interest to epidemiologists and public health professionals.

742. WINKELSTEIN, Warren, Jr., James A. Wiley, Nancy S. Padian, Michael Samuel, Stephen Shiboski, Michael S. Ascher, Jay A. Levy. "The San Francisco Men's Health Study: Continued decline in HIV seroconversion rates among homosexual/bisexual men." *American Journal of Public Health* **78** (1988): 1472-1474.

Reports on the decline in the practice of high risk behaviors and the decline of HIV seroconversion rates among a cohort of homosexual/bisexual men.

Research

The incidence of infection by HIV has been monitored since 1984 in a probability sample of homosexual/bisexual men in the San Francisco area where the epidemic of AIDS has been most severe. HIV seroconversion rates in previously uninfected cohort members have declined by 88% from 5.9% during the first six months of 1985 to 0.7% in the last six months of 1987. Sexual behaviors associated with HIV transmission have declined concurrently by 80%.

Of interest to health educators and public health professionals.

d. Dissertations

743. BRADFORD, Judith Baynard. "Reaction of gay men to
      A.I.D.S.: A survey of self-reported change." Ph.D.
      dissertation, Virginia Commonwealth University, 1986.

Two research questions were of major interest: 1) the sources of
information about AIDS, and the amount, type, and accuracy of knowledge gained by participants; and 2) the self-reported changes in
behavior that have resulted from this knowledge and from other
identifiable factors.

Research

Although studies in other cities indicated that most gay men had
modified their sexual behavior because of AIDS, the current findings
were contradictory; only about one in four reported sexual behavior
change. Findings about the relative importance of various sources of
information were also unexpected. Earlier studies demonstrated that
the source of information about a particular health threat was not a
significant factor. In the current study, sources of information did
matter. Those who had secured information from specialized sources
were more likely to have changed their behavior and were also less
afraid than were participants who had not had contact with these
sources.

Of interest to health educators and behavioral scientists.

744. CHARLES, Kenneth Alan. "Factors in the primary prevention
      of AIDS in gay and bisexual men." Ph.D. dissertation,
      California School of Professional Psychology, Berkeley, 1985.

This study applied health psychology principles to primary prevention
of AIDS.

Research

Perceived threat, response efficacy, and personal efficacy were
examined with measures of social skills, peer support, belief in AIDS
health guidelines, and self-esteem to determine the extent to which
each predicted sexual risk-taking. Respondents were 824 gay and
bisexual men in San Francisco. Personal efficacy and belief in health
guidelines emerged as strong predictors of sexual risk taking.
Partial support was found for the hypothesis that perceived threat,
response efficacy, and self-esteem were also significantly related to
risk behaviors. Social skills and peer support did not emerge as
significant factors.

Of interest to social and behavioral scientists and mental health
counselors.

745. MONTGOMERY, Susanne Boeckmann. "Behavioral change in a
      cohort of homosexual men at risk for AIDS." Ph.D.
      dissertation. The University of Michigan, 1987.

The magnitude and predictors of behavioral change are reported in a cohort of homosexual men at risk for AIDS.

Research

Significantly related to behavior change were perceived stress, social norms, knowledge, and education. Race and age were inversely related to behavior change. Perceived risk was negatively related to positive behavior change. Personality characteristics, such as mastery and self-esteem, were important predictors of change. Findings indicate a strong potential for differentiating "profiles" of respondents who are at low risk, those who show recidivism, and those who are unable to change their behavior in a positive way.

Of interest to health educators and behavioral scientists.

B. IV DRUG USERS

a. Books

746. GREENWICH House, Inc. *AIDS Education for Substance Abusers.* New York, 1988.

A knowledge, opinion, and practice study of substance abusers in treatment at Greenwich House.

Research

The overall knowledge gain among respondents indicated that AIDS education seemed to have some effect. However, this did not seem to alter, substantially, the sexual and drug use practices of the sample.

Of interest to health professionals and the general public.

747. ROBERTSON, Roy. *Heroin, AIDS and Society.* London: Hodder and Stoughton, 1987.

A book based on the author's experience in a Scottish general practice not previously involved with drug takers other than those on drugs prescribed by the Health Service. With the occurrence of the heroin epidemic, a unique opportunity to observe individuals from the start of their drug taking presented itself.

Text

The nine chapters include such topics as heroin, social consequences, patterns of drug use, illness and death, AIDS, prescribing, treatment, and new directions. The book is written as a series of discussions in order to stimulate debate as to why health professionals and the public behave as they do.

Of interest to health professionals in general, and to the layman.

b. Articles

748. BALL, John C., W. Robert Lange, C. Patrick Myers, Samuel R.
      Friedman. "Reducing the risk of AIDS through methadone
      maintenance treatment." *Journal of Health and Social
      Behavior* 29 (1988): 214-226.

A study conducted principally to ascertain the effectiveness of
methadone maintenance treatment in reducing IV drug use and
concomitant needle sharing among addicted patients.

Research

Treatment was found to be effective in reducing IV drug use and needle
sharing among most heroin addicts. Of 338 patients who remained in
treatment for one year or more, 71% ceased IV use. Conversely, 82% of
patients who left treatment rapidly relapsed to IV drug use.   HIV
seropositivity among high risk drug users is related to frequency of
injections and needle sharing. Effective methadone treatment can stop
these practices.

Of interest to drug treatment and counseling personnel and social and
behavioral scientists.

749. BATTJES, R.J., C.G. Leukefeld, P.W. Pickens, H.W.
      Haverkos. "The acquired immunodeficiency syndrome and
      intravenous drug abuse." *Bulletin on Narcotics* 40 (1989):
      21-33.

Presents an overview of AIDS in IV drug abusers and a strategy for
prevention.

Discussion

Intravenous drug abusers (IVDAs) constitute 25% of the AIDS cases in
the U.S. and 21% of such cases in Europe. The potential for the rapid
spread of HIV among IVDAs exists because such persons commonly share
injection equipment. The heterosexual and perinatal spread of AIDS is
largely associated with IVDAs. The primary AIDS prevention strategy
must be to help addicts stop using drugs. It is suggested that drug
abuse treatment resources be expanded and outreach programs be
developed to encourage more IVDAs to enter treatment.

Of interest to drug counselors, mental health professionals,
policymakers, and the public.

750. CURTIS, James L., F. Carolyn Crummey, Stanley N. Baker,
      Rogelio E. Foster, Cyril S. Khanyile, Robert Wilkins. "HIV
      screening and counseling for intravenous drug abuse
      patients." *Journal of the American Medical Association* 261
      (1989): 258-262.

A questionnaire about knowledge, attitudes, and behavior concerning AIDS was answered anonymously by 79% of the clinical staff and 67% of the patients at a drug abuse clinic.

Research

Approximately 90% of the staff and 72% of the patients thought that a voluntary HIV screening program should be offered to all patients. Almost all staff (98%), but only 50% of the patients, thought the HIV test results should be known to physicians, nurses, and counselors at the clinic. Few staff members (15%) believed that patients had changed their sexual behavior; more (48%) thought that needle sharing was reduced. Patients believed methadone patients, in general, had changed their sexual behavior and reduced needle sharing to prevent becoming infected.

Of interest to drug abuse counselors and mental health professionals.

751. DES JARLAIS, Don C., and Samuel R. Friedman. "AIDS prevention among IV drug users: Potential conflicts between research design and ethics." *IRB: A Review of Human Subjects Research* 9, no. 1 (1987): 6-8.

Identifies potential ethical conflicts in AIDS research among IV drug users and suggests strategies for minimizing conflicts.

Descriptive

Conflicts between the requirements of rigorous research design and ethical considerations involve: using HIV seroconversion as an outcome measure; using individuals as the unit of analysis; the advocacy of "AIDS-safe" drug injection; and choosing whether to use limited resources for AIDS prevention or research. Strategies for minimizing conflicts include: promoting public awareness of the conflicts, developing better methodology in AIDS prevention research, and conceptual analysis of the conditions that promote risk reduction.

Of interest to substance abuse counselors, researchers, health educators, and public health officials.

752. ———, Cathy Casriel, Alan Kott. "AIDS and preventing initiation into intravenous (IV) drug use." *Psychology and Health* 1 (1987): 179-194.

Discusses risk reduction for AIDS among drug users.

Research/Theoretical

Reviews limitations on current risk reduction efforts among IV drug users, and suggests the need for a long-term strategy of limiting initiation into IV drug use. Summarizes the results of a pilot study of conditions for such initiation among youth aware of AIDS, and describes a program for preventing initiation into drug use.

Of interest to public health professionals, drug abuse counselors, and health educators.

753.   ———, William Hopkins.   "Risk reduction for the acquired immunodeficiency syndrome among intravenous drug users." *Annals of Internal Medicine* 103 (1985): 755-759.

Reports on the perceptions of AIDS risk among intravenous drug users in New York City and the increased demand for new needles.

Descriptive

In the absence of effective treatment or vaccines, control of the AIDS epidemic among intravenous drug users will rely on efforts to reduce needle sharing. Risk perceptions of IV drug users are hindered by the long latency period of AIDS, other causes of death, and the ambiguity of AIDS-related symptoms, lowering their motivations for behavior change. However, there has been a sustained increase in demand for new, unused needles in New York City.

Of interest to substance abuse counselors, public health officials, and public policymakers.

754.   ———, Rand L. Stoneburner.   "HIV infection and intravenous drug use: Critical issues in transmission dynamics, infection outcomes, and prevention." *Reviews of Infectious Diseases* 10 (1988): 151-158.

Reviews five emerging critical issues regarding HIV infection among IV drug users.

Review

It is clear that simply providing information about AIDS is not likely to lead to enough risk reduction to stop HIV transmission among IV drug users. The success of "beyond basic education" prevention efforts will be critical for controlling transmission of HIV through shared drug-injection equipment and through heterosexual transmission in both the U.S. and Europe.

Of interest to virologists and infectious disease specialists.

755.   DRUCKER, Ernest.   "AIDS and addiction in New York City." *American Journal of Drug and Alcohol Abuse* 12 (1986): 165-181.

Outlines the projected dimensions of the AIDS epidemic among intravenous drug abusers in New York City and its implications for hospital utilization and local health care expenditures.

Review

Drug treatment programs must be the nucleus for developing any effective intervention in the addict community. Increased accessibility to existing drug treatment programs and expansion of their capacity is essential to attract and retain a much larger share of the addict population. The premise of drug treatment services must shift from cure to care.

Of interest to substance abuse counselors and mental health professionals.

756. FRIEDMAN, Samuel R., Don C. Des Jarlais, Jo L. Sotheran, Jonathan Garber, Henry Cohen, Donald Smith. "AIDS and self-organization among intravenous drug users." *International Journal of the Addictions* 22 (1987): 201-219.

Compares the two major risk groups for AIDS--gays and IV drug users--in terms of their responses and their social organization, and considers whether the lesser degree of individual behavior change among drug injectors might be due to their lesser degree of self-organization.

Descriptive

It is suggested that collective self-organization can lead to peer support for risk reduction and that this can help IV drug users to reduce their risks on an ongoing basis. Difficulties that face IV drug users' attempts to organize collectively, and examples of IV drug user collective organization to deal with AIDS and other problems are discussed.

Of interest to mental health professionals, counselors, and health educators.

757. GALEA, Robert P., Benjamin F. Lewis, Lori A. Baker. "A model for implementing AIDS education in a drug abuse treatment setting." *Hospital and Community Psychiatry* 39 (1988): 886-890.

Describes an AIDS education program at Spectrum House, a private, non-profit facility providing comprehensive treatment for substance abuse.

Descriptive

Two years after the beginning of Spectrum's AIDS education efforts, the treatment milieu remains more open to information about HIV, ARC, and AIDS. Several patients who tested positive for the virus but who have remained asymptomatic have shared the information, feelings, and experiences with their peers. Currently, about 98% of Spectrum's clients request HIV testing during their treatment stay, and 15% are found to be seropositive. Because of staff and patient turnover, the discovery of new information regarding HIV infection, and recurring concerns among staff, AIDS education is now provided to staff on an on-going basis through frequent inservice seminars. The development and implementation of educational modules for the IV drug user will continue to be important. The development of reliable means of assessing the results of AIDS education of drug users remains an area for further investigation.

Of special interest to drug counselors.

758. ————. "Voluntary testing for HIV antibodies among clients in long-term substance abuse treatment." *Social Work* 33 (1988): 265-268.

A discussion of HIV testing among persons in residential substance abuse treatment programs.

Descriptive

The attitudes of the clients in this study indicated that testing for exposure to HIV among members of this population may prove beneficial to treatment outcome. However, such testing should be implemented within treatment settings where knowledge about HIV has been disseminated among staff and clients to allow a supportive reaction to the presence of HIV-positive individuals. It is also important that clients be provided with intensive pre- and post-test counseling and access to support groups throughout the course of their treatment.

Of particular interest to substance abuse counselors and health professionals caring for drug abusers.

759. GHODSE, A.H., G. Tregenza, M. Li. "Effect of fear of AIDS on sharing of injection equipment among drug abusers." *British Medical Journal* 295 (September 19, 1987): 698-699.

A questionnaire investigating the injection practices of drug abusers was completed anonymously by 232 drug users attending three London drug dependence treatment units.

Research

Despite the risk of AIDS, a hard core of drug abusers continue to share syringes. There are two overlapping groups: those who use syringes after someone else and those who allow others to use their syringes. The discrepancy in numbers between the two groups suggests that those in the second group have been sharing with drug abusers not receiving treatment and, thus, a policy of providing clean syringes should logically extend to those not attending treatment units, although this might encourage more drug abusers to start injecting.

Of interest to health professionals, public health personnel, drug counselors, and public policymakers.

760. HUBBARD, Robert L., Mary Ellen Marsden, Elizabeth Cavanaugh, J. Valley Rachal, Harold M. Ginzburg. "Role of drug-abuse treatment in limiting the spread of AIDS." *Reviews of Infectious Diseases* 10 (1988): 377-384.

Examines the role of drug-abuse treatment in the AIDS epidemic by investigating the extent to which use of major drugs decreases following treatment.

Research

Drug-abuse treatment results in substantial declines in the use of heroin, cocaine, prescription psychotherapeutic drugs, and other drugs in the year after treatment. Declines are closely related to the length of time spent in treatment; treatment of more than six months has a significant impact on drug use after treatment. The potential impact of drug-abuse treatment in combatting the AIDS epidemic is discussed.

Of interest to drug abuse counselors, public health officials, and health professionals in general.

761. KRAMER, Thomas H., Frank R. Cancellieri, Gennaro Ottomanelli, Jo Ann Mosely, James Fine, Bernard Bihari. "A behavioral measure of AIDS information seeking by drug and alcohol inpatients." *Journal of Substance Abuse Treatment* 6 (1989): 83-85.

AIDS information seeking behavior of patients on four drug and alcohol inpatient units at a large public hospital in New York City was measured, using a nonreactive, observational research method.

Research

Results showed only 23 inquiries from 271 male and female patients over a six-week interval. Possible explanations and implications of these results are discussed.

Of interest to public health officials, substance abuse counselors, and health educators.

762. LEWIS, Benjamin F., and Robert P. Galea. "A survey of the perceptions of drug abusers concerning the acquired immunodeficiency syndrome (AIDS)." *Health Matrix* 4, no. 2 (1986): 14-17.

Forty-nine adult clients in a drug-free residential treatment program were surveyed to determine their knowledge, attitudes, and beliefs about AIDS and to identify appropriate risk-reduction interventions.

Research

While most of the respondents had some knowledge about the transmission of HIV, many were confused about how to avoid infection. Most believed that they were at high risk of infection, more than 50% believed they had been exposed to HIV, and 90% wanted to be tested. Most believed that they should curtail sharing needles and sex with individuals suspected of being exposed to AIDS, yet a majority indicated that they would continue to associate with them despite the fact that they could not control their activities at the time of "shooting dope." The greatest possibilities for prevention were believed by the respondents to be in education and in testing programs. The personal level of anxiety and hopelessness reflected by this population was quite high.

Of interest to substance abuse counselors, mental health professionals, and health educators.

763. MAGURA, Stephen, Joel I. Grossman, Douglas S. Lipton, Kenneth R. Amann, James Koger, Kevin Gehan. "Correlates of participation in AIDS education and HIV antibody testing by methadone patients." *Public Health Reports* 104 (1989): 231-240.

Factors associated with methadone patients' decisions about participating in a clinic-based AIDS prevention protocol were examined.

Research

Despite the offer of incentives, only 27% of the patients attended AIDS education classes, and only 12% obtained voluntary HIV tests. However, AIDS education classes were attended by proportionately more of those who were at highest risk for AIDS because of current IV drug use. The availability of HIV testing neither encouraged nor discouraged participation in AIDS education. Patients who were more likely to choose HIV testing were older, had been or were married, had plans to have children, believed the test to be useful, and believed that their counselors supported their decision to be tested. Implications for implementing AIDS prevention measures in methadone programs are discussed.

Of interest to substance abuse counselors, mental health professionals, and health educators.

764. MAGURA, Stephen, Joel I. Grossman, Douglas S. Lipton, Qudsia Siddiqi, Janet Shapiro, Ira Marion, Kenneth Amann. "Determinants of needle sharing among intravenous drug users." *American Journal of Public Health* 79 (1989): 459-462.

Data from 110 IV drug abusers in methadone maintenance were analyzed to determine the correlates of needle sharing.

Research

Needle sharing was directly related to peer group behavior, attitudes, economic motivation, not owning injection equipment, and fatalism about developing AIDS. Sharers were aware of their AIDS risk. Measures to reduce needle sharing include positive peer support groups to help resist pressures to share, legal and free access to fresh injection equipment, education on the utility of risk reduction, and increased treatment options for IV cocaine users.

Of interest to substance abuse counselors, mental health professionals, health educators, public health officials, legislators, and public policymakers.

765. MAGURA, Stephen, Janet L. Shapiro, Joel I. Grossman, Douglas S. Lipton. "Education/support groups for AIDS prevention with at-risk clients." *Social Casework* 70 (1989): 10-20.

Describes how an education/support group with methadone patients was effective as part of an AIDS prevention demonstration project.

Descriptive

Not all methadone patients are willing to participate in voluntary groups, even with incentives. Others are too emotionally distressed or have too many other needs to be able to participate successfully in a group. Such patients can usually benefit from intensive individual counseling. One advantage in establishing AIDS prevention groups is that counselors' time for such patients can be increased because group participants usually require less individual attention.

Of interest to substance abuse counselors and mental health professionals.

766 POWER, Robert, Richard Hartnoll, Emmanuelle Daviaud. "Drug injecting, AIDS, and risk behaviour: Potential for change and intervention strategies." *British Journal of Addiction* 83 (1988): 649-654.

Examines a sample of 127 regular illicit drug users in terms of injecting and needle sharing patterns, and investigates the impact of concern about AIDS upon those behaviors.

Research

Among those that have ever injected, it was found that 54% had substantially reduced their risk behavior in that they either no longer injected, or no longer shared injecting equipment. A further 32% had, to some extent, reduced their risk behavior, and 14% stated that they had been unaffected by concern about AIDS. Those who were in contact with agencies were more likely to have reduced, substantially, their risk behavior than those not in contact with agencies.

Of interest to substance abuse counselors.

767. SKIDMORE, C.A., J.R. Robertson, J.J.K. Roberts. "Changes in HIV risk-taking behaviour in intravenous drug users: A second follow-up." *British Journal of Addiction* 84 (1989): 695-696.

Interviews were conducted in Edinburgh, in 1988, to identify changes in risk-taking behavior in a sample of randomly selected IV drug users whose needle-sharing and drug use had been studied twice previously.

Research

All aspects of drug and needle use had changed positively. Overall, the addicts were injecting less frequently, 35% said they never shared equipment, and those who were still sharing were doing so less frequently and with fewer people than in 1987. Infected and uninfected users reported fewer sexual contacts. In both groups, the trend was toward single, long-term relationships or marriage.

Of interest to substance abuse counselors and public health officials.

768. SORENSON, James L., Steven L. Batki, Paul Good, Kenneth Wilkinson. "Methadone maintenance program for AIDS-affected opiate addicts." *Journal of Substance Abuse Treatment* 6 (1989): 87-94.

Describes a program that provides methadone maintenance treatment to opiate addicts who have been diagnosed with AIDS, ARC, or other significant symptoms of HIV infection.

Descriptive

The program aims to protect the health of patients and of the general public by slowing the spread of HIV. This article describes its history and goals, referral and patient admission process, methods of assessment and treatment planning, medical care, counseling procedures, tolerance for misbehavior, philosophy toward eventual detoxification, and procedures that maintain confidentiality.

Of interest to substance abuse counselors and other mental health professionals.

769. VALDISERRI, Edwin V., Alan J. Hartl, Catherine A. Chambliss. "Practices reported by incarcerated drug abusers to reduce risk of AIDS." *Hospital and Community Psychiatry* 39 (1988): 966-972.

A pilot study comparing the degree to which intravenous and nonintravenous drug users in a county jail are informed about AIDS and assessing their AIDS risk-reducing behaviors.

Research

Fifty-eight county jail inmates--27 IV drug users and 31 nonintravenous drug users--completed three survey instruments to determine AIDS knowledge, drug-related behavior, and locus of control. IV drug users were more fearful about getting AIDS than non-IV drug users. Less than half of either group knew that asymptomatic HIV-infected persons were infectious. IV drug users who reported no longer sharing needles or no longer shooting drugs were more likely to believe that individuals had control over events.

Of interest to correctional officials, and health educators.

770. WEDDINGTON, William W., and Bsrry S. Brown. "Acceptance of HIV-antibody testing by persons seeking outpatient treatment for cocaine abuse." *Journal of Substance Abuse Treatment* 5 (1988): 145-149.

Describes the author's experience with a group of persons who sought outpatient treatment for cocaine abuse and were recommended to undergo voluntary HIV testing as part of a routine medical evaluation.

Research

Twelve of 100 applicants tested HIV positive; eight of these had injected drugs with syringes and needles used by other addicts and four had never taken drugs intravenously. There were no significant differences between the HIV positive and negative applicants regarding the percentages who completed the evaluation, began treatment, and completed four weeks of treatment. The authors conclude that on-site, voluntary HIV testing for drug abusing patients entering treatment appears feasible and is not a deterrent to persons entering and continuing in treatment for drug abuse.

Of interest to drug abuse counselors, mental health professionals, and public health officials.

771. WODAK, Alex, Kate Dolan, Allison A. Imrie, Julian Gold, Jael Wolk, Bruce M. Whyte, David A. Cooper. "Antibodies to the human immunodeficiency virus in needles and syringes used by intravenous drug abusers." *Medical Journal of Australia* 147 (September 21, 1987): 275-276.

A pilot sterile needle and syringe exchange program was established in an inner city neighborhood in Sydney in an attempt to reduce needle and syringe sharing among IV drug abusers. Exchanged equipment was tested for presence of HIV.

Research

Both ELISA and Western blot methods were used for testing the contents of exchanged syringes for antibody to HIV. Of a sample of 300, three (1%) needles and syringes were confirmed positive and potentially infectious. Since only 70% of known positive-control syringes were detected, the proportion of infectious injection equipment returned may have been underestimated. These findings highlight the importance of removing used needles and syringes from circulation and supplying sterile equipment if HIV transmission among drug abusers is to be reduced. It is suggested that this method of monitoring exchanged needles and syringes may be used as a means of evaluating measures to control the spread of infection.

Of interest to public health officials and health professionals working in drug abuse programs.

C. MINORITIES

b. Articles

772. AMARO, Hortensia.   "Considerations for prevention of HIV
      infection among Hispanic women."   *Psychology of Women
      Quarterly* 12 (1988): 429-443.

Identifies important considerations for designing programs to prevent
HIV infection among Hispanic women.

Discussion

Because the risk of HIV infection varies among different Hispanic
groups, the incidence and characteristics of HIV infection are
important factors to consider in designing a prevention program.
Sociocultural and psychological characteristics are also important
factors.   Recommendations are made for research and prevention
programs.

Of interest to health educators and health care providers working with
Hispanic women.

773. BOUKNIGHT, Reynard R., and LaClaire G. Bouknight.
      "Acquired immunodeficiency syndrome in the black community:
      Focusing on education and the black male."   *New York State
      Journal of Medicine* 88 (1988): 638-641.

Discusses the impact of AIDS on the black community and the need for
education and prevention programs.

Descriptive

Black men must begin to act more responsibly with regard to their
sexuality and IV drug use.   Targeted programs for AIDS prevention are
needed for black men who engage in homosexual activity, and for blacks
of either sex who engege in other high-risk behavior, including IV
drug abuse.   This identifies a central role for minority professional
and community organizations in providing education about AIDS and its
prevention in the black community.

Of interest to health educators and public health officials.

774. FLASKERUD, Jacquelyn H., and Adeline M. Nyamathi.   "An
      AIDS education program for Vietnamese women."   *New York
      State Journal of Medicine* 88 (1988): 632-637.

A study to determine the effect of an AIDS education program for
Vietnamese women on the knowledge, attitudes, and practices of the
participants.

Research

Significant differences occurred in the experimental group in pretest/posttest items measuring knowledge, attitudes, and practices. Significant gains occurred in knowledge, and positive changes occurred in attitudes and intended practices. The most dramatic changes occurred in attitudes and intended changes in practice. The findings demonstrate that a didactic program can result in changes in knowledge levels and also in attitudes and intended behavior.

Of interest to health educators and social scientists.

775. GINZBURG, Harold M., Mhairi Graham MacDonald, James William Glass. "AIDS, HTLV-III diseases, minorities, and intravenous drug abuse." *Advances in Alcohol and Substance Abuse* 6, no. 3 (1987): 7-21.

Reviews the available data on AIDS and its causative agent, HIV, among minorities with a history of IV drug use.

Review

Eighty percent of heterosexual male and female AIDS patients are black or Hispanic. The development and implementation of effective prevention and education programs for these individuals rests upon an understanding of the less traditional approaches, which may be necessary to reach these groups. The general public must be made aware of the hazards of HIV and the risk of infection. Minorities are at high risk because of the drug abuse that exists among them.

Of interest to health educators and substance abuse counselors.

776. JIMENEZ, Richard. "Educating minorities about AIDS: challenges and strategies." *Family and Community Health* 10, no. 3 (1987): 70-73.

Discusses educating blacks and Hispanics about AIDS in culturally sensitive, cognitively appropriate ways.

Discussion

To effectively teach minority groups, it is necessary to take cultural differences into account when planning curricula and implementing educational strategies. AIDS education should be congruous with the language, values, and traditions of each group. The teaching style should be matched to the group's preferred cognitive learning style.

Of interest to educators, counselors, and social workers.

777. RICHWALD, Gary A., Margarita Schneider-Muñoz, R. Burciaga Valdez. "Are condom instructions in Spanish readable? Implications for AIDS prevention activities for Hispanics." *Hispanic Journal of Behavioral Sciences* 11 (1989): 70-82.

This study used three readability formulas designed for use with Spanish language materials to determine the reading grade level necessary to understand the Spanish instructions provided with condoms.

Research

Only half of the manufacturers of condoms available in Los Angeles provided instructions in Spanish. Seven different Spanish texts were identified from the 13 marketed brands. Readability tests indicate that these texts pose difficulties in comprehension for anyone whose reading skills are below the ninth grade level. These instructions inadequately serve the majority of the Hispanic community whose limited reading skills inhibit comprehension of high school level materials.

Of interest to health educators and public health officials.

778. RICKERT, E.J. "Differing sexual practices of men and women screened for HIV (AIDS) antibody." *Psychological Reports* 64 (1989): 323-326.

Describes the results of a survey of all persons screened for antibodies to HIV at a county health department during a three month period.

Research

Findings suggest that stronger educational efforts are needed to disseminate information to women and blacks who are at risk for HIV infection.

Of interest to health educators and public health officials.

779. ROGERS, Martha F., and Walter W. Williams. "AIDS in blacks and Hispanics: Implications for prevention." *Issues in Science and Technology* 3, no. 3 (1987): 89-94.

Examines the reasons for the disproportionately high incidence of AIDS among blacks and Hispanics.

Commentary

The authors warn that AIDS is likely to spread at much higher rates among these minorities than among whites and argue that this neglected aspect of the disease has important implications for controlling and slowing its spread, especially among the heterosexual community.

Of interest to laymen.

780. SCHILLING, Robert F., Steven P. Schinke, Stuart E. Nichols, Luis H. Zayas, Samuel O. Miller, Mario O. Orlandi, Gilbert J. Botvin. "Developing strategies for AIDS prevention research with black and Hispanic drug users." *Public Health Reports* 104 (1989): 2-11.

Considers the nature and extent of AIDS among ethnic/racial minorities and the cultural aspects of drug use and sexual behavior related to HIV transmission.

Descriptive/Analytical

Studies are needed that: 1) describe the phenomena of drug use and sexual behavior among ethnic/racial minority populations; 2) establish the efficacy of culturally specific AIDS prevention strategies in drug treatment and community settings; and 3) demonstrate new ways of recruiting, treating, and reducing relapse among drug users.

Of interest to public health officials, epidemiologists, and social and behavioral scientists.

D. WOMEN

a. Books

781. KAPLAN, Helen Singer. *The Real Truth About Women and AIDS: How to Eliminate the Risks Without Giving Up Love and Sex.* New York: Simon and Schuster, 1987.

The author, a sex therapist, clarifies every woman's unique risks and choices and explodes the myths about AIDS.

Guide/Sourcebook

Designed to give women facts and information about AIDS and about how to reduce their risks of contracting the disease. Also about female sex and sexuality. Appendices and references are provided.

Of interest to the general public, especially women.

782. NORWOOD, Chris. *Advice for Life: A Woman's Guide to AIDS Risks and Prevention.* New York: Pantheon Books, 1987.

An examination of the AIDS tragedy and ways in which women can protect themselves.

Text

The nine chapters include the following information: transmission and symptoms of AIDS, which men have AIDS, personal prevention, education and testing, prostitution and the heterosexual connection, giving and getting blood, who will tell the kids, after a diagnosis, and the caring woman. A questionnaire for assessing one's own risks is provided along with several appendices and references.

Of interest to the general public, especially women.

783. PATTON, Cindy, and Janis Kelly. *Making It: A Woman's Guide
      to Sex in the Age of AIDS.* Ithaca, NY: Firebrand Books,
      1987.

Designed to present the facts relevant to coping with AIDS and help
promote an understanding of how coping differs for each woman. Contains suggestions for implementing the changes that are necessary for
survival.

Guidebook

This book, written in two parts—one in Spanish and one in English—
offers practical advice about AIDS: who gets it, how it is spread, and
its prevention.

Of interest to women.

b. Articles

784. CARPENTER, Charles C.J., Kenneth H. Mayer, Alvan Fisher,
      Manish B. Desai, Linda Durland. "Natural history of
      acquired immunodeficiency syndrome in women in Rhode
      Island." *American Journal of Medicine* 86 (1989): 771-775.

In an effort to determine whether the natural history and clinical
course may be different, the authors documented the clinical courses
of the first 24 known cases of AIDS in women in Rhode Island.

Research

More information on the natural history of HIV infection in North
American women is needed. If more extensive data from other
geographic areas confirm the observations in this study, the optimal
approach to prophylaxis against opportunistic infections in women with
AIDS may be substantially different from that which is most
appropriate for males.

Of interest to health professionals, especially infectious disease
physicians.

785. DONOVAN, Patricia. "AIDS and family planning clinics:
      Confronting the crisis." *Family Planning Perspectives* 19,
      no. 3 (1987): 111-114, 138.

Discusses the challenges facing family planning clinics as a result of
the AIDS epidemic.

Review

Family planning clinics have a unique opportunity to provide patient
education about AIDS and behavior that puts women at risk to their
clients. In-depth counseling and treatment programs are also options
that deserve serious consideration. Speakers at the meeting of the

Planned Parent Federation of America, held in Arlington in June 1987, urged family planning clinics to accept the ethical, moral, and legal responsibility to exploit their opportunities to slow the spread of disease among heterosexuals, particularly the drug-using population, by expanding their role "beyond birth control to disease control."

Of interest to family planning providers, counselors, and health educators.

786. MINKOFF, Howard L., and Sheldon H. Landesman. "The case for routinely offering prenatal testing for human immunodeficiency virus." *American Journal of Obstetrics and Gynecology* 159 (1988): 793-796.

Argues the case for HIV testing for all pregnant patients with appropriate counseling, consent, and confidentiality instead of testing only patients assumed or self-reported to be at risk.

Clinical Opinion

Testing all pregnant patients for HIV will enable women to make informed choices about whether to continue or terminate their pregnancies. It will also allow physicians to manage the treatment of infected women in a more effective and timely way. As the incidence of HIV infection continues to increase among heterosexuals, the distinctions between groups at risk and non-risk groups will blur and make it less likely that infected persons have been tested.

Of particular interest to obstetricians/gynecologists.

787. MONDANARO, Josette. "Strategies for AIDS prevention: Motivating health behavior in drug dependent women." *Journal of Psychoactive Drugs* 19 (1987): 143-149.

Reviews some of the basic issues concerning women and AIDS as well as some intervention techniques that may be responsive to the particular needs of women.

Review

Contaminated needles are now the major source of AIDS for women, newborns, prisoners, and minorities, and the only present hope for control is education and prevention. AIDS prevention and educational materials need to be specifically tailored to drug dependent women in order to increase their knowledge of the disease and change their attitudes and health behaviors.

Of interest to mental health professionals, social workers, and others involved in drug abuse programs.

788. SHAW, Nancy Stoller. "Preventing AIDS among women: The role of community organizing." *Socialist Review* 18, no. 4 (1988): 76-92.

Explores the challenge of preventing AIDS among women through community organizing.

Discussion

Community organization projects are complex and their study requires
appropriate methodology. One goal of AIDS prevention research should
be comparison of the effectiveness of different organizing strategies
in controlling the AIDS epidemic. Research could be done in several
black and Latino communities within one large metropolitan area or
state in order to control for epidemiological and/or political factors. Several organizing techniques could be studied. Interventions
could include not only the community organizing per se, but a variety
of AIDS prevention techniques, such as support groups, media messages,
behavior modification, counseling, etc.

Of interest to community organizers, health educators, and social
scientists.

789. VALDISERRI, Ronald O., Frank A. Bonati, Donna Proctor,
     Dolores A. Glaser. "HIV antibody testing in a family
     planning clinic setting." *New York State Journal of Medicine*
     88 (1988): 623-625.

Self-reported risk factors and HIV serostatus were determined for 433
women attending two family planning clinics in western Pennsylvania
between April 1987 and April 1988.

Research

Only one of the 433 women had a positive ELISA test, and she was
negative by Western blot analysis. However, a substantial number of
the women reported high risk behaviors. AIDS education and identification of infected women should be provided at family planning
clinics.

Of interest to family planning personnel and public health officials.

E. CHILDREN AND ADOLESCENTS

a. Articles

790. BLOKZIJL, M.L. "Human immunodeficiency virus infection in
     childhood." *Annals of Tropical Paediatrics* 8 (1988): 1-17.

Describes transmission, the clinical picture, and immunological
abnormalities of HIV infection in children in general, and the special
problems of AIDS in African children.

Review

HIV infection in children presents with failure to thrive, pulmonary interstitial pneumonitis, hepatosplenomegaly, and recurrent bacterial infections. These are common manifestations of diseases prevalent in children in Africa, where malnutrition and recurrent parasitic infections already cause immunosuppression. Supportive treatment and relief of pain and suffering are the only means of management at present. Prevention of spread of the illness to infants and young children is, therefore, of paramount importance.

Of interest to epidemiologists, public health officials, and virologists.

791. BROWN, Larry K., and Gregory K. Fritz. "Children's knowledge and attitudes about AIDS." *Journal of the American Academy of Child and Adolescent Psychiatry* 27 (1988): 504-508.

Knowledge, attitudes, and coping skills were surveyed in 908 seventh and tenth grade students.

Research

The majority of students knew that AIDS was transmitted by sexual rather than casual contact. Correlations between knowledge and behavioral attitudes were minimal, so the impact of increasing knowledge about AIDS would seem unpredictable. A subgroup of least tolerant students could be distinguished from the other students only by differences in coping strategies.

Of interest to psychologists, health educators, school science teachers, and school nurses.

792. DEKKER, Anthony H. "The impact of AIDS in the pediatric and adolescent populations." *Journal of the American Osteopathic Association* 88 (1988): 629-633.

Attempts to sensitize the physician and other health care workers to the prevalence, problems, complications, and emotional aspects of HIV infections in the pediatric and adolescent populations.

Descriptive

As there appears to be no effective treatment for these patients, an aggressive, preventive approach is needed. The diagnosis and symptomatology of pediatric AIDS differ from those of the adult population. Vaccination protocols for symptomatic HIV-infected children differ from those of their uninfected peers. Adolescent issues of sexual activity, sexual exploitation, and chemical abuse raise the probability of spread in this population.

Of particular interest to pediatricians and child health care professionals.

793. HEIN, Karen. "AIDS in adolescents: A rationale for concern."
    New York State Journal of Medicine 87 (1987): 290-295.

Discusses why teenagers are an important group for targeted
interventions to prevent further spread of AIDS.

Theoretical

It is hypothesized that the "sexual adventurers" among adolescents,
who have been a reservoir for other sexually transmitted diseases, are
most likely to be the entry of HIV infection into the teenage
population. Adolescents are a proximal group that may become rapidly
infected in the near future and, therefore, require the immediate
attention of health policy and health care agencies. Special
attention should be paid to adolescents in developing more effective
treatments and primary preventive measures against HIV.

Of interest to public health officials and health policymakers.

794. ———. "Commentary on adolescent acquired immunodeficiency
    syndrome: The next wave of the human immunodeficiency
    virus epidemic?" *Journal of Pediatrics* 114 (1989):
    144-149.

Discusses degrees of HIV risk and rates of HIV infection among
adolescents, and offers eight recommendations to reduce the spread of
AIDS among adolescents.

Commentary

There are special needs and opportunities related to AIDS in adolescence. Thoughtful, but quick action is the goal. If we cannot
determine and deter the AIDS risk for adolescents now, we are likely
to face massive morbidity and mortality rates among young adults in
the near future.

Of interest to pediatricians and child development specialists.

795. JAFFE, Leslie R., and Richard N. Wortman. "The fear of
    AIDS: Guidelines to the counseling and HTLV-III antibody
    screening of adolescents." *Journal of Adolescent Health
    Care* 9 (1988): 84-86.

A discussion of guidelines to the counseling and HTLV-III antibody
screening of adolescents.

Editorial

Biologic, psychosocial, ethical, and legal issues preclude a
categorical stance by the physician about serotesting for HTLV-III
antibody. Caution should be used in doing antibody testing.
Considerable counseling time and effort are needed to prevent AIDS
virus spread among those at high risk.

Of special interest to pediatricians.

796. KASTNER, Ted and Deborah Friedman. "Pediatric acquired immune deficiency syndrome and the prevention of mental retardation." *Journal of Developmental and Behavioral Pediatrics* 9 (1988): 47-48.

AIDS is a cause of mental retardation and developmental disabilities. However, the severity of the AIDS epidemic and its impact on the provision of services to handicapped children has been generally underappreciated.

Commentary

We must redouble our efforts in the prevention of AIDS, not only for the good of children with AIDS, but for the good of all children with mental retardation and developmental disabilities who must be served in a society where there already is a limited supply of services.

Of particular interest to pediatricians.

797. MELTON, Gary B. "Adolescents and prevention of AIDS." *Professional Psychology: Research and Practice* 19 (1988): 403-408.

Identifies factors that are likely to affect the success of AIDS prevention among adolescents, suggests corollary actions by government to reduce the threat of HIV infection, and outlines a program of behavioral research necessary for a well-designed prevention program.

Discussion

For adolescents to learn to avoid behavior that increases the risk of HIV infection, educational programs must increase the personal salience of such risks. Information about risks should be complemented by problem-solving programs designed to counteract social inhibitions on the use of contraception and environmental manipulations designed to increase access to condoms. Market-based regulatory strategies show some potential to decrease needle sharing. There exists a compelling need for a large behavioral research initiative to develop a body of knowledge necessary for prevention of HIV infection.

Of interest to psychologists, social and behavioral scientists, and health educators.

798. OLIVA, Geraldine E., George W. Rutherford, Moses Grossman, Janet Shalwitz, Abigail English, Frances Taylor, David Werdegar. "Guidelines for the control of human immunodeficiency virus infection in adolescents." *Western Journal of Medicine* 148 (1988): 566-589.

Guidelines were developed that emphasize education and medical care and deemphasize antibody testing.

Descriptive

Descriptive

For adolescents known to be infected with HIV, the authors recommend
no restrictions on access to educational or treatment programs except
when their health providers recommend such restrictions to protect
them from exposure to opportunistic infections. For adolescents of
unknown antibody status with a possible previous exposure to HIV, the
authors recommend that as long as the incidence of HIV infection and
clinical AIDS remains low, there should be no restrictions on residential placement and on routine antibody testing.

Of special interest to pediatricians and child care personnel.

799. OVERBY, Kim J., Bernard Lo, Iris F. Litt. "Knowledge and
     concerns about acquired immunodeficiency syndrome and their
     relationship to behavior among adolescents with hemophilia."
     Pediatrics 83 (1989): 204-210.

A questionnaire and interview were administered to 26 adolescent
hemophiliacs, aged 13 to 19, to determine the relationship between
knowledge of and concerns about AIDS and sexual behavior.

Research

Although participants demonstrated a high level of factual knowledge
about AIDS and awareness of the importance of using condoms, those who
were sexually active did not practice safe sex. Restriction in the
use of heat-treated clotting factor because of concern about AIDS
frequently was reported. Professionals providing AIDS education and
counseling should focus on the social and situational pressures
confronting teenagers with hemophilia.

Of interest to health educators and counselors.

800. SUNENBLICK, Mary Beth. "The AIDS epidemic: Sexual
     behaviors of adolescents." *Smith College Studies in Social
     Work* 59 (1988): 21-37.

Examines the association between levels of knowledge about AIDS,
concern about personal susceptibility to AIDS, and sexual behaviors of
late adolescents.

Research

Students demonstrated a high level of knowledge about the cause,
transmission, and treatment of AIDS. Those with higher levels of
knowledge showed less concern about personal susceptibility. There
was no significant relationship between knowledge perception of
susceptibility, and sexual behaviors. The author recommends that
clinicians and educators work together to encourage adolescents to
avoid sexual or needle-sharing risk taking.

Of interest to educators and health professionals.

b. Dissertation

801. HUSZTI, Heather Christine. "The effects of educational programs on adolescents' knowledge and attitudes about acquired immunodeficiency syndrome (AIDS)." Ph.D. dissertation, Texas Tech University, 1987.

This study examined the effectiveness of two different types of AIDS education programs for adolescents.

Research

The effects of a lecture, a film presentation, and no program were compared. Knowledge about AIDS, attitudes towards AIDS patients, and attitudes toward practicing preventive behaviors were assessed one week before the program, immediately after the program, and one month after the program in 448 tenth grade students who had been divided into three groups. The subjects in the two groups which attended the lecture or film presentation exhibited a significant increase in knowledge, positive attitudes toward AIDS patients, and positive attitudes toward practicing preventive behavior; those in the lecture group demonstrated the greatest gains. Subjects in both treatment groups retained some of their gains in knowledge and positive attitudes towards AIDS patients over the follow-up period, but neither group maintained positive attitudes about prevention practices. The no-program group showed significant decreases in knowledge and attitudes toward practicing preventive behaviors over time, and no changes in attitude towards AIDS patients. Females had significantly higher knowledge scores and more positive attitude scores than males.

Of interest to teachers and health educators.

F. OTHER

a. Articles

802. BAER, Jay W., Priscilla C. Dwyer, Susan Lewitter-Koehler. "Knowledge about AIDS among psychiatric inpatients." *Hospital and Community Psychiatry* 39 (1988): 986-988.

Reports on an assessment of AIDS knowledge among psychiatric inpatients.

Research

Ninety psychiatric inpatients were given a 10-item true-false test on AIDS plus a demographic questionnaire on age, race, education, work history, and sources of information about AIDS three days prior to discharge. Patients were then interviewed and their charts reviewed. Only 40% of patients reported having learned about AIDS with staff help, but other sources were reported. The results suggest that persons with major psychiatric illness can learn about AIDS, and the authors recommend that hospital staff teach them.

Of interest to psychiatric educators.

803.   BALDWIN, John D., and Janice I. Baldwin. "Factors affecting AIDS-related sexual risk-taking behavior among college students." *Journal of Sex Research* 25 (1988): 181-196.

Questionnaires were mailed to a random sample of students at a university in Southern California to assess factors affecting AIDS-related sexual risk-taking behavior among college students.

Research

The results revealed that, for the most part, students were engaging in few activities that would protect them from contracting HIV. Findings led the authors to conclude that AIDS-related education must not rely solely on programs designed to relay AIDS information only, but must also stress the value of certain lifestyle habits, social responsibility, and caution in the face of risky activities.

Of interest to counselors, college administrators, and health educators.

804.   CATANIA, Joseph A., Heather Turner, Susan M. Kegeles, Ron Stall, Lance Pollack, Thomas J. Coates.   "Older Americans and AIDS: Transmission risks and primary prevention research needs." *Gerontologist* 29 (1989): 373-381.

Reviews the incidence and transmission of HIV among Americans, 50 years of age or older, and suggests research areas.

Review

Ten percent of the AIDS cases in the United States have been reported in persons, age 50 and older, and as many as 125,000 may be infected. Between 1982 and 1987, the largest segment of the AIDS cases were in homosexual and bisexual men, although the percentage of transfusion-related cases increased from 5.3% to 17.3%. HIV infection is more common among older spouses of transfusion-infected persons than among younger ones and those who have sex infrequently. The authors call for research to determine population-based HIV seroprevalence, sexual and IV drug behaviors, and AIDS knowledge and beliefs of older individuals.

Of interest to gerontologists, geriatricians, public health officials, and health educators.

805.   CHIKWEM, John O., T. Oyebode Ola, Wadzani Gashau, Susan D. Chiwem, Mary Bajami, Salmatu Mambula. "Impact of health education on prostitutes' awareness of and attitudes to acquired immune deficiency syndrome (AIDS)." *Public Health* 102 (1988): 439-445.

Results of a study initiated to gain information concerning prostitutes' motives and activities as well as to evaluate their awareness of and attitudes to HIV infection are presented.

Research

Results showed that about 75% of the prostitutes surveyed in Maiduguri are below 30 years of age, about 44% are divorced, most (74%) have children, and 27% are foreigners. Each prostitute has an average of 3.3 customers per day. Results showed that prostitutes are receptive to health education and that a majority of them advocate some form of restriction of HIV carriers in order to protect the general public from HIV infection.

Of interest to public health officials, health educators, and social and behavioral scientists.

806. KEETER, Scott, and Judith B. Bradford. "Knowledge of AIDS and related behavior change among unmarried adults in a low-prevalence city." *American Journal of Preventive Medicine* 4 (1988): 146-152.

Interviews regarding AIDS knowledge and related behavior change were conducted with a random sample of 409 married individuals, 18-39 years of age, in Richmond, Virginia.

Research

Sixty-five percent of sexually active nonmonogamous individuals reported changing their behavior because of concern about AIDS; an additional eight percent reported that they were already being careful. Fifty-two percent of those who changed their behavior reported having fewer sexual partners, and 51% were learning more about potential partners than before the AIDS crisis. Thirty-seven percent were using condoms to minimize risk. The level of concern for self was strongly associated with behavior change. The amount of knowledge about AIDS did not distinguish between those who had changed and those who had not. The level of concern was the most influential independent variable.

Of interest to health educators, physicians specializing in preventive medicine, public health officials, and behavioral scientists.

807. McMILLAN, A. "HIV in prisons." *British Medical Journal* 297 (1988): 873-874.

Calls for AIDS education and the issuance of condoms to prisoners.

Editorial

Issuing condoms to prisoners is the only alternative to isolating or closely supervising those who are seropositive if HIV transmission in prisons is to be decreased. Prisoners should be educated about the risks of injecting drugs. The effect of issuing sterile needles to prisoners should be studied.

Of interest to prison administrators, policymakers, and ethicists.

808. MATHEWS, William Christopher, and Lawrence S. Linn. "AIDS
      prevention in primary care clinics: Testing the market."
      Journal of General Internal Medicine 4 (1989): 34-38.

To assess attitudes toward educational programs about AIDS, 540
patients and 36 of their medical providers in primary care clinics
were systematically sampled to ascertain what age groups should be
exposed to a pamphlet entitled, "Am I at Risk for AIDS?"

Research

Although fewer than 10% of patients and providers opposed asking both
teenagers and adults to read a pamphlet listing risk groups and
practices, 24% of patients and 51% of providers opposed exposing
children to the pamphlets. Only six percent of patients and none of
the providers opposed all posters about AIDS, but 30% of patients and
44% of providers opposed posters listing risk groups. Opposition was
even greater to posters describing safe sex.

Of interest to health educators and public health professionals.

809. MOROKOFF, Patricia J., Elizabeth Holmes, Carol Silva Weisse.
      "A psychoeducational program for HIV seropositive persons."
      Patient and Education Counseling 10 (1987): 287-300.

Describes a psychoeducational program for individuals who are seropositive for HIV to help patients understand their medical condition,
prevent transmission of the virus, and alter lifestyles that may
compromise health.

Descriptive

Gives background information on the prevalence of AIDS, cofactors for
the development of AIDS, and how the virus is transmitted. Describes
the HIV program at Naval Hospital Bethesda, including the contents of
eight classes that provide patients with information on the medical
nature of HIV infection and AIDS, the psychological impact of HIV
infection, Navy career implications, how stress affects the immune
system, how to reduce stress, how to prevent transmission of HIV
through safer sex, religious issues connected with being at high risk
for a fatal disease, and alcohol and drug issues. The emotional
issues faced by the HIV-seropositive person are illustrated in a case
presentation.

Of particular interest to health educators and counselors.

810. MURRAH, Valerie A., and Genevieve A. Scholtes. "Antibody
      testing and counseling of dental patients at risk for human
      immunodeficiency virus (HIV) infection and associated clinical
      findings." *Oral Surgery, Oral Medicine, and Oral Pathology*
      66 (1988): 432-439.

Reports the results of HIV antibody screening of 206 high-risk patients at the University of Minnesota School of Dentistry from July 1985 through July 1987.

Research

Two hundred and six dental patients were tested for antibodies to HIV when a review of their medical histories revealed a high risk for infection. Serologic results are correlated with soft tissue and osseous findings recorded during routine head and neck and radiographic examination. Counseling recommendations for use in association with testing are outlined. A more active role for the dentist as a preventive agent is advocated to control the spread of AIDS.

Of interest to dentists and dental hygienists.

811. SOLOMON, Mildred Z., and William DeJong. "Preventing AIDS and other STDs through condom promotion: A patient education intervention." *American Journal of Public Health* **79** (1989): 453-458.

Reports on two studies that assessed the impact of a soap-opera style videotape on inner city STD patients' knowledge about and attitudes toward condom use, and willingness to redeem coupons for free condoms.

Research

Participants in the first study who viewed the videotape had higher knowledge scores and more accepting attitudes than subjects who did not. The intervention was most effective among the relatively poorly educated and, to a lesser extent, among those who reported less frequent use of condoms and fewer sexual partners. In the second study, the intervention group participants were more likely than those in the control group to redeem coupons, although both groups exhibited a high level of interest in free condoms. The authors argue that education and accessibility to free condoms both can increase condom use and that health care providers have a vital role in promoting this form of STD prevention.

Of interest to STD counselors, health educators, public health officials, and public policymakers.

b. Dissertations

812. DeROSE, Joseph Anthony. "A study of AIDS-related complex patients." Ph.D. dissertation. United States International University, 1986.

The sexual activities practiced by ARC patients one year prior to diagnosis and subsequent to diagnosis were investigated.

Research

Findings showed that the majority of subjects had changed their sexual practices since the diagnosis of ARC. The subjects' perceived understanding of "safe" and "unsafe" sexual practices has resulted in the need for additional educational programs geared toward educating high-risk groups.

Of interest to health educators and behavioral scientists.

813.   HERNANDEZ, Jeanne T. "The variable effect of AIDS education programs on college students." Ph.D. dissertation, North Carolina State University, 1988.

To determine the differential effects of three prevention strategies and two presented risk factors within AIDS education programs, on the attitudes, intentions, and behaviors of college-age adolescents, 388 students were presented one of three multimedia programs, administered a personality inventory, and completed questionnaires on sexual and dating attitudes and behaviors before and after the program presentations.

Research

The programs stressing abstinence and encouraging decision-making resulted in an increase in condom buying and use, while the program that instructed in condom use and safe sex practices resulted in a general decrease in condom buying and use. Subjects high on sensation seeking were the most sexually active, but after the programs were more likely to improve their safe sex practices. The highly anxious and the sexually inactive, who endorsed safe sex practices less than their counterparts before the programs, appeared to endorse them more after the programs. Overall, subjects exhibited high baseline levels of precautionary dating and safe sex intentions. The results indicate the need for further research.

Of interest to behavioral scientists and health educators.

5.   HEALTH PROFESSIONALS

a. Books

814.   BARR, Charles E. and Michael Z. Marder. *AIDS: A Guide for Dental Practice.* Chicago: Quintessence, 1987.

Provides information on AIDS and specific treatment guidelines for dentists.

Text

Discusses the epidemiology, etiology, and immunology of AIDS. Describes barrier techniques and methods of treating the more common oral manifestations of AIDS. Discusses the control of the dentist office environment to provide safe and fruitful encounters for both dentist and patient, and considers the ethical, legal, and social responsibilities of the dentist.

Of interest to all providers of dental care.

815. GREENSPAN, Deborah, Jens J. Pindborg, John S. Greenspan, Morten Schiodt. *AIDS and the Dental Team.* Chicago: Year Book Medical Publishers, 1986.

Provides information to help members of the dental team understand the problems of AIDS as they relate to their jobs.

Text

Contains an up-to-date introduction to the viral and epidemiologic aspects of AIDS, a detailed description of what is known about oral manifestations of HIV infection, and a chapter on the principles and practice of AIDS infection control in dentistry.

Useful to dentists, dental hygienists, dental assistants, and dental laboratory technicians.

816. *The HIV Epidemic and Medical Education: A Report of the AAMC Committee on AIDS and the Academic Medical Center.* Washington, DC: Association of American Medical Colleges, February 1989.

Addresses the educational challenges posed by HIV/AIDS.

Report

The report is based on the Committee's examinations of the likely impact of the epidemic on future medical practice; its review of medical school efforts to introduce HIV/AIDS into the medical school curriculum; its judgment regarding the knowledge, skills, and attitudes physicians need to care for HIV-infected persons and to help prevent further spread of the infection; its conclusions as to resources needed to achieve desired objectives; and its analysis of special issues for academic medicine.

Of interest to educators focusing on general professional education in medicine, medical student education, and early residency training.

817. OTTER, Jean (Ed.). *The Current Status of HTLV-III Testing.* Arlington, VA: American Association of Blood Banks, 1985.

Provides information and guidelines to individuals involved in the many aspects of AIDS testing.

Monograph

Addresses the economic, legal, scientific, logistic, and ethical issues encountered in testing for AIDS in both the blood center and transfusion service. Covers the impact of AIDS testing on the transfusion service; the impact of AIDS testing on the donor center; test

methodologies; risk to health care workers; and donor notification.
Contains a post-test, and may be used as a self-study course for
earning .2 credit hours in continuing medical education.

Of particular interest to health care workers involved in blood
banking.

818.   PROCEEDINGS of Multidisciplinary Curriculum Development
       Conference on HIV Infection. Washington, DC: Health
       Resources and Services Administration, Public Health
       Service, U.S. Department of Health and Human Services,
       November 1987.

Identifies the major issues of concern to seven health professions and
makes recommendations for educating students and professionals in the
care of HIV-infected persons.

Conference Proceedings

Includes the conference objectives, keynote speeches, reports of
single-discipline task forces, and proposed procedures. The appendices contain detailed reports by task forces for physicians, dentists,
nurses, physician assistants, emergency medical technicians, social
workers, and public health practitioners.

Of interest to educators developing AIDS curricula for health
professionals.

b. Articles

819.   ANDERSON, Peter, and Richard Mayon-White. "General practi-
       tioners and management of infection with HIV." *British
       Medical Journal* 296 (1988): 535-537.

Two hundred and eighty general practitioners were sent a questionnaire
inquiring about their education, knowledge, current practice, and
attitudes in relation to managing infections with HIV.

Research

Of the 235 (84%) general practitioners who replied, nine out of 10
were giving advice about infection with HIV to their patients. One or
two were testing patients for such infection, and one in four were
caring for infected patients. Nevertheless, uncertainty remained
about the risks of transmission of infection with HIV, and general
practitioners' knowledge of educational activities for their patients
could be improved.

Of interest to general practitioners and family physicians.

820.   ATCHISON, Kathryn A., Teresa A. Dolan, Harriet K. Meetz.
       "Have dentists assimilated information about AIDS?" *Journal
       of Dental Education* 51 (1987): 668-672.

A random sample of 396 general dentists, oral surgeons, and periodontists in Los Angeles was interviewed, in 1986, to determine their experience in treating patients infected with HIV.

Research

One-third of the dentists reported treating a known or suspected AIDS patient, and 56% indicated that they would not or could not treat patients with AIDS. Dentists displayed little knowledge of the oral and systemic signs and symptoms of AIDS. Dentists who reported attending continuing education were found to have only slightly greater knowledge of diagnostic signs. After two or more lectures on AIDS, 31% still named no oral signs or symptoms of AIDS.

Of interest to dentists, public health officials, and health educators.

821. BOR, Robert, Jonathan Elford, Lucy Perry, Riva Miller. "AIDS/HIV in the work of family therapy trainees." *Journal of Family Therapy* 10 (1988): 375-382.

The views and knowledge of 37 family therapy trainees regarding people with HIV and AIDS were investigated.

Research

Two-thirds of the trainees depended upon the media as their primary source of information about HIV infection. They demonstrated adequate knowledge regarding the risk of transmission, but inadequate information on virus inactivation, drug therapy for AIDS patients, and occupational risks of infection. Family therapists need up-to-date information on AIDS as well as appropriate counseling skills.

Of interest to family therapists and other mental health professionals.

822. BOWLES, L. Thompson. "The AIDS epidemic." *Journal of Medical Education* 62 (1987): 541.

Discusses the importance of the AIDS epidemic and its biopsychosocial elements in the education of medical students, housestaff, and faculty members as well as the general public.

Editorial

Medical centers need to review carefully their programs for treating AIDS patients and consider their preparation of students and housestaff to deal with those individuals. Support programs will be needed for professionals providing medical care to young patients with fatal illnesses. A policy is needed by academic medical centers that will serve both the institution and AIDS patients when those patients may include medical students, housestaff members, or members of the professional staff.

Of interest to medical educators and hospital administrators.

823. DARROW, William W. "A framework for preventing AIDS."
      American Journal of Public Health 77 (1987): 778-779.

Discusses the formulation of a compassionate, comprehensive and
effective approach to controlling and preventing further transmission
of AIDS.

Editorial

More attention must be given to the effective education of health care
providers regarding the transmission of AIDS, as well as proper
diagnostic approaches and appropriate patient management techniques.
Interventions must transcend the traditional limits of medicine to
address the societal problems associated with the transmission of the
HIV virus.

Of interest to health educators and physicians.

824. DUERFELDT, William F. "Preparing an AIDS policy for colleges
      of osteopathic medicine." *Journal of the American Osteo-
      pathic Association* 89 (1989): 95-103.

Reviews the approach taken by the Ohio University College of Osteopathic Medicine to establish and implement an AIDS policy.

Descriptive

In a survey of osteopathic colleges, an AIDS task force identified the
most important issues to consider in setting policy; these included
mandatory HIV testing, AIDS education, confidentiality, the obligation
of students and faculty to care for HIV-positive patients, and
measures to prevent occupational transmission of HIV. Once the AIDS
policy had been established, a copy was provided to all departments of
the college and the osteopathic medical center. Summary statements
were distributed to all students prior to their initial clinical
rotations and later, to all entering students. One session on AIDS is
conducted for preclinical students each year.

Of interest to health professions educators, administrators of schools
for health professionals, and hospital administrators.

825. GERBERT, Barbara. "AIDS and infection control in dental
      practice: Dentists' attitudes, knowledge, and behavior."
      Journal of the American Dental Association 114 (1987):
      311-314.

A random sample of 541 dentists in California was surveyed to
determine dentists' attitudes toward AIDS, their role in relation to
AIDS, their knowledge about AIDS, their behaviors in regard to
screening for AIDS, and their use of infection-control measures.

The results showed that dentists believe they have a responsibility to care for patients with AIDS, but prefer not to do so; are moderately knowledgeable about AIDS and AIDS-related issues; and are inconsistent in their use of infection-control measures.

Of interest to dentists and dental educators.

826. ————, Bryan Maguire, Victor Badner, David Altman, George Stone. "Fear of AIDS: Issues for health professional education." *AIDS Education and Prevention* 1, no. 1 (1989): 39-52.

Examines how fear of AIDS has been managed in the health care system; describes the extent of this fear among health care professionals; analyzes strategies used to address fear of AIDS in this group; documents its persistence; and offers explanations for its continuation.

Descriptive

The authors describe the impact of the fear of AIDS among health care professionals on health care delivery. They describe four strategies that have been used to allay fears and explain why these strategies have failed. Persons involved in the training of health professionals are encouraged to attend to the pitfalls described in this paper when designing interventions.

Of interest to health professionals of all types.

827. GILES, Gordon Muir, and Mary Elisabeth Allen. "AIDS, ARC and the occupational therapist." *British Journal of Occupational Therapy* 50, no. 4 (1987): 120-123.

Suggests precautions to be taken around individuals infected with HIV.

Descriptive

Infection control and health risks, which are of relevance to the occupational therapist in the hospital and in a domiciliary setting, are discussed. The importance of safe sex for the total population is emphasized. Counseling issues are discussed.

Of particular interest to occupational therapists.

828. GOLDMAN, Jonathan D. "An elective seminar to teach first-year students the social and medical aspects of AIDS." *Journal of Medical Education* 62 (1987): 557-561.

Description of a comprehensive seminar covering the biological, psychological, and social aspects of acquired immune deficiency syndrome.

Descriptive

A television movie; documentary film; reading materials and lectures
on the pathology, epidemiology, and history of AIDS; roundtable discussions with AIDS patients, volunteers who coordinate support and
advocacy for persons with AIDS, and health professionals involved in
the care of AIDS patients; and monitoring and discussion of radio and
television reporting on AIDS all form part of a seven-week elective
seminar for freshman medical students. Students report the seminar to
be valuable in helping them overcome their fear of AIDS, develop
empathy for patients with catastrophic diseases, and understand a
comprehensive approach to a complex disease.

Valuable for medical educators.

829. HIRSCH, Martin S., Gary P. Wormser, Robert T. Schooley,
      et al.   "Risk of nosocomial infection with human T-Cell
      lymphotropic virus III (HTLV-III)." *New England Journal of
      Medicine* 312 (1985): 1-4.

The risk of nosocomial infection with HTLV-III was evaluated among
hospital employees, including victims of needle-stick exposure,
endoscopists, and pathologists, by testing for antibodies to HTLV-III.

Research

Enzyme-linked immunosorbent assay and electrophoretic (Western blot)
techniques were performed to determine the serologic status of hospital employees considered at high risk of infection. Although 22
AIDS patients and 6 of 7 with ARC tested positive when both assays
were employed, none of 85 hospital employees with nosocomial exposure
to specimens from patients were positive for HTLV-III antibody.
Although these studies must be regarded as preliminary, they suggest
that when current hospital isolation procedures are employed, the risk
of nosocomial infection with HTLV-III is low.

Of interest to epidemiologists, virologists, hospital administrators,
and hospital employees exposed to the blood and body fluids of
patients with AIDS and ARC.

830. HUGHES, James M., Julia S. Garner, Ruthanne Marcus, Harold
      W. Jaffe. "AIDS: Epidemiological lessons from the health care
      setting." *Journal of Hospital Infection* 11, Supplement A
      (1988): 209-217.

Reviews the epidemiology of AIDS in the U.S., three recent reports on
the AIDS epidemic in the U.S., the results of several studies to
assess the magnitude of risk of HIV infection to health care workers,
and current CDC recommmendations for preventing and controlling HIV
transmission in the health-care setting.

Review

. It is known that the risk following needle-stick exposures to the blood of HIV infected patients is less than 1%, transmission following exposure to blood rarely occurs in the absence of a needle-stick injury, and an acute illness is common in those who become infected. There is no evidence of casual transmission in the health-care setting. Blood and body fluids from all patients should be treated as potentially infective. The prevalence of infection in groups with extensive blood exposure is not known, nor are the efficacy of "extraordinary" precautions in further minimizing the risk of transmission to health-care workers, the most effective methods for ensuring compliance with existing recommendations, or the impact of knowledge of serological status of patients on the compliance of health care workers.

Of interest to hospital administrators, health care workers, and infection control specialists.

831. JUKASH, Judy. "AIDS: The disease and its implications for dentistry." *Journal of the American Dental Association* 115 (1987): 394-403.

A discussion of AIDS and its implications for dentistry.

Descriptive

Discusses the history of AIDS, future of the disease, virology and immunology, clinical manifestations of HIV infection, oral manifestations of HIV infection, and office treatment. Offers a list of information resources on AIDS. A brief section on legal and ethical issues for dentists is also presented.

Of interest to dentists and dental hygienists.

832. KLEIN, Robert S., Joan A. Phelan, Katherine Freeman, Charles Schable, Gerald H. Friedland, Norman Trieger, Neal H. Steigbigel. "Low occupational risk of human immunodeficiency virus infection among dental professionals." *New England Journal of Medicine* 318 (1988): 86-90.

The authors studied 1,309 dental professionals without behavioral risk factors for AIDS to determine their occupational risk for HIV.

Research

Despite infrequent compliance with recommended infection-control precautions, frequent occupational exposure to persons at increased risk for HIV infection, and frequent accidental puncturing of the skin with sharp instruments, dental professionals are at low occupational risk for HIV infection.

Of interest to dentists, dental hygienists, and assistants.

833. KRACHMAN, Samuel, and Gilbert E. D'Alonza. "Acquired immunodeficiency syndrome and the health care worker." *Journal of the American Osteopathic Association* 88 (1988): 749-754.

Provides information for the osteopathic physician on the risks and prevention of HIV infection for the health care worker.

Descriptive

Physicians and health care workers must be informed and prepared to answer questions regarding the most effective methods to prevent the transmission of HIV to the health care worker. The physician must also be able to instruct the health care worker in the proper management of accidental parenteral and mucosal exposure to the blood and body fluids of a patient.

Of general interest to health care workers.

834. KUHLS, Thomas L., Susan Viker, Nancy B. Parris, Alice Garakian, John Sullivan-Bolyai, James D. Cherry. "Occupational risk of HIV, HBV and HSV-2 infections in health care personnel caring for AIDS patients." *American Journal of Public Health* 77 (1987): 1306-1309.

A prospective study of 246 female health care workers, some with high exposure, some with low exposure, and some with no exposure to AIDS patients.

Research

No health care workers had clinical, serologic, or immunologic evidence of HIV infection, and none seroconverted to cytomegalovirus. One health care worker in the high exposure group seroconverted to hepatitis B virus and another to herpes simplex virus type 2, although all three groups were similar with respect to hepatitis B virus and herpes simplex virus type 2 seropositivity.

Of interest to health care personnel, especially nurses, physicians, and other health professionals in direct patient care.

835. LEWIS, Charles E., and Howard E. Freeman. "The sexual history taking and counseling practices of primary care physicians." *Western Journal of Medicine* 147 (1987): 165-167.

As part of a statewide survey of experiences related to the acquired immunodeficiency syndrome and competencies of a random sample of primary care physicians in California, done in early 1986, 1000 internists, family, and general practitioners were interviewed about their sexual history-taking and counseling practices.

Research

Less than 4% have patients complete a history form that includes questions about sexual orientation or practices, and only 10% ask new patients questions specific enough to identify those at high risk of exposure to the HIV virus. Internists, women and younger physicians, and those expressing little discomfort in dealing with gay men more often took adequate sexual histories and gave appropriate advice. Among those physicians with patients at risk of becoming infected, only half recommended the use of condoms, and 60% advised a reduction in the number of partners. More than 15% recommended abstention from sexual intercourse, and 8% suggested these patients should switch to a heterosexual lifestyle.

Of interest to physicians and other health professionals.

836. LOSCHEN, D.J. "Protecting against HIV exposure in family practice." *American Family Physician* 37 (1988): 213-219.

Addresses the concerns of family physicians regarding the protection of health care workers from exposure to HIV, misconceptions about the possible modes of spread to these workers, and specific measures for protecting them.

Commentary/Guide

Primary care physicians, and particularly family physicians, are being called upon to provide more of the routine care of patients with AIDS or ARC. The prospect of assimilating these patients into their practices has become a source of concern, and, in some cases, unwarranted alarm among family physicians and their staffs. While physicians must ensure that reasonable precautions are taken to prevent accidental exposure to HIV, they also have the responsibility of educating themselves and their staffs so that the myths and misconceptions surrounding the epidemiology of AIDS will be minimized and patients can receive the care they need. Specific measure for the prevention of infection are described.

Of interest to primary care physicians.

837. MANTELL, Joanne E., Lawrence C. Schulman, Mary F. Belmont, Howard B. Spivak. "Social workers respond to the AIDS epidemic in an acute care hospital." *Health and Social Work* 14 (1989): 41-51.

Social work staff responsiveness to caring for people with AIDS, workload requirements, staff education and training, and the implications for social work organizational changes, program and service delivery, and psychosocial care of people with AIDS are presented.

Descriptive

The findings suggest the need for a more effective integration of social work clinical expertise, service design and delivery, health and social policy, and ethical codes of practice. Concomitant with the delivery of quality clinical services, social work's professional support of and advocacy for people with AIDS must continue to accelerate. Social workers must provide leadership in expanding resources for communities.

Of special interest to social workers.

838. MILLER, Patti J., and Barry M. Farr. "A survey of SHEA
      members on universal precautions and HIV screening."
      Infection Control and Hospital Epidemiology 9 (1988): 163-166.

Members attending a meeting of The Society of Hospital Epidemiologists
in October 1987 were surveyed to determine their opinions and their
hospitals' actual practices with regard to universal precautions
recommended by the CDC, HIV screening, and informed consent.

Research

Of 198 questionnaires distributed, 134 were returned, a response rate
of 68%. Respondents were from 121 different institutions in 36 states
and one foreign country. Results indicate that infection control
professionals overwhelmingly support the concept of universal
precautions applied to all patients, but support for elimination of
the category of blood and body fluids is modest (54%) and there is no
agreement as to how it should be accomplished. A majority of the
respondents oppose routine HIV screening of low-risk patients and
agree that when HIV testing is done, informed consent should be
obtained. Sixty-nine percent of the institutions represented have
adopted universal barrier precautions, at least 95% do not screen
routinely for HIV, and a majority require informed consent before
testing. The survey results are discussed.

Of interest to hospital personnel and public health officials.

839. MILNE, R.I.G., and S.M. Keen. "Are general practitioners
      ready to prevent the spread of HIV?" British Medical
      Journal 296 (1988): 533-535.

A survey of 196 general practitioners was carried out to assess their
readiness to undertake health education to prevent the spread of HIV
infection.

Research

One hundred and thirty-two physicians responded to the questionnaire.
Sixty-four of them expressed little interest in health education about
HIV.   Only 75 of them had initiated discussions about HIV with
patients. Moreover, many underestimated the risks from heterosexual
sex while exaggerating the risks from non-sexual contact.

Of interest to general practitioners, family physicians, and health
educators.

840. MOORE, Fredric A. "The dentist and AIDS." Journal of
      Prosthetic Dentistry 59 (1988): 236-241.

Provides basic information important to all health care personnel.

Review

Provides an overview of AIDS, including definitions; morbidity, mortality, and high risk groups; epidemiology and transmission; and needlestick injuries. Covers signs, symptoms, and diagnosis, and provides information on infection control for prevention of transmission, including clinical and laboratory precautions that are particularly appropriate for dentists.

Of particular interest to dentists, but may also be useful to other health care personnel.

841. PENZIEN, Donald B. "The acquired immunodeficiency syndrome (AIDS): Essential information for mental health practitioners." *Behavior Therapist* 6 (1986): 117-120.

Presents a brief summary of the essential information that mental health practitioners should know about AIDS.

Descriptive

The description and epidemiology of AIDS are given along with the pathogenesis, transmission, and medical treatment. In addition, psychosocial issues are briefly addressed. References for further reading are provided along with information on how to contact agencies offering support to AIDS patients.

Of interest to mental health professionals and counselors.

842. PETERMAN, Thomas A. Willard Cates, Jr., James W. Curran. "The challenge of human immunodeficiency virus (HIV) and acquired immunodeficiency syndrome (AIDS) in women and children." *Fertility and Sterility* 49 (1988): 571-581.

Discusses the need for everyone to learn about the modes of transmission of HIV.

Review

The number of AIDS cases will continue to increase for years, and, unless a cure is found, those who are infected with HIV will probably remain at risk for AIDS for their entire lives. For every person with AIDS, several more have ARC, and an even larger number are asymptomatic carriers. Everyone must learn about the modes of transmission, and physicians, in particular, need to learn about the disease so that they can care for the increasing numbers of HIV-infected patients and educate patients on ways to avoid infection. Physicians concerned with reproductive health care have a special interest in reducing HIV infection in women and decreasing perinatal transmission.

Of interest to physicians, particularly obstetricians and gynecologists.

843. ROYSE, David, and Barbara Birge. "Homophobia and attitudes
      towards   AIDS   patients   among   medical,   nursing,   and
      paramedical   students."   *Psychological   Reports* 61 (1987):
      867-870.

A study was undertaken to explore attitudes towards AIDS victims,
using an available sample of students training for health careers.

Research

For a previously developed 28-item questionnaire and a sample of
students training for careers in health professions, homophobia was
inversely associated with empathy for AIDS victims. Homophobia was
also a better predictor of fear of AIDS than age, sex, mental status,
or desired health career. It was concluded that students in the
health professions may need additional instruction related to AIDS and
homosexuality.

Of interest to educators in health professional schools.

844. SEARLE, E. Stephen. "Knowledge, attitudes, and behavior of
      health professionals in relation to AIDS."   *Lancet* 1,
      no. 8523 (1987): 26-28.

A survey of health professionals' knowledge, attitudes, and behavior
in relation to AIDS.

Research

The results demonstrate an eagerness to serotest patients, especially
those in high-risk groups, before hospital admission. Apart from
those professionals who wished to test their patients for safety
reasons, a sizeable proportion wished to identify seropositive
patients so as to refer them elsewhere. Staff education about HIV
infection is needed at all levels.

Of interest to health educators and health professionals in general.

845. SHANSON, D.C.   "Controversies about guidelines to prevent
      transmission of human immunodeficiency virus in hospitals in
      Britain."   *Journal of Hospital Infection* 11, Supplement A
      (1988): 218-222.

Summarizes the current risks of transmission of HIV in British
hospitals, and discusses some controversial issues that have been
proposed to protect health care workers and patients.

Review

Widespread screening of donors of blood, semen, and organs has contributed to prevention of the spread of HIV to patients in British
hospitals, and the chances of acquiring HIV from a transfusion are now
estimated at less than one in one million. The wider use of HIV

antibody tests to identify infected patients and rationalize additional precautions to protect staff is controversial. The risks of infection of hospital staff are very low if a high standard of hygiene is maintained and inoculation injuries are avoided. However, screening HIV antibody tests, preferably with consent, can help the smooth running of operating theaters in areas where many "high risk" patients require surgery, eliminating the need for unnecessary precautions when patients are HIV negative. All prenatal patients should be screened to prevent vertical transmission and facilitate the rational use of extra precautions to protect health care workers.

Of interest to health care workers and hospital administrators.

846. TREIBER, Frank A., Darlene Shaw, Robert Malcolm. "Acquired immune deficiency syndrome: Psychological impact on health personnel." *Journal of Nervous and Mental Disease* 175, no. 8 (1987): 496-499.

Eight nurses and four physicians responded to three self-report measures that assessed the psychological distress associated with caring for a patient with AIDS and for a matched non-AIDS patient.

Research

Increased anxiety, greater interference in non-work activities, more frequent negative ruminations, and more negative perceptions regarding the patient's behavior were experienced by the physicians and nurses while working with the AIDS patient than with the non-AIDS patient. Psychological and educational interventions are needed to reduce staff's fear and concerns when providing care to AIDS patients and to facilitate optimal care of AIDS patients.

Of interest to medical and nursing educators, mental health professionals, and health care providers and administrators.

847. UNITED States Public Health Service Centers for Disease Control. "Recommendations for prevention of HIV transmission in health-care settings." *Morbidity and Mortality Weekly Report* 36, S2 (1987): 3S-18S. Reprinted in *New York State Journal of Medicine* 88 (1988): 25-31.

The recommendations presented have been developed for use in health-care settings and emphasize the need to treat blood and other body fluids from all patients as potentially infective.

Guidelines

Presents universal precautions to prevent transmission of HIV, and discusses environmental considerations for HIV transmission, precautions to prevent transmission of HIV, and the management of infected health-care workers.

Of interest to all health care workers.

848. VLAHOV, David, and B. Frank Polk. "Transmission of human
     immunodeficiency virus within the health care setting."
     Occupational Medicine 2, no. 3 (1987): 429-450.

Reviews the epidemiology of HIV infection and evaluates the data
regarding the risk to health care workers.

Review

Discusses modes of transmission, risk of infection in health care
workers, prevention of transmission, and the management of infectious
waste, sterilization, and disinfection. Finally, the management of
health care workers with HIV infection or AIDS is discussed.

Of interest to health care administrators.

849. WALLACK, Joel J. "AIDS anxiety among health care profes-
     sionals." *Hospital and Community Psychiatry* 40 (1989):
     507-510.

In 1985, house staff physicians and nurses at a major New York City
teaching hospital completed a questionnaire designed to assess AIDS
anxiety, fear of contagion, and personal attitudes about
homosexuality.

Research

Sixty-three percent of 172 respondents did not believe assurances by
experts that health care workers were at minimal risk of contracting
AIDS if they observed safety guidelines. Minority respondents were
significantly less trusting and were more uncomfortable with
homosexual patients. Twenty-six percent of all respondents feared
that they would become victims of AIDS if they continued their work,
yet 97% expressed a firm commitment to caring for AIDS patients. The
author suggests that instructors in AIDS training and educational
programs for health care professionals should consider their cultural
backgrounds and psychosocial needs.

Of interest to health professions educators.

850. WHALEN, James P. "Participation of medical students in the
     care of patients with AIDS." *Journal of Medical Education* 62
     (1987): 53-54.

Discusses the responsibilities of medical students in regard to the
care of patients with AIDS.

Discussion

The author cites a case in which a third year medical student refused
to draw blood from an AIDS patient as an example of the need for a
policy addressing the issue of student responsibility. He states that
the real issue behind whether students should work with AIDS patients

is whether they are professional enough to subject themselves to the unknown risks attendant on being a health care professional. Medical students, like licensed professionals, must display the essential professional characteristics of any fully qualified health care worker. It therefore follows that students should be expected to work with patients with AIDS and to perform all procedures commensurate with their technical skills.

Of interest to medical students and medical educators.

851. "WHAT are your odds of getting AIDS from patients?" *Emergency Medicine* 19, no. 16 (1987): 68-74, 79-85.

Discusses the risk to the primary care physician of being infected by patients who are HIV positive.

Commentary

Studies have shown the actual risk of infection when treating HIV positive patients is very low, considerably less than that of such diseases as hepatitis B. However, since it does exist, the precautions recommended by the CDC should be taken. While the physician should not overreact, thereby promoting undue hysteria, neither should he/she minimize the risk. It is unnecessary to wear protective clothing unless particular medical procedures justify doing so, but the physician should be aware of his/her own physical condition and take such sensible precautions as protecting chapped hands from contact with body fluids.

Of interest to all clinicians.

852. WILEY, Katherine, Linda Heath, Marvin Acklin. "Care of AIDS patients: Student attitudes." *Nursing Outlook* 36 (1988): 244-245.

A questionnaire was developed to identify curricular changes in nursing necessitated by the AIDS epidemic.

Research

Graduate nurses and junior and senior undergraduate nursing students did not differ in their worry about exposure to HIV or their use of protective measures. More than half of the students felt that health care workers should be allowed to refuse to treat seropositive patients.

Of special interest to nurse educators.

c. Dissertation

853. KAGAN, Lois S. Levine. Baccalaureate nursing students' attitudes toward patients with acquired immunodeficiency syndrome. Ed.D. dissertation. Columbia University Teachers College, 1986.

The attitudes of baccalaureate nursing students toward patients who acquired AIDS in three different ways were investigated.

Research

The intravenous drug user was evaluated significantly more negatively than the other patients. The intravenous drug user was significantly more fear-producing than the homosexual. The homosexual was rated significantly less potent than the blood transfusion recipient with AIDS and than the patient without AIDS. Thus, the mode of transmission was a significant independent variable.

Of particular interest to nursing educators and nurses caring for AIDS patients.

6. SCHOOLS

a. Books

854.   FLYNN, Eileen P.   *Teaching About AIDS*.   Kansas City, MO: Sheed & Ward, 1988.

A practical guide for teaching young people about AIDS.

Guidebook

Divided into two sections: background material that teachers need to understand before they can instruct students about AIDS; and a collection of lesson plans and materials which can be used in teaching about AIDS. There are lesson plans for use with parents as well as lesson plans for students in grades 6-8 and 9-12.

Written for the classroom teacher.

855.   KAUS, Danek, and Robert D. Reed.   *Teaching About AIDS: A Teacher's Guide*.   Saratoga, CA: R & E, 1987.

A guide to help teachers with pertinent, factual, and valuable information and resources in educating children about AIDS.

Text

Contains vital information that teachers and administrators must share with their students. Explains the nature of the disease, how it is transmitted, and the course of action that each individual must take to ensure his or her own safety. Also included are recommendations from public health officials for dealing with AIDS victims in the schools and a list of resources for further study and research for any teacher or student who wishes to investigate this disease and its global implications in greater depth.

A guide for teachers in junior high and high schools.

856. KEOUGH, Katherine E. *Dealing with AIDS: Breaking the Chain of Infection.* Arlington, VA: American Association of School Administrators, 1988.

Intended to stimulate and provide a framework for local discussion leading to the development of an AIDS education program consistent with local needs and standards.

Booklet/Guide

Sets out ways to develop an AIDS education program, describes the purposes of an AIDS education program, lists criteria for evaluating an AIDS education program, and presents sample learner outcomes. Sample lesson plans are provided for early elementary school, middle school, junior high, and high school. A glossary and list of resources are presented.

For school administrators and teachers.

857. KIRP, David L., with Steven Epstein, Marlene Strong Franks, Jonathan Simon, Douglas Conaway, John Lewis. *Learning by Heart: AIDS and Schoolchildren in America's Communities.* New Brunswick, NJ: Rutgers University Press, 1989.

A series of closely linked stories about AIDS, communities, and children.

Social History

Scientific evidence regarding casual transmission of AIDS suggests the risk of spreading AIDS in the classroom or the schoolyard to be infinitesimally small. However, small is not nonexistent; knowing that life is full of risks, people must calculate the risks to which their children are to be exposed and consider the lessons they wish their children to be taught. Faced with the prospect of HIV infected children or children with AIDS attending local schools, some towns turn themselves into communities of exclusion, while others become communities of openness. This book tells the true stories of infected schoolchildren in seven different American towns or cities and of the ways that the communities in which they live responded to their presence.

Of interest to a general audience.

858. QUACKENBUSH, Marcia, and Pamela Sargent. *Teaching AIDS: A Resource Guide on Acquired Immune Deficiency Syndrome.* Santa Cruz, CA: Network Publications, 1986.

A curriculum for teaching middle and high school students about AIDS.

Resource Book

Designed to help teachers, effectively and thoroughly, to present teenagers with accurate information about AIDS. Divided into four sections: the curriculum, teaching plans, teaching materials, and background materials.

A valuable guide for high school and middle school teachers.

859. WACHTER, Oralee.   *Sex, Drugs, & AIDS: A Candid and Practical Guide.* **New York:** Bantam, 1987.

A concise, illustrated text, based on the film of the same name, to provide young people with accurate, clear, and honest information about AIDS.

Text

Answers questions, which young people may ask, about what AIDS is, how it is and is not spread, who is at risk, and how it can be prevented. Concludes with a list of available information resources.

A useful textbook for teenagers and young adults.

860. WEINER, Roberta.   *AIDS: Impact on the Schools.*   Arlington, VA: Education Research Group, Capital Publications, 1986.

A special report, designed to clear up the misconceptions about AIDS.

Text

The seven chapters cover AIDS facts, the effect of AIDS on schools, AIDS litigation, policies about AIDS in the school and workplace, and problems facing colleges and universities in dealing with AIDS. Recommendations are scattered throughout the book to help schools and administrators deal with AIDS.

Of special interest to educators and administrators of schools and colleges.

861. YARBER, William L.   *AIDS Education: Curriculum and Health Policy.*   Bloomington, IN: Phi Delta Kappan Educational Foundation, 1987.

Designed to provide educators with some guidelines for developing an AIDS curriculum and for formulating school health policies about AIDS.

Pamphlet

In the absence of a vaccine, preventive educational programs are the best defense against the spread of AIDS. The risk of AIDS for young people is high, since many adolescents are sexually active and use IV drugs. Information about ways to protect their health should be given to students in school before they unknowingly make behavioral choices that put them at risk for AIDS. It is also imperative that all schools adopt policies for handling persons with AIDS attending school. Covered in this booklet are: background information on AIDS; an approach for teaching about AIDS; instructor qualifications for AIDS education; community involvement in AIDS education; and school health policies for persons with AIDS.

Of interest to teachers, school administrators and policymakers, and school health personnel.

b. Articles

862. ALDRIDGE, Jerry, Gypsy Clayton, Rhoda Chalker. "AIDS education and policies among Southern Baptist church leaders in the state of Texas." *Psychological Reports* 64 (1989): 493-494.

During a statewide meeting on AIDS of the Southern Baptist Convention of Texas, a survey was conducted to assess the knowledge and attitudes of preschool and children's church school directors.

Research

After attending a three day program on AIDS, more than 90% of the 67 participants correctly answered 14 of 15 knowledge items and exhibited positive attitudes. No pre-test was reported. Although 90% believed that AIDS education should be provided in public schools, only 50% believed it was appropriate in Sunday schools. Forty of the participants completed a second survey on policies regarding AIDS. All indicated that their churches had no policy for admitting children with AIDS to their programs, and only 15% indicated that discussion had been held about the development of such policies.

Of interest to church educators and administrators and health educators.

863. ALLENSWORTH, Diane DeMuth, and Cynthia Wolford Symons. "A theoretical approach to school-based HIV prevention." *Journal of School Health* 59 (1989): 59-65.

Describes a proactive, educationally sound approach to school-based AIDS education.

Descriptive

To develop effective school-based programs to prevent the spread of AIDS, programmers must apply principles related to learning and behavior change and use a multidisciplinary approach. Health promotion efforts should include policy mandates, direct intervention, instruction, environmental support, media, role modeling, and social support. Consistent, continuous messages through multiple channels and by multiple agents need to be provided. Examples of appropriate intervention strategies that may be employed by professionals working in the school and the community are provided.

Of interest to educators, school administrators, parents, and public policymakers.

864. BLACK, Jeffrey L. "AIDS: Preschool and school issues." *Journal of School Health* 56 (1986): 93-95.

Reviews the epidemiological, clinical, and public health aspects of AIDS in the pediatric population, emphasizing modes of transmission, and presents guidelines to assist school staff in the educational management of children infected with HIV.

Review

AIDS challenges the health education resources of school health professionals. Fear and misinformation regarding AIDS transmission are rampant in the general population, and school boards, teachers, and parents have responded inappropriately to AIDS-afflicted students. Children also lack sufficient information about AIDS. Informed school health personnel can play an important role in correcting misconceptions about HIV infection. Heightened public interest in children with AIDS provides the impetus for school-based programs of community education. Accurate knowledge and appropriate beliefs about AIDS can be promoted through in-service education for staff and appropriate health education curricula for students. Medically sound policy decisions could be promoted by periodic provision of the latest scientific information to members of school boards and administrations.

Of interest to school health educators, teachers, and administrators.

865. BOWER, Wilma, Kay Kane, Alice West.   "Infectious diseases: Current issues in school and community health." *Thrust* 16, no. 3 (1986): 15-20.

Discusses infectious diseases, including AIDS, and the need for schools to teach primary disease prevention.

Descriptive

Gives information about the transmission, symptoms, incubation, and treatment of AIDS, hepatitis A and B, cytomegalovirus, and herpes simplex, types I and II. Advocates teaching students and staff about good health practices, maintaining a sanitary school environment, and requiring special accommodations for those who do not practice proper hygiene. Warns school officials about legal liabilities.

Of interest to school administrators and teachers.

866. BROWN, J.S., W.G. Irwin, K. Steele, R.W. Harland. "Students' awareness of and attitudes to AIDS." *Journal of the Royal College of General Practitioners* 37, no. 303 (1987): 457-458.

Students' attitudes to and knowledge and awareness of AIDS were assessed by questionnaire.

Research

Students between the ages of 18 and 24 were generally aware that AIDS was not associated with social contact, but there was confusion about the risk of infection from donating or receiving blood. Most of the students were aware that the condom reduces the risk of the spread of AIDS sexually, but there was no indication of widespread condom use among the students who admitted they were sexually active. Almost half of the sample wished to have their blood tested for the AIDS virus. A high proportion of the sample believed that AIDS victims should be cared for at home or in a special hospice.

Of special interest to high school, college, and health educators.

867. CARUSO, Barbara Ann, and John R. Haig. "AIDS on campus: A survey of college health service priorities and policies." *Journal of American College Health* 36 (1987): 33-36.

Health service departments from 47 Philadelphia area colleges were surveyed concerning 1) their judgment of how campus AIDS programs should really be run, and 2) their institutions' current activities related to the AIDS situation.

Research

Respondents expressed a clear preference for providing AIDS education to on-campus groups over those less centrally related to the campus. Respondents also expressed strong approval for providing special on-campus counseling for "risk groups," but preferred to refer individuals off campus for medical testing. There were discrepancies between respondents' conceptualization of an ideal AIDS program and what had actually occurred on these campuses to date. Approximately two-thirds of these institutions had received professional AIDS-related guidelines, established a campus AIDS task force, purchased and/or distributed brochures to the campus community, and expressed interest in joining an AIDS coalition.

Of interest to college administrators and health educators.

868. CENTERS For Disease Control, Center for Health Promotion and Education. "Guidelines for effective school health education to prevent the spread of AIDS." *Journal of School Health* 58 (1988): 142-148.

Guidelines for persons who are responsible for planning and implementing appropriate and effective strategies for teaching young people how to avoid HIV infection.

Descriptive

Guidelines are offered regarding the preparation of education personnel; the purpose and content of AIDS education in early elementary school, middle school, and senior high school; curriculum time and resources; and program assessment.

Of interest to health educators and school administrators.

869. DiCLEMENTE, Ralph J. "Prevention of immunodeficiency virus infection among adolescents: The interplay of health education and public policy in the development and implementation of school-based AIDS education programs." *AIDS Education and Prevention* 1, no. 1 (1989): 70-76.

Presents the rationale and scope of school-based AIDS education.

Commentary

The prevalence rates of pregnancy and sexually transmitted diseases among adolescents indicate that a coordinated, systematic school-based education program is needed. HIV prevention programs should include standardized curricula, adequate teacher training, and short and long-term evaluation. Curricula should be age-appropriate, culturally sensitive, and adaptable to local needs. Although adolescents cannot be coerced into behavior change, they may reduce or eliminate high-risk behaviors if provided with developmentally appropriate HIV information.

Of interest to school boards, teachers, and administrators; parents; and public policymakers.

870. ———, Cherrie B. Boyer, Edward S. Morales. "Minorities and AIDS: Knowledge, attitudes, and misconceptions among black and Latino adolescents." *American Journal of Public Health* 78 (1988): 55-57.

Data were collected from 261 white, 226 black, and 141 Latino adolescents in the San Francisco Unified School District as part of a needs assessment of knowledge about the cause, transmission, and treatment of AIDS.

Research

White adolescents were more knowledgeable than blacks, and blacks were more knowledgeable than Latinos about the cause, transmission, and prevention of AIDS. Black and Latino adolescents were twice as likely as whites to have misconceptions about the casual transmission of AIDS. Less knowledge and prevalent misconceptions about AIDS were associated with greater levels of perceived risk of contracting the disease.

Of interest to educators in general and health educators in particular and to public health professionals.

871. ———, Cheri A. Pies, Elizabeth J. Stoller, Christie Straits, Geraldine E. Olivia, Joan Haskin, George W. Rutherford. "Evaluation of school-based AIDS education curricula in San Francisco." *Journal of Sex Research* 26 (1989): 188-198.

Three hundred and eighty-five students in three middle schools and 254 students in three high schools in San Francisco participated in the evaluation of an AIDS education curriculum.

Research

Classes within schools were designated as either intervention or nonintervention classes. Students in intervention classes received three class periods of AIDS instruction with a newly developed curriculum, while students in nonintervention classes received no special AIDS instruction. All students completed a pretest and posttest AIDS knowledge and attitude survey. Results indicated that AIDS instruction classes demonstrated significantly greater knowledge than nonintervention classes, as well as a change in attitudes (e.g., reflecting greater tolerance for attending class with AIDS or HIV infected students).

Of interest to educators and school administrators.

872. ———, Jim Zorn, Lydia Temoshok. "Adolescents and AIDS: A survey of knowledge, attitudes, and beliefs about AIDS in San Francisco." *American Journal of Public Health* 76 (1986): 1443-1445.

To assess adolescents' knowledge, attitudes, and behavior about AIDS, data were obtained from 1,326 adolescents in San Francisco.

Research

There was a marked variability in knowledge across informational items, particularly about the precautionary measures to be taken during sexual intercourse that may reduce the risk of infection. The authors conclude that development and implementation of school health education programs on AIDS and other sexually transmitted diseases are needed for this population.

Of interest to health educators, school teachers, and public health officials.

873. DORMAN, Steven M., and Barbara A. Rienzo. "College students' knowledge of AIDS." *Health Values* 12, no. 4 (1988): 33-38.

University students enrolled in health classes were asked to respond to a series of AIDS-related knowledge and attitude questions and to rate themselves on a "worry index."

Research

While the level of knowledge of students is better than in previous surveys, a major gap in knowledge of particular AIDS issues continues to exist. Prejudicial inclinations towards AIDS-related attitude statements were also found to exist. Students' level of worry was stronger for AIDS than for any other health condition mentioned.

Of special interest to university and college administrators, teachers, and health educators.

874. FLYGARE, Thomas J. "Judge orders children with AIDS virus back into the classroom." *Phi Delta Kappan* 69 (1988): 381-382.

Reports a significant legal decision regarding the admission of HIV positive children to the classroom.

Case Report

After Robert, Richard, and Randy Ray were excluded from the classrooms of two different communities when school officials were informed that the three young hemophiliacs tested positive for HIV although all were asymptomatic, their parents filed suit in U.S. district court. U.S. District Court Judge Elizabeth Kovachevich issued an injunction returning the children to the classroom with a series of restrictions on their personal conduct, which would minimize the possibility of risk to others. Although this case represents a significant legal precedent with respect to the placement of students infected with HIV in regular public school classrooms, this will continue to be a difficult area of law and public policy as long as the epidemic of AIDS continues to spread and the accompanying fear and prejudice continue to intensify. Coping with the problem will require sensitivity and respect for the rights of everyone involved, tolerance, diplomacy, and courage on the part of school officials.

Of interest to educators, school administrators, lawyers, and policymakers.

875. FORREST, Jacqueline Darroch, and Jane Silverman. "What public school teachers teach about preventing pregnancy, AIDS and sexually transmitted diseases." *Family Planning Perspectives* 21, no. 2 (1989): 65-72.

Reports on a survey of American teachers to determine the extent and content of sex education in the public schools.

Research

Of 9,800 public school teachers of biology, health education, home economics, physical education, and school nursing in grades seven to 12, 93% reported that sex education or AIDS education was offered in their schools. Almost all believed prevention of pregnancy, AIDS, and other sexually transmitted diseases should be taught in the public schools no later than in grades seven to eight. However, sex education usually is not offered before the eight grade. Virtually all of the teachers believed that sexual decision making, abstinence, and birth control methods should be taught, but only about 82% worked in schools that included those topics in the curriculum. Birth control was the subject least likely to be taught.

Of interest to teachers, administrators, public health officials, and policymakers.

876. FREIMUTH, Vicki S., Timothy Edgar, Sharon L. Hammond. "College students' awareness and interpretation of the AIDS risk." *Science, Technology, & Human Values* 12, no. 60 & 61 (1987): 37-40.

Reports data providing insight on the attitudes of college students concerning their own risk of HIV infection and need for risk reduction behavior change.

Research

A questionnaire was sent to 1250 randomly selected students at the University of Maryland's College Park campus. The 458 (approximately 37%) who responded, when compared to the entire university population, were found to be a fairly representative sample. Results suggest that most students are knowledgeable about AIDS, but there is little personalization of risk or behavior change as a result of this knowledge. Certain sources of information, such as the gay community, are not trusted by students. Students rate the chances of infection with HIV during a single unprotected encounter higher than is actually probable, but rate their own risk as very low, while experts believe college students to be a potentially high risk group. The vast majority of students have not been tested for antibodies to HIV. The importance of getting baseline data about a target audience before developing risk reduction strategies is pointed out.

Of interest to health educators, college educators, and public health professionals.

877. GOODWIN, Megan P. "AIDS: Students' knowledge and attitudes at a Midwestern university." *Journal of American College Health* 36 (1988): 214-222.

To understand the educational needs and concerns of young people better, 495 college students were surveyed and their knowledge and attitudes concerning AIDS and the relationships between their acceptance of homosexual behavior and their knowledge and fear of AIDS were examined.

Research

Results suggest these college students possess moderate knowledge regarding AIDS prevalence, high-risk groups, modes of transmission, and symptoms. They demonstrate some concern (fear) about the transmission of AIDS and are highly nonaccepting of homosexual behavior. More males than females were found to possess negative attitudes toward homosexuality, and those who were highly accepting of homosexual behavior were least fearful of contracting AIDS.

Of interest to college administrators and health educators.

878. "GUIDELINES for effective school health education to prevent the spread of AIDS." *Morbidity and Mortality Weekly Report* 37, no. S-2 (January 29, 1988): 1-14.

Guidelines have been developed to help school personnel and others plan, implement, and evaluate educational efforts to prevent unnecessary morbidity and mortality associated with AIDS and other HIV-related illnesses.

Special Issue/Descriptive

The guidelines provide information that should be considered by persons who are responsible for planning and implementing appropriate and effective strategies to teach young people about how to avoid HIV infection. These guidelines are not rules, but rather a source of guidance.

Of special interest to school administrators, teachers, and health educators.

879. HAFFNER, Debra W. "AIDS and adolescents: School health education must begin now." *Journal of School Health* 58 (1988): 154-155.

An appeal for school health education programs to educate adolescents about AIDS.

Descriptive

Discusses teenagers' risk of infection. Existing school-based AIDS education programs are inadequate. AIDS education should be integrated into existing comprehensive health or sexuality education programs, and should emphasize how AIDS is transmitted, how AIDS is not transmitted, and how to protect oneself from HIV.

Of interest to health educators.

880. HAVEN, Grant G., and Jeffrey W. Stolz. "Students teaching AIDS to students: Addressing AIDS in the adolescent population." *Public Health Reports* 104 (1989): 75-79.

Describes a project called Students Teaching AIDS to Students (STATS), which was designed to help medical students educate teenagers in schools, churches, and youth organizations about AIDS.

Descriptive

The proposed project involves the preparation and distribution of a package of materials that can be used by medical students to initiate a STATS program. Included are a manual, which explains how to start a youth health education project and how to gain community support, and age-appropriate curricula, tailored for presentation to students over two school-class periods, with basic AIDS information and exercises. Also included are a slide show for explaining STATS to school boards, parent groups, and the leaders of other youth organizations, other audiovisual material, reference articles, and sample press releases. The program is available through the Americal Medical Student Association.

Of interest to medical students, teachers, school administrators, and health educators.

881. HELGERSON, Steven D., Lyle R. Petersen, and the AIDS Education Study Group. "Acquired immunodeficiency syndrome and secondary school students: Their knowledge is limited and they want to learn more." *Pediatrics* 81 (1988): 350-355.

A survey regarding the knowledge of AIDS of 657 junior and senior high school students was conducted in two Connecticut school districts.

Research

Most students had some factual knowledge about the AIDS virus, but many were misinformed about methods of transmission, high risk groups, and methods of avoiding infection, and most did not recognize the existence of a carrier state. Responses of students of different grades, ages, sexes, races, and school districts differed rarely and without apparent pattern. Students reported learning about AIDS from television or radio (57%), magazines or newspapers (16%), parents (6%), or teachers (4%). Seventy-four percent of students said they wanted to learn more about AIDS, and 49% said they wanted to learn it in school. Results indicate that students' knowledge about AIDS is inadequate, students wish to learn more, and information about AIDS should be presented in public schools.

Of interest to educators and school administrators.

882. HORAN, Patricia F., and Ronald A. Sherman. "School psychologists and the AIDS epidemic." *Professional School Psychology* 3 (1988): 33-49.

Provides an overview of what is known about AIDS, AIDS transmissibility, and the modes of transmission.

Review

The impact of the AIDS epidemic on the nation's school systems and the importance of AIDS education in altering the course of the epidemic are described. The opportunity and responsibility for school psychologists to assume leadership positions in this crisis, and possible psychoeducational interventions and research topics, are discussed.

Of interest to school psychologists.

883. HOWLAND, Jonathan, Diane Baker, Julie Johnson, James Scaramucci. "Teaching about AIDS in public schools: Characteristics of early adopter communities in Massachusetts." *New York State Journal of Medicine* 88 (1988): 62-65.

This study attempted to determine whether or not there are attitudes that would predict the likelihood of a community's integrating AIDS information into the public school curriculum.

Research

The authors conclude that there are other factors, as yet unidenti-
fied, that explain why some towns teach about AIDS while others do
not. Further research is necessary.

Of interest to educators, especially those in public schools.

884. ISHII-KUNTZ, Masako.   "Acquired immune deficiency syndrome
      and sexual behavior changes in a college student sample."
      Sociology and Social Research 73 (1988): 13-15.

Reports on a study conducted at the University of California, River-
side examining how knowledge and concern about AIDS affect perceived
change in sexual behavior among a sample of undergraduate college
students.

Research

Results indicate that students' concern about AIDS is strongly related
to their perceived change in sexual behavior. However, more accurate
knowledge of sexual transmission does not seem to encourage such
change. Encouraging students to practice "safe sex" involves raising
their concern by means of formal or informal information. Prevention
efforts should be directed, not only to provide an accurate knowledge
about AIDS, but to increase students' concern about AIDS transmission.

Of interest to health educators and public health officials.

885. JOHNSON, Jeffrey A., J. Frank Sellew, Ann E. Campbell,
      Edward G. Haskell, Aaron A. Gay, Brian J. Bell.   "A
      program using medical students to teach high school
      students about AIDS."   *Journal of Medical Education* 63
      (1988): 522-530.

Describes a pilot program, in Norfolk, Virginia, in which 20 medical
students taught high school students about AIDS.

Descriptive

All participating high school seniors completed a 15-item knowledge
test about AIDS prior to the intervention and an equivalent post test
after the program was completed. T-test analysis revealed a significant increase in knowledge by students at all five high schools.
Responses to 10 subjective post test questions indicated that the high
school students were interested in learning about AIDS and having
medical students as their teachers.

Of interest to school administrators, medical students, medical
educators, and other health professionals.

886. *JOURNAL of School Health* 58, no. 8 (1988): 311-347.

Devoted to AIDS education in the schools.

Special Journal Issue

Following a summary of the results of the American School Health Association's AIDS Education Needs Assessment, this special issue contains five articles dealing with AIDS education in the schools, a commentary on the consequences of the AIDS crisis for the health education profession, techniques for teaching about AIDS and the immune system, and an article on the impact of AIDS on school health services.

Of interest to school administrators, teachers, health service personnel, and health educators.

887. KANE, William M. "The physician and AIDS in the schools." *Journal of the American Osteopathic Association* 88 (1988): 634-636.

Provides the physician with information regarding health curricula and resources that commonly exist in schools.

Descriptive

Outcome objectives, teaching and learning strategies, and material for implementing a five-day, school-based AIDS education program are identified. Guidelines and recommendations to assist in preparing for the role of "guest speaker" in the schools are suggested.

Of interest to health educators and physicians engaged in AIDS education.

888. KANN, Laura, Gary D. Nelson, Jack T. Jones, Lloyd J. Kolbe. "Establishing a system of complementary school-based surveys to annually assess HIV-related knowledge, beliefs, and behaviors among adolescents." *Journal of School Health* 59 (1989): 55-58.

Describes a cooperative effort to develop a data base for planning an effective HIV education program for youth living in areas with a high incidence of AIDS.

Descriptive

In 1987, 14 states and nine local education agencies serving areas with a high incidence of AIDS worked with the CDC to develop a common set of data items to be used in assessing HIV-related knowledge, beliefs, and behaviors among adolescents. Surveys were administered in 1988 to representative samples of adolescents in each partici-pating state and city. The results from this complementary system of school-based surveys will be used as a guide in planning HIV educa-tion, setting program priorities, allocating resources, and monitoring cognitive and behavioral change.

Of interest to educators, school administrators, and public health professionals.

889. KEELING, Richard P.   "Risk communication about AIDS in
     higher education." *Science, Technology, & Human Values* 12,
     no. 60 & 61 (1987): 26-36.

Discusses the importance of education as the primary response of higher education to the AIDS epidemic, the issues that bear on AIDS education on college campuses, and the important features of AIDS education programs.

Review

College and university students are at particular risk for the transmission of HIV, and institutes of higher education have the responsibility of protecting their students by helping them to assess and reduce their risk of HIV infection. Many have implemented AIDS education activities combining the building of awareness with the acceptance of risk in order to motivate changes in behavior. The role of education in preventing HIV infection, effective risk reduction education, and the risk to the institution that is incorporated in the decision to educate about AIDS and in the resulting risk reduction program are discussed.   The author suggests that colleges and universities assess and address the concerns and fears of those who govern and fund them and aggressively market the need for AIDS education and the explorational programming it requires in a manner that clarifies its place within the overall goals of the institution.

Of interest to college and university educators and to health educators.

890. KENNEY, Asta M., Sandra Guardado, Lisanne Brown.   "Sex
     education and AIDS education in the schools: What states
     and large school districts are doing."   *Family Planning
     Perspectives* 21, no. 2 (1989): 56-64.

All of the states and 203 large school districts in the United States were surveyed to determine the extent and nature of AIDS and sex education in the public schools.

Research

Support for sex education and AIDS instruction was strong. About 80% of the states and 90% of the large school districts either require or encourage sex education in the public schools. All but four states, and virtually every large school district, support the provision of instruction about AIDS and sexually transmitted diseases. Encouragement of sexual abstinence is generally recommended. Fewer states and districts (two-thirds and four-fifths, respectively) require or encourage the schools to teach about pregnancy prevention. Districts also offer local educators more support (through curricula, training, and other activities) than do states. AIDS education is better funded by states and local school districts than is sex education.

Of interest to school administrators, teachers, school nurses, and health policymakers.

891. KEOUGH, Katherine E., and George Seaton. "Superintendents' views on AIDS: A national survey." *Phi Delta Kappan* 69 (1988): 358-361.

A survey of school administrators, focusing on their attitudes towards and perceptions of the AIDS crisis.

Research

Results indicated that school administrators are not well-equipped, at the present time, to deal with the AIDS crisis. School administrators are much less inclined to endorse mandatory testing for AIDS than either current federal officials or the general public. Superintendents said that their districts should have a policy on AIDS, should help students who seek information on AIDS testing, should work closely with community health agencies to meet the needs of students with AIDS, and should include AIDS education in their curricula.

Of interest to teachers and school administrators.

892. KING, Alan J.C., Richard P. Beazley, Wendy K. Warren, Catherine A. Hankins, Alan S. Robertson, Joyce L. Radford. "Highlights from the Canada Youth and AIDS Study." *Journal of School Health* 59 (1989): 139-145.

Summarizes findings from a national study to determine the knowledge, attitudes, and behavior regarding AIDS and sexually transmitted diseases of 38,000 Canadians in grades 7, 9, 11, and the first year of college.

Research

Most young Canadians know how HIV is transmitted, but only one quarter of those who are sexually active protect themselves most of the time by using condoms and spermicides. Dropouts and street youth are the group most uninformed about AIDS and most likely to take risks. Mass media is the major source of information about AIDS, but schools are the major source of information about other STDs. A considerable proportion of young people indicated that they have negative feelings toward people with HIV infection. Recommendations for education and further research are given.

Of interest to educators, school administrators, and public health officials.

893. KIRP, David L., and Steven Epstein. "AIDS in America's schoolhouses: Learning the hard lessons." *Phi Delta Kappan* 70 (1989): 585-593.

Uses the examples of two different communities' attitudes towards AIDS to illustrate the debate between isolation and openness in America's classrooms with respect to AIDS.

Descriptive/Analytical

Contrasts two different community models. Ocilla, Georgia has defined itself as a community of isolation; for them, AIDS is to be avoided and the virus and those who have it are to be contained. The Chicago neighborhood served by Pilsen Academy has proved to be a model of openness; for them, the solution to the AIDS crisis lies in education, individual empowerment, collective decision-making, and an ethic of cooperation.

Of interest to educators, public school administrators, and teachers.

894. KJOLLER, Susanne, Bente Hansen, Erling Segest. "Free condoms in the schools of Copenhagen, Denmark." *Journal of School Health* 59 (1989): 66-68.

A questionnaire assessing attitudes toward using condoms as a preventive measure against AIDS was administered to 438 ninth grade students and 28 teachers in Copenhagen.

Research

Results demonstrated that messages regarding safe sex were well understood. However, 42% of the sexually active students reported not using condoms during their last sexual intercourse, and many indicated difficulty in using condoms, suggesting that a continuing need exists for advice to the young. An information campaign with distribution of free condoms was well accepted by students and teachers. Almost all (94%) pupils indicated they will use condoms more frequently in the future. Pupils suggested that free condoms be available where advice can be obtained, and teachers suggested distributing them at discotheques.

Of interest to educators, school administrators, and school board members.

895. KOOP, C. Everett. "Teaching children about AIDS." *Issues in Science and Technology* 4 (1987): 67-70.

The Surgeon General's view on AIDS education and prevention.

Commentary

In the absence of a vaccine or any miracle drug to stop AIDS, the best thing society can do to contain this epidemic is to present scientifically accurate and personally sensitive information about AIDS to our children. The objective is to make them a lot more responsible in their relationships than their elders have been. In fact, before AIDS education begins, every child should be given information relative to his or her own sexuality.

Of interest to the general public, health professionals, and, in particular, teachers and school administrators.

896. LANDEFELD, C. Seth, Mary-Margaret Chren, Judith Shega, Theodore Speroff, Edward McGuire. "Students' sexual behavior, knowledge, and attitudes relating to the acquired immunodeficiency syndrome." *Journal of General Internal Medicine* 3 (1988): 161-165.

Five hundred and ninety students receiving primary care in a university health service were surveyed anonymously in 1985-1986 to determine their self-reported sexual behavior and knowledge and attitudes about AIDS.

Research

Most students (75%) were heterosexual and 32% had two or more sexual partners in the past year. Only 23% had changes their sexual prac- tices because of AIDS. Some students who engaged in high risk sexual behavior were not very knowledgeable. Overall, less knowledgeable students had more personal concerns about AIDS. The authors conclude that many students receiving primary care engage in sexual behavior that could spread HIV, and less knowledgeable students have particular concerns and attitudes about AIDS.

Of interest to health educators, student health staff, and educators.

897. LAREAU, Annette P., and Llewellyn Hendrix. "The spread of AIDS among heterosexuals: A classroom simulation." *Teaching Sociology* 15 (1987): 316-319.

A classroom simulation was designed to teach students about the transmission of the AIDS virus, particularly in the heterosexual population.

Descriptive

An evaluation one week after the simulation showed that students' attitudes were generally positive. Almost three-fourths felt that it had stimulated their thinking on AIDS as a public health problem and had heightened their awareness of their own chances of getting AIDS. Nearly four-fifths agreed that the stimulation was interesting; even more said it was helpful in visualizing the spread of AIDS. A few students felt awkward and embarrassed by the simulation, and a few found the simulation confusing.

Of interest to college teachers of the social and behavioral sciences.

898. McDERMOTT, Robert J., Michele J. Hawkins, John R. Moore, Susan K. Cittadino. "AIDS awareness and information sources among selected university students." *Journal of American College Health* 35 (1987): 222-226.

A questionnaire to assess knowledge of and sources of information about AIDS was constructed and distributed to 161 selected university students.

Research

Overall knowledge of AIDS-related facts was high, but 37.3% of the sample was unclear about AIDS' lethal potential, 35.4% did not recognize AIDS-associated opportunistic diseases, and 31.7% did not relate risk of contracting AIDS with indiscriminate sexual behavior. The three leading reported sources of AIDS information were television, newspapers, and magazines, respectively; no respondent cited "physicians" as the major source. Although media attention to AIDS abounds, certain misconceptions still are held by young adults.

Of interest to educators and public health officials.

899. MILLER, Leslie. "AIDS: What you and your friends need to know--a lesson plan for adolescents." *Journal of School Health* 58 (1988): 137-141.

The AIDS knowledge and attitudes of students attending an urban high school in Seattle were pretested and posttested after an intervention.

Research

Significant increases in knowledge about AIDS, and parallel changes in tolerant and compassionate beliefs about people with AIDS were observed. Learning outcomes were retained at retesting eight weeks after instruction.

Of interest to high school teachers, school officials, and health educators.

900. PRICE, James H., Sharon Desmond, Gary Kukulka. "High school students' perceptions and misperceptions of AIDS." *Journal of School Health* 55, no. 3 (1985): 107-109.

Examines the knowledge, beliefs, and sources of information of junior and senior high school students concerning AIDS.

Research

A convenience sample of 118 male and 132 female students, 16 to 19 years of age, from four local high schools were administered a 29-item questionnaire on AIDS. Results indicated that the students had a very limited knowledge of AIDS, although the males were more knowledgeable than the females, and the majority were not concerned about contracting the disease. The primary sources of information were TV, newspapers, magazines, and radio. Schools were mentioned least often as a source of information.

Should interest educators in general and health educators in particular as well as public health professionals.

901. REED, Sally. "Children with AIDS: How schools are handling the crisis." *Phi Delta Kappan* 69 (1988): K1-K12.

Discusses how various school districts have responded to the admission of children with AIDS to the classroom, and why public schools must be involved in dealing with the AIDS problem.

Review/Commentary

Some school systems have rejected children with AIDS until placed under court order, while others have quietly and effectively accepted them, and some groups of parents, children, and educators have banded together to protect children with AIDS, while others have vigorously protested their admission to school. After giving examples of the ways in which some school districts have averted or resolved the problems associated with the admission of infected children to school, the author discusses the variety of measures being taken to ensure AIDS education in the schools at both state and local levels; how various school districts are responding to the crisis; and why it is so important that public schools become involved in dealing with the AIDS problem.

Of interest to educators, school administrators, legislators, and public policymakers.

902. REID, D.A. "Knowledge of schoolchildren about the acquired immune deficiency syndrome." *Journal of the Royal College of General Practitioners* 38 (1988): 509-510.

A questionnaire survey of the knowledge and sources of information about AIDS was carried out on 232 15 year-olds at a school in Fife.

Research

The results showed that this younger age group is well-informed about AIDS, particularly methods of transmission of the virus, and that the majority of information was obtained from TV (95%) and leaflets (85%).

Of interest to health educators.

903. REMAFEDI, Gary J. "Preventing the sexual transmission of AIDS during adolescence." *Journal of Adolescent Health Care* 9 (1988): 139-143.

A discussion of the need for AIDS education to focus on youth.

Descriptive

Learning about AIDS is most likely to effect behavioral change when accompanied by other programs to build social supports, self-esteem, and positive identity. The ethical and rational use of HIV antibody testing may be a helpful adjunct to education for certain adolescents. Preventive education should particularly target gay and other homosexually active young men.

Of interest to pediatricians, health educators, and public health officials.

904. SHAYNE, Vivian T., and Barbara J. Kaplan. "AIDS education
      for adolescents." *Youth and Society* 20, no. 2 (1988):
      180-208.

Reviews adolescent attitudes toward AIDS, current efforts to change
attitudes, school efforts, the media, targeted educational programs,
and education for professionals who work with youth.

Descriptive

The authors describe the magnitude of the AIDS epidemic for youth.
Although there is little research addressing this specific problem,
available evidence suggests many youths are still ill informed. Youth
at risk are especially hard to reach. Adolescents in high-risk groups
targeted for intervention may require special consideration. Such
youths may know even less than other adolescents or they may be more
anxious and defensive about what information they do have.

Of interest to health educators, pediatricians, school administrators, and teachers.

905. SILIN, Jonathan G. "The language of AIDS: Public fears,
      pedagogical responsibilities." *Teachers College Record* 89,
      no. 1 (Autumn 1987): 3-20.

Discusses the moral, ethical, and educational challenges that face
educators in the midst of the AIDS epidemic.

Essay

Students not only need the practical knowledge that will prevent them
from getting and giving AIDS, they also need to understand and grapple
with the social implications of the disease. Teachers can encourage
free expression out of which shared understandings of social good,
public virtue, and civic responsibility may emerge.

Of interest to all educators.

906. SKEEN, Patsy, and Diane Hudson. "AIDS: What adults should
      know about AIDS (and shouldn't discuss with very young
      children)." *Young Children* 42, no. 4 (1987): 65-71.

Presents an epidemiological overview of AIDS and recommendations for
educating young children about AIDS.

Discussion

Information is provided on the origin, incidence, transmission,
treatment, and prevention of HIV and AIDS. Recommendations are made
for dealing with children whose parents have AIDS and children who ae
infectd with HIV. Very young children should be reassured that they
are in very little danger of getting AIDS, not told about the medical
ramifications of AIDS or the sexual/drug related behaviors of

adolescents and adults. Teachers should respond to questions about AIDS-related death and grief with simple, direct answers.

Of interest to early childhood educators.

907. TURNER, Charlotte, Peter Anderson, Ray Fitzpatrick, Godfrey Fowler, Richard Mayon-White. "Sexual behavior, contraceptive practice, and knowledge of AIDS among Oxford University students." *Journal of Biosocial Science* 20 (1988): 445-451.

Presents findings from a mail survey of 374 Oxford students about their sexual behaviors, use of contraceptives, and knowledge of AIDS.

Research

About two-thirds of the respondents were sexually active. Fifteen percent of the sexually active females reported that they did not use adequate contraception in the four weeks prior to the survey. The use of barrier contraceptives had increased over the past five years, and the use of oral contraceptives had decreased. Most students were well informed about AIDS. Many reported that they were more likely to use condoms because of AIDS.

Of interest to health educators and university health service professionals.

908. WALKER, David W., and Mary B. Hulecki. "Is AIDS a biasing factor in teacher judgment?" *Exceptional Children* 55 (1989): 342-345.

The effect of teacher bias on the placement of children with AIDS in special rather than regular classes was examined.

Research

AIDS was not found to be a biasing factor in the judgments of 130 third grade teachers in public schools in Indiana regarding the need of a hypothetical student for special education placement, expectations of academic functioning, and peer relationships. The findings may be due to teachers' awareness of the national publicity resulting from the Ryan White case or to their sensitivity to the needs and rights of students with AIDS.

Of interest to teachers, school administrators, and school board members.

909. WARWICK, Ian, Peter Aggleton, Hilary Homans. "Constructing common sense--young people's beliefs about AIDS." *Sociology of Health and Illness* 10 (1988): 213-233.

Reports findings from a series of in-depth interviews carried out with young people participating in local authority youth provision, voluntary sector youth groups, and youth training schemes in England.

Research

An examination of some of the complexities and contradictions within
young people's beliefs about HIV infection and AIDS made it clear
that mainstream medical explanations are, at best, moderately well
understood.   Young people do not seem to be especially confused or
ignorant about the issues; in many ways, their lay beliefs are comparable to those identified among segments of the adult population.
However, findings suggest that for many of the young people studied,
mainstream medical information on HIV and AIDS may be insufficient to
allay anxiety about risk.

Of interest to health educators, public health officials and school
teachers.

910.   WIDEN, Helen A.   "The risk of AIDS and the defense of
       disavowal: Dilemmas   for   the   college   psychotherapist."
       Journal of American College Health 35 (1987): 268-273.

Reviews 21 out of 800 cases in which mental health staff at Northwestern University conducted psychotherapy with students in which
AIDS was an issue, and summarizes seven cases to illustrate the
spectrum of AIDS concerns and therapist interventions.

Review

The review of cases revealed a tendency to separate the knowledge of
risk from the apprehension of the meaning and emotional significance
of one's behavior, a tendency to disavowal that also occurred in
therapists.   The psychological, medical, and psychiatric literature on
AIDS is reviewed to provide a context for the case review.   Some of
the psychotherapeutic and psychoeducational issues faced by therapists
in their work with students during the developing AIDS epidemic are
examined together with the concommitant consciousness raising that is
occurring.

Of interest to mental health professionals and university educators
and administrators.

911.   WINSLOW, Robert W.   "Student   knowledge   of   AIDS
       transmission."   *Sociology   and   Social   Research* 72 (1988):
       110-113.

A San Diego State University AIDS survey of students' knowledge of how
the AIDS virus is transmitted.

Research

The term, "casual contact," may not be a unidimensional variable.   The
findings suggest that students largely agree that they cannot
contract HIV through "dry" contact with AIDS virus carriers, but
disagree regarding "wet" contact.   Thus, the term, "casual contact"
in education campaigns may be confusing and may provoke ambivalent
reactions.

Of interest to health educators and public health officials.

c. Dissertations

912. PARDINI, Brenda Joyce. "Content analysis of policy statements concerning acquired immunodeficiency syndrome at universities and colleges." Ph.D. dissertation, University of Pittsburgh, 1987.

Compares policy statements of universities and colleges to recommendations formulated by the American College Health Association (ACHA); explores medical and legal issues confronting administrators dealing with the AIDS epidemic; and provides recommendations for developing policy statements.

Research/Analysis

Approximately 66% of the 241 responding institutions have developed AIDS policies or are in the process of doing so. Of 70 policies analyzed, approximately half incorporated the recommendations of the ACHA. All 70 administrators, interviewed by phone to determine their perception of their policies, strongly recommended the development of AIDS policies, and the majority recommended following the ACHA guidelines. Administrators must bear in mind the rights of individuals with AIDS or ARC, the rights of the community regarding safeguards against transmission, and the role of the institution. Institutions of higher education must make critical and conscientious decisions regarding the AIDS crisis. Through education, higher education can perform the only major intervention now available for limiting the consequences of AIDS, primary prevention.

Of primary interest to college administrators.

913. SEATON, George Merle, II. "Views of school superintendents on schools and acquired immune deficiency syndrome." Ed.D. dissertation, Virginia Polytechnic Institute and State University, 1988.

Describes the personal views of superintendents and their opinions of their school boards' views regarding schools and AIDS.

Research

There was a high degree of concurrence between superintendents' views and their beliefs of their school boards' views regarding schools and AIDS. Only the issue of condom distribution in schools indicated an anticipated conflict in opinion.

Of interest to educators and school administrators.

914. WALLS, Wemme Ensor. "An analysis of the medical and legal aspects related to the educational placement in the public schools of children with human immunodeficiency virus infection." Ed.D. dissertation, Virginia Polytechnic Institute and State University, 1988.

The salient medical and legal aspects related to the educational placement in the public schools of children with HIV infection were examined and analyzed.

Research/Analysis

Awareness of sound medical evidence to support educational decision-making provides a means of projecting a solid grounded policy to the school population and to the community. There is no medical evidence to support the exclusion of children from regular school attendance based on the suspicion or identification of HIV infection. In cases of accident or injury, health care precautions should be taken and routine procedures established for the removal of blood and/or body fluids.

Of interest to school administrators, school nurses, and teachers.

915. YOUNG, Marilyn McSpadden. "The development of a programmed instruction resource unit for AIDS education." Ed. D. dissertation, Delta State University, 1988.

An instructional resource unit, utilizing current information on the symptoms, transmission, and prevention of AIDS, was developed and a pilot study conducted in selected classes of three high schools to provide data on the effectiveness of the resource unit in terms of student achievement and to determine attitudes of teachers and students toward the method and materials used.

Research

Data analysis revealed significant gains in terms of knowledge of AIDS in the ninth, tenth, eleventh, and twelfth grades. Responses from both students and teachers revealed satisfaction with the format as an instructional method. Analysis of data did not point out any major flaws in content or construction of the materials. Those comments considered negative related primarily to the length of the unit. Comments from both students and teachers formed the basis for program revision.

Of interest to teachers and school administrators.

Chapter 5

SERVICES FOR PERSONS AFFECTED BY AIDS

1. CLINICAL CARE OF THE AIDS PATIENT

a. Books

916. MILLER, David, Jonathan Weber, John Green (Eds.). *The Management of AIDS Patients.* London: Macmillan, 1986.

An integrated, problem-oriented approach to the management of AIDS patients and those with AIDS-related disorders.

Book of Readings

Provides information on the clinical management of AIDS and HIV infection; immunology; virology; venereology; AIDS-related problems in managing hemophilia; nursing; psychology, AIDS, ARC, and PGL; counseling HIV seropositives; the worried well; risk reduction in high risk groups; and hospital counseling. An appendix provides useful addresses for members of high risk groups.

Useful to doctors, nurses, laboratory staff, and counselors.

917. O'CONNOR, Tom, with Ahmed Gonzalez-Nunez. *Living with AIDS: Reaching Out.* San Francisco: Corwin, 1987.

A very readable, realistic, and excellent coverage of aspects of AIDS that are often ignored or forgotten.

Text

The 16 chapters and appendices cover topics such as: learning about health, nurturing health, drugs, components of a good diet, viruses and parasites, and body manipulation. The appendices address drugs used in AIDS; nutritional approach to the treatment of AIDS; food additives, allergy tests, and rotation diets.

Of special interest to laymen.

918.   SANDE, Merle A., and Paul A. Volberding (Eds.).   *The Medical
        Management of AIDS.*   Philadelphia: W.B.   Saunders,   1988.

Addresses the clinical issues commonly encountered by physicians
treating AIDS patients, as well as the controversies related to HIV
testing and the health care worker's professional responsibility to
provide care.

Book of Readings

Twenty-seven chapters are divided into the following sections: The
virus and its transmission; AIDS controversies that affect the
physician; direct consequences of HIV infection: clinical spectrum
and patient management; diagnosis and management of the secondary
opportunistic infections; the malignancies associated with AIDS; and
special problems of the AIDS epidemic.   Concludes with a chapter on
an integrated approach to caring for the patient with AIDS.

Should interest all health professionals who care for AIDS patients.

b. Articles

919.   ABRAMS, Donald I., James W. Dilley, Linda M. Maxey, Paul A.
        Volberding.   "Routine care and psychosocial support of the
        patient with the acquired immune deficiency syndrome."
        Medical Clinics of North America 70, no. 3 (1986): 707-720.

Focuses on routine medical care and psychosocial support of the
patient with AIDS.

Descriptive

A description of the cooperative AIDS program of San Francisco
Hospital, the city of San Francisco, and the University of California
--a comprehensive, community-based organization for providing medical
care and psychosocial support.

Of interest to virologists, oncologists, psychiatrists, nurses, social
workers, allied health professionals, and counselors.

920.   ANDERSON, Gary R.   "Children and AIDS: Implications for
        child welfare."   *Child Welfare* 63 (1984): 62-73.

Discusses current (1984) findings on AIDS and children with AIDS and
how the child welfare field can respond.

Commentary

Although the discovery of AIDS in children provided further impetus
for government support of research, little money has been allocated

for the care of victims. The number of children with AIDS or similar deficiencies is small, but may be growing or, frequently, undetected. Child welfare agencies, torn between the need to protect foster families and the need to respond to children in acute need of special care, are challenged to identify, train, and intensively support a designated group of foster parents or to develop an appropriate alternate placement for children with AIDS who are at risk of isolation, neglect, and abandonment.

Of particular interest to child welfare workers.

921. ATKINSON, J. Hampton, Jr., Igor Grant, Caroline J. Kennedy, Douglas D. Richman, Stephen A. Spector, J. Allen McCutchan. "Prevalence of psychiatric disorders among men infected with human immunodeficiency virus." *Archives of General Psychiatry* 45 (1988): 859-864.

The authors used structured diagnostic interviews and rating scales to assess lifetime prevalence of psychiatric disorders among an unselected sample of 56 ambulatory homosexual men who had AIDS, ARC, or were asymptomatic for HIV.

Research

The data suggest that there may be a higher prevalence of anxiety disorder and major depressive illness in homosexual men when compared with sociodemographically matched heterosexual men, and that the psychiatric morbidity may have preceded the onset of the AIDS epidemic. These findings indicate that awareness of psychiatric history is necessary to comprehensive medical care of men at high risk for AIDS, even among relatively healthy outpatients.

Of interest to mental health professionals, social workers, and counselors.

922. BAER, J.W., Joanne M. Hall, Kris Holm, Susan Lewitter-Koehler. "Challenges in developing an inpatient psychiatric program for patients with AIDS and ARC." *Hospital and Community Psychiatry* 38 (1987): 1299-1303.

Describes the experience of admitting 36 AIDS and ARC patients to a locked psychiatric inpatient unit at San Francisco General Hospital over an 18 month period.

Descriptive

The presence of AIDS and ARC patients on the psychiatric unit required the education and adaptation of both staff and other patients. The authors discuss the reaction of staff to patients with terminal illness who need increased physical care, the need for milieu management that takes into account the limitations of AIDS patients suffering from dementia, diagnostic complications arising from mixed psychopathology in some AIDS patients, and the increased susceptibility of AIDS patients to side effects and toxicity from psychotropic medication.   Issues relating to infection control, ethical concerns, the needs of friends and family, and disposition planning are also discussed.

Of particular interest to physicians, nurses, and mental health professionals working in psychiatric hospitals and hospital units.

923. BUCKINGHAM, Stephan L. (Ed.). "AIDS: Bridging the gap between information and practice." *Social Casework* 69, no. 6 (1988): Entire Issue.

A collection of informative, practice-oriented articles about AIDS covering a broad range of special concerns.

Special Journal Issue

Topics covered are: legal and ethical issues; integrating safer sex counseling into social work practice; women and AIDS: countertransference issues; children and AIDS; parallel issues for AIDS patients, families, and others; rural community strategies in response to AIDS; critical issues involving AIDS and the inner city; practice implications of AIDS-dementia complex; inpatient care of persons with AIDS; AIDS and terminal illness; case management practice in an AIDS service organization; and AIDS education.   Concludes with a list of information resources.

Intended for social workers, but should interest all health care professionals.

924. CALABRESE, Leonard H.   "The physician's role in a community-based effort against the AIDS epidemic." *Cleveland Clinic Journal of Medicine* 54 (1987): 473-474.

Discusses the role of the physician in community based prevention efforts against AIDS.

Editorial

The physician-patient relationship provides an ideal forum for discussing prevention because it is not restricted by the social standards applied to the schools or the mass media.   Every patient under the care of a physician has a need and a right to be informed about AIDS.

Of general interest to physicians.

925. CAMPBELL, Robert.   "AIDS: The general practitioner's concern." *Journal of the American Osteopathic Association* 88 (1988): 371-380.

Identifies major concerns of general practitioners regarding the treatment of patients who may be infected with HIV.

Provides information on addressing HIV/AIDS problems, examining personal attitudes towards AIDS, taking thorough histories from those at risk of HIV, being aware of findings suggestive of HIV, working up patients for HIV complications, and advising/counseling patients on the findings.

Of interest to primary care physicians.

926. CECCHI, Robert Lee. "Health care advocacy for AIDS patients." *Quality Review Bulletin* 12 (1986): 297-303.

Describes the need for advocacy for AIDS patients and the role of the Gay Men's Health Crisis (GMHC) ombudsman.

Descriptive

Insufficient resources for the required level of care, denial of services due to health care professionals' fears or prejudices, misinterpretation of infection control policies, lack of adequate needs assessment, and minimal patient and family education all contribute to the problems encountered by AIDS patients in an inpatient setting. These issues are compounded by homophobia, a negative attitude toward chemical dependency, racism, and withdrawal from the terminally ill. AIDS has created a need to educate health professionals as well as the general public. Discrimination against AIDS patients can lead to patient abuse, neglect, mistreatment, and apathy. In response to the need for a central clearinghouse for complaint documentation, problem resolution, and resource identification, the GMHC, with support from a state service organization grant, created a patient advocate's position to provide a link between the AIDS patient and the health care system. Development of the ombudsman position may help solve the problems of mistreatment and social stigma that now plague AIDS patients.

Of interest to health professionals and social service workers.

927. CLEMENTS. C.J., C.F. Von Reyn, J.M. Mann. "HIV infection and routine childhood immunization: A review." *Bulletin of the World Health Organization* 65 (1987): 905-911.

Reviews some significant studies regarding the efficacy and safety of the usual childhood immunizations for HIV-infected children, which provide a current data base for decisions about immunization of these children.

Review

Summarizes current experience with immunization of HIV-infected children, relevant data on the immunization of HIV-infected adults, and in vitro studies with vaccine antigens and HIV-infected cells. Discusses theoretical concerns about the possible effects of repeated antigenic stimulation on the course of HIV infection, and reviews available information on the course of vaccine preventable diseases in HIV-infected children.

Of particular interest to pediatricians and family physicians.

928.   COHEN, Mary Ann, and Henry W. Weisman. "A biopsychosocial approach to AIDS." *Psychosomatics* 27, no. 4 (1986): 245-249.

Describes the Multidisciplinary AIDS Program (MAP), which was developed to improve the care of persons with AIDS.

Descriptive

Coping capacities of AIDS patients are undermined and their sense of alienation and expendability increased by the severe and devastating illnesses of the disease. A comprehensive multidisciplinary program to coordinate services, educate staff members, and improve communication has been organized at Metropolitan Hospital Center in New York City. Its goal is to improve the care of AIDS patients by means of a biopsychosocial approach to the multiple aspects of the disease, bringing the patients coordinated care and treatment with dignity.

Of interest to physicians, nurses, social workers, and mental health professionals.

929.   DENTON, Rick.   "AIDS: Guidelines for occupational therapy intervention."   *American Journal of Occupational Therapy* 41 (1987): 427-432.

Reviews the current facts regarding AIDS, and presents guidelines for occupational therapy assessment and treatment, including general precautions and recommended intervention strategies.

Review

Therapists treating AIDS patients need to be knowledgeable about the disease and the necessary precautions for health care workers. Persons with AIDS encompass a broad illness-wellness spectrum, and intervention depends on where in the spectrum the patient fits. Physical, as well as psychosocial, assessments are necessary for evaluating the patient, since multiple AIDS-related neuromotor and neuropsychiatric deficits have been observed. Occupational therapy services may include direct service and consultation as well as assessment.

Useful to occupational therapists.

930.   DEUCHER, Neil.   "AIDS in New York City with particular reference to the psychosocial aspects."   *British Journal of Psychiatry* 145 (1984): 512-619.

A discussion of the psychiatric and psychosocial problems of AIDS.

Descriptive

New York Metropolitan Hospital Center has developed a comprehensive program for people with AIDS.   Its goal is to develop a "biopsychosocial" approach, which maintains the view that each individual is a member of a family and community and deserves a coordinated approach to medical care, and treatment with dignity. The program includes maintenance of a multidisciplinary treatment team, provision of on-going psychological support for patients and families, and education and support for hospital staff. As such, it is clearly a good example of consultation-liaison psychiatry.

Of interest to mental health professionals and to hospital administrators as well as all health professionals treating AIDS patients.

931. ELFORD, Jonathan. "Moral and social aspects of AIDS: A medical students' project." *Social Science and Medicine* 24 (1987): 543-549.

The implications for health service workers of a purported increase in the number of AIDS cases in Great Britain was assessed.

Descriptive

A group of preclinical students at the Royal Free Hospital School of Medicine, London, undertook a project in which they explored some of the sociological and epidemiological aspects of AIDS.   Particular attention was paid to any stigma that may surround the disease. It is suggested that the management of AIDS patients and those who are HIV-positive will require both health care staff and students to carefully consider their own beliefs regarding the disease and those most at risk.

Of interest to medical educators, social and behavioral scientists, and health educators.

932. GRAVES, Edmund J., and Mary Moien. "Hospitalizations for AIDS, United States, 1984-85." *American Journal of Public Health* 77 (1987): 729-730.

Data from the National Hospital Discharge Survey on hospitalizations for AIDS were analyzed for 1984-85.

Research

During 1984, an estimated 10,000 discharges from short-stay hospitals had a diagnosis of AIDS. In 1985, this figure more than doubled to 23,000. Ninety-seven percent of all AIDS discharges were male, and 85% were between the ages of 25 and 44. Hospitalizations accounted for 510,000 days of hospital care and lasted an average of 15.6 days each.

Of interest to hospital administrators and health economists.

933. HELEY, Andrew.   "AIDS: What to do."   *The Practitioner* 232
      (1988): 133-138.

A practical approach to AIDS, giving advice to general practitioners
in Britain about what to do and what not to do.

Descriptive

Discusses what is not to be done, what cannot be done, and what should
be done by general practitioners regarding AIDS.

Of use to general practitioners and family physicians.

934. HELGERSON, Steven D.   "AIDS project in Seattle Washington."
      American Journal of Public Health 74 (1984): 1419.

Describes the AIDS Project in Seattle and the AIDS Assessment Clinic.

Descriptive

Describes the surveillance system, educational activities, and AIDS
assessment clinic in Seattle.

Of interest to public health officials.

935. KAPLAN, Robert M., John P. Anderson, Albert Wu, Wm.
      Christopher Mathews, Franklin Kozin, David Orenstein.
      "The Quality of Well-Being Scale: Application in AIDS,
      cystic fibrosis, and arthritis." *Medical Care* 27, no. 3,
      Supplement (1989): 527-543.

Describes how the Quality of Well-Being Scale was used to evaluate
outcomes in three different clinical conditions.

Research

The authors conclude that the scale has substantial validity as a
general health outcome measure, and that the scale can be used with
different populations.

Of interest to physicians, public health professionals, and health
educators.

936. LEWIS, Charles E., Howard E. Freeman, Christopher R. Corey.
      "AIDS-related competence of California's primary care
      physicians." *American Journal of Public Health* 77 (1987):
      795-799.

A random sample of primary care physicians practicing throughout the
state of California was surveyed by telephone to determine their
AIDS-related experiences and competencies.

Research

Data reflected increased incidence of AIDS in Los Angeles and San Francisco, and the proportion of physicians in rural areas who evaluated possible cases (17%) and counseled patients at risk (50%) indicated the generalized nature of the problem. Levels of competency in diagnosing and treating AIDS-related disorders increased in Los Angeles compared to similar data obtained in 1984. However, a majority of those interviewed statewide lacked the AIDS-related knowledge and skills for dealing with the disease.

Of interest to public health professionals, physicians, and medical educators.

937. LINN, Lawrence S., and Katherine L. Kahn. "Physician attitudes toward the 'laying on of hands' during the AIDS epidemic." *Academic Medicine* 64 (1989): 408-409.

Attitudes of 227 faculty and 148 housestaff physicians toward touching patients were studied in relationship to sociodemographic and job characteristics, previous exposure to and concern about HIV infection, and attitudes toward glove-wearing.

Research

Although a majority of the physicians felt that touching patients was personally satisfying, facilitated healing, and established rapport, such positive attitudes were more likely to be expressed by younger physicians and by those who worked longer hours, spent more time in primary care, and spent less time teaching. Positive attitudes were also related to less favorable attitudes toward glove-wearing and greater belief that more frequent glove use would have a negative effect on patient care.

Of interest to all health professionals.

938. LOPEZ, Diego J., and George S. Getzel. "Helping gay AIDS patients in crisis." *Social Casework* 65 (1984): 387-394.

Describes a crisis intervention program and uses a case example to show the clinical phases of AIDS as well as the program's intervention strategies and case advocacy.

Discussion

The biopsychosocial consequences of AIDS, as observed by social workers and volunteers working for the Gay Men's Health Crisis, Inc., are presented. Special attention is given to a description of the implications of AIDS for gay patients' varied historical and current lifestyles.

Of interest to health professionals, especially counselors and therapists.

939. McGUIRK, Kathleen, and Terry Miles. "Establishing a dedicated AIDS unit." *Journal of Nursing Administration* 17, no. 6 (1987): 25-30.

Describes the establishment of a dedicated unit for AIDS patients at St. Clare's Hospital in New York.

Descriptive

In 1985, St. Clare's Hospital in New York City opened the first separate dedicated unit for AIDS patients on the East Coast. The hospital lacked the financial resources, facilities, or AIDS patient caseload of larger, well-known medical institutions in New York, but through the perseverance of its staff, the obstacles to the establishment of the unit were overcome. The authors described the reasons for proposing such a unit and how the enthusiasm of the staff, the positive feedback from the patients and their significant others, the experiential hospital education, the commitment of the administration, and the involvement of the community worked together to bring it about. The lessons learned at St. Clare's can be applied anywhere.

Of interest to health professionals, hospital personnel, and hospital administrators.

940. PASCARELLI, Emil F., and Anne S. Holtzworth. "Developing an ambulatory care program for AIDS patients." *Journal of Ambulatory Care Management* 10 (1987): 44-55.

Identifies the ambulatory care needs of AIDS patients and defines useful guidelines for a program that will enable agencies and institutions to fulfill these needs.

Descriptive

Describes how to identify ambulatory care needs; how to plan and develop an AIDS ambulatory care facility, including structure, staffing, space, equipment, and community liaisons; and how to assess the costs and identify cost savings of ambulatory care.

Of interest to all health professionals.

941. PINDARO, Carole M. "Alternatives to hospitalization: AIDS home care." *Journal of the Louisiana State Medical Society* 137, no. 9 (1985): 57-59.

Describes an array of home health care services for AIDS patients.

Descriptive

Home health care, using community volunteers, respite care, Medicare/Medicaid, and private insurance, is outlined.

Of interest to nurses and home health care providers.

942 POLAN, H. Jonathan, David Hellerstein, Jess Amchin. "Impact of AIDS related cases on an inpatient therapeutic milieu." *Hospital and Community Psychiatry* 36 (1985): 173-176.

Presents case vignettes of four patients with AIDS related problems admitted to a voluntary acute-stay ward of a teaching hospital.

Case Studies

The largely indifferent reaction of the other ward patients to the AIDS-related patients, the tense and fearful reactions of the staff, and the subsequent interruption of the usual functioning of the therapeutic milieu are discussed. To develop an optimal management plan, the authors recommend attention to specific principles of patient and milieu assessment.

Of interest to psychiatrists, psychologists, and mental health professionals working with AIDS patients.

943. PROBART, Claudia K. "Guidelines for nutrition support in AIDS." *Journal of School Health* 59 (1989): 170-171.

Summarizes recommendations of the Task Force on Nutrition Support in AIDS.

Review

Because of the effects of malnutrition on the immune system, restoring an AIDS patient's nutritional status may be a useful adjunct to therapy. Complications including oral/esophageal problems, diarrhea and malabsorption, anorexia, and psychosocial factors have a direct negative impact on nutritional status. It is recommended that nutrition support be initiated at the first sign of symptomatic HIV infection and continued throughout. Intravenous nutrition should be reserved for cases where the gastrointestinal tract cannot be used.

Of interest to physicians, nurses, and dieticians.

944. RICHARDSON, Jean L., Thomas Lochner, Kimberly McGuignan, Alexandra M. Levine. "Physician attitudes and experience regarding the care of patients with acquired immunodeficiency syndrome (AIDS) and related disorders (ARC)." *Medical Care* 25 (1987): 675-685.

A survey of 314 heterosexual and homosexual physicians in Los Angeles County was conducted to determine their willingness and perceived ability to care for patients with AIDS.

Research

Results indicated that most physicians believe that special clinics staffed by physicians who have a particular expertise in caring for AIDS patients should be established. Many of the physicians surveyed indicated that concern about the risk of contagion is a deterrent to treating AIDS patients. Current evidence indicates this concern to be unfounded. There is a need for more clinically based training opportunities for physicians who would like to provide care for AIDS patients.

Of interest to physicians and all other health professionals.

945. ROBERTSON, J. Roy. "Coming to terms with AIDS." *Practitioner* 231 (1987): 1079-1080.

Discusses the difficulties of managing the day to day problems associated with HIV positivity and AIDS.

Editorial

Managing the psychological and physical problems associated with HIV infection and AIDS requires all the experience and commitment of the doctor and is likely to involve most of the primary care team. The anxiety about personal safety can be overcome only by managing patients and the passage of time. Doctors and other health care workers must handle each case with sensitivity, doing their best to respect the patient's confidentiality while protecting others at risk. Primary prevention by reducing sexual spread of the disease to those unaware of their partner's risk status is within the doctor's scope, as is the provision of support to distressed patients who badly need it.

Of interest to physicians and other health care workers.

946. "SYMPOSIUM on AIDS, Part I." *The Practitioner* 232 (1988): 379-405.

A series of articles offering practical guidelines for general practitioners becoming involved in HIV.

Symposium

The five articles in this series are based on the experience of a team of health care professionals who work together in one district. They include discussions of the "worried well;" of the issues to explore in preparing patients for HIV antibody tests, including some guidance on how best to do so, of community care for HIV-positive patients; and constructive comments and the personal views of an HIV-positive man. Concludes with a list of HIV/AIDS resources in the United Kingdom.

Of particular interest to primary care physicians.

947. "SYMPOSIUM on AIDS, Part II." *The Practitioner* 232 (1988): 445-469.

Part two of a symposium offering practical guidelines for general practitioners becoming involved in HIV.

Symposium

The four articles in this section cover: the management of HIV symptomatic patients in general practice; how AIDS affects women and children; terminal care; and AIDS and injecting drug users. Concludes with a reprint of the resource list contained in part one.

Useful to primary care physicians.

948. TURNER, Barbara J., Joyce V. Kelly, Judy K. Ball. "A severity classification system for AIDS hospitalizations." *Medical Care* 27 (1989): 423-437.

Describes the development of a model for classifying hospitalized AIDS patients according to the severity of their illness.

Descriptive

Based on clinical literature and expert opinion, a model indicating the relative severity of AIDS complications was formulated. After being tested empirically by mortality data from more than 6000 adult AIDS hospitalizations in New York State during 1985, the model was revised to reflect a continuum of increasing likelihood of death in the hospital. The final classification system for AIDS hospitalizations has 20 substages, grouped in three stages with inpatient mortality rates increasing from six percent to 60%. The automated system can be applied to different AIDS populations to analyze resource use and outcomes of hospital care.

Of interest to physicians, nurses, hospital administrators, policymakers, and economists.

949. TURNER, Norma Haston, and M. Jean Keller. "Therapeutic recreation practitioners' involvement in the AIDS epidemic." *Therapeutic Recreation Journal* 22, no. 3 (1988): 12-20.

Describes the implications of the AIDS epidemic for therapeutic recreation practitioners in various settings.

Descriptive

Therapeutic recreation practitioners have traditionally responded to the health and well-being of special populations. The AIDS epidemic presents a new challenge to these practitioners. Issues regarding the types of services that will be needed by persons with AIDS, and whether policies that will allow therapeutic practitioners to provide equitable services can be developed, are discussed.

Of special interest to therapeutic recreation specialists.

950. VALDISERRI, R.O., G.M. Tama, M. Ho. "A survey of AIDS patients regarding their experiences with physicians." *Journal of Medical Education* 63 (1988): 726-728.

To determine the training needs of health professionals from the viewpoint of persons with AIDS, the authors undertook a survey of AIDS patients who were being evaluated for enrollment into an experimental study of anti-HIV treatment.

Research

A majority of patients did not feel they were given an accurate explanation of what to expect throughout the course of their illness. Only a small percentage of the physicians recommended that their patients' partners be referred for counseling and HIV antibody testing. A majority of the physicians did not discuss precautions that should be taken with sexual partners or household members. Of those patients who did receive information on preventing sexual transmission, most reported that their physicians had advised the use of condoms for vaginal and/or anal intercourse, but this was often accompanied by a message to stop having sex.

Of interest to all physicians, health educators, and public health officials.

951. VOLBERDING, Paul. "Supporting the health care team in caring for patients with AIDS." *Journal of the American Medical Association* 261 (1989): 747-748.

Discusses the issues evoked by AIDS, the difficulties of AIDS care for the medical community, and the implications for the health care system.

Commentary

The complexities of AIDS care force us to reconsider our health care systems, question whether they are functioning well, and be prepared to revise them when needed to enable medical providers to deal with the medical, psychosocial, and ethical problems of AIDS. AIDS poses severe and chronic stress for health care providers, causing many physicians to avoid assuming an AIDS care role. Health care providers must be provided with the resources needed to reduce those stresses if they are to maintain their own health and continue to provide effective care. Some of the burdens and stresses accompanying AIDS care can be addressed by intensified professional education, but others may require new regulations or standards of conduct within the medical profession.

Of interest to health professionals, medical educators, and medical ethicists.

952. WACHTER, Robert M., Molly Cooke, Philip C. Hopewell, John M. Luce. "Attitudes of medical residents regarding intensive care for patients with the acquired immunodeficiency syndrome." *Archives of Internal Medicine* 148 (1988): 149-152.

A survey was conducted of medical house staff at the University of California at San Francisco to elicit their attitudes toward intensive care for patients with AIDS.

Research

The results suggest that the intensity of exposure to patients with AIDS determines the assessment of prognosis, and that one or both of these factors strongly influence attitudes toward intensive care. Of interest to medical educators, house staff, and medical students.

953. WARD, Matthew, and Maxine A. Papadakis. "Untrapping the metaphor of AIDS." *American Journal of Medicine* 83 (1987): 1135-1138.

Presents an AIDS patient's perceptions of his needs, tempered by his doctor's evaluation of which needs can be and which needs must be filled by the physician.

Editorial

AIDS must be viewed as a disease caused by a virus, not as a form of "moral contagion." Doctors must work to overcome their prejudices or excuse themselves from treating patients with AIDS. They cannot distance themselves from their patients, but must treat them with humanity and convey upon them a sense of self-worth.

Intended for primary care physicians treating AIDS patients.

954. YABROV, Alexander. "New approach to treatment of AIDS and AIDS related complex." *Medical Hypotheses* 27 (1988): 81-82.

A new approach to the treatment of AIDS is suggested.

Theoretical

The author suggests isolating the patient's blood, removing anti-T-cell substance from the plasma, treating the cells with an anti-viral agent, and then returning the blood to the patient.

Of interest to virologists and physicians.

2. NURSING CARE

a. Books

955. DURHAM, Jerry D., and Felissa Lashley Cohen (Eds.). *The Person with AIDS: Nursing Perspectives.* New York: Springer, 1987.

An informative, comprehensive sourcebook for nurses who are caring for patients with AIDS.

Book of Readings

Includes: an overview of the AIDS epidemic, including its history, epidemiology, etiology, and clinical pathology; a discussion of the issues regarding the control and treatment of infection in institutional settings; information on the prevention and treatment of AIDS;

a discussion of the psychosocial and ethical dimensions of AIDS, and public and private sector responses to AIDS; guidelines for acute and sustained nursing care for AIDS patients; information on the prevention and treatment of AIDS; and a discussion of children with AIDS.

Intended for nurses, but should be useful to all health care providers.

956. EIDSEN, Ted (Ed.). *The AIDS Caregiver's Handbook.* New York: St. Martin's Press, 1988.

A compilation of material that is presented in a two and a half day training seminar to those who decide to become volunteer caregivers or those who have a personal relationship with an AIDS or ARC patient.

Handbook

Designed to accomplish two ends: to tell you what you must know to assist a person with AIDS or ARC; and to tell you where to find more information when you have the time and desire. The handbook is akin to a first aid manual, easily read and easily referenced. Chapters cover all aspects of AIDS--scientific, medical, nutritional, psychological, interpersonal, and spiritual. Included is a list of organizations, hotlines, and information sources.

Directed to the individual caregiver.

957. GEE, Gayling, and Theresa A. Moran (Eds.). *AIDS: Concepts in Nursing Practice.* Baltimore: Williams & Wilkins, 1988.

A comprehensive guide to AIDS information and AIDS nursing care for nurses.

Book of Readings

The introductory section of this book offers an overview of the epidemic and a review of issues relevant to women, children, and hemophiliacs who have HIV infection. The second section begins with an immunologic review of the effects of HIV on the body's defense mechanisms. Each chapter on the disease processes reviews the pathophysiology and clinical manifestations of the disease as well as appropriate nursing assessments and diagnoses. The third section covers specific nursing management concerns. The final section covers the ethical issues surrounding AIDS care, psychosocial issues facing individuals with HIV infection, and the impact on their families and caregivers. Support and self-care strategies are offered for both patients and care providers.

Of special interest to nurses.

958. PRATT, Robert J. *AIDS: A Strategy for Nursing Care.* London: Edward Arnold, 1986.

Information, guidance, and support for nurses caring for AIDS patients.

Text

Contains general information on the epidemiology, etiology, nature, transmission, and presenting illnesses of AIDS and specific information on the need for and nature of strategic nursing care of AIDS patients in various settings, issues and management of strategic nursing care, and medical treatment of HIV infection. Stresses the health education aspects of AIDS.

Specifically written for nursing personnel, but may also interest physicians, hospital administrators, and health educators.

959. ROYAL College of Nursing AIDS Working Party. *Nursing Guidelines on the Management of Patients in Hospital and the Community Suffering from AIDS.* London: Royal College of Nursing, 1985.

A guide for giving safe, effective, and meaningful care to the patient suffering from the effects of acquired immune deficiency syndrome, while protecting the caregiver from accidental infection.

Text/Manual

Divided into sections on staff protection; guidelines for care; and psychosocial support for nurses, patients, and significant others.

Useful to nurses and other health care providers.

b. Articles

960. BARIL, Marianne T., and Suzanne K. Jaser. "Living with AIDS." *RN* 51, no. 3 (1988): 81-88.

Provides guidance to the nurse who is providing home care for AIDS patients.

Guide

With the advent of new antiviral agents and improved treatment for opportunistic infections, the need for regular nursing assistance for AIDS patients at home, for longer periods of time, will continue to increase. The authors use two case examples to demonstrate how nurses may provide patient education, clinical care, and support for AIDS patients and their families.

Of particular interest to home care nurses.

961. BENNETT, Jo Anne. "Nurses talk about the challenge of AIDS." *American Journal of Nursing* 87 (1987): 1150-1155.

A dialogue between several nurses about getting information about AIDS, advocacy, and home care.

Descriptive

A factual, direct series of comments from nurses who have cared for AIDS patients.

Of particular interest to nurses.

962. FLASKERUD, Jacquelyn H.   "AIDS: Psychosocial aspects."
      Health Values 12, no. 4 (1988): 44-52.

Assesses the psychosocial impact of AIDS and discusses the effect of the unique series of stresses generated by the disease.

Review

AIDS generates unique stresses for patients, their lovers/spouses and family members, and health care professionals and creates serious problems for everyone with whom the patient has close contact, including friends and employers. The problems confronting people with AIDS, and the fear engendered by the disease, affect every aspect of a patient's life. Nursing care of AIDS patients requires special attention to the psychosocial aspects of the disease. Nurses need also be concerned with the stresses experienced by the lovers and families of AIDS patients and the stresses they, themselves, experience in caring for these patients.

Of interest to nurses and other caregivers.

963. ───── (Ed.). "AIDS: The Psychosocial Dimension." *Journal of Psychosocial Nursing and Mental Health Services* 25, no. 12 (1987): Entire Issue.

Deals with the challenges presented by the medical, psychological, and social consequences of AIDS to the practice, education, and research of mental health nurses.

Special Journal Issue

The six articles in this special issue cover: the challenges of the AIDS client to mental health nurses; the psychosocial stresses of AIDS on patients, family, friends, and nurses; nursing assessment of CNS complications; a model for a community AIDS task force; how therapists can help clients with AIDS confront the reality of disease; and how the spread of AIDS will affect the next generation.

Intended specifically for mental health nurses, but should prove useful to all nurses, therapists, and mental health professionals.

964. GRADY, Christine. "Ethical issues in providing nursing care to human immunodeficiency virus-infected populations." *Nursing Clinics of North America* 24, no. 2 (1989): 523-534.

Discusses ethical behavior in caring for HIV infected persons.

Review

Although an incredible body of knowledge regarding HIV infection and its ramifications has accumulated in the past few years, many questions regarding proper conduct toward persons who are HIV infected still exist. Nurses have an obligation to be informed about HIV infection, its clinical manifestations, treatments, and the care of infected persons. They must help their patients to know their needs and options, listen to them, and advocate for them. Nurses caring for patients with AIDS require courage to face risks and impartiality to temper prejudice. In addition, they need a strong sense of caring, compassion for fellow human beings, and a conviction that they can make a difference in promoting a person's welfare and preserving his or her dignity.

Of interest to nurses and other health professionals caring for AIDS patients.

965. ———, and Linda C. Andrist (Eds). "AIDS." "Sexually transmitted diseases." *Nursing Clinics of North America* 23, no. 4 (1988): 683-987.

A symposium on AIDS and sexually transmitted diseases.

Symposium Proceedings

The 22 papers in this issue are divided into two sections, each preceded by the editor's preface. Part I includes: the epidemiology of HIV; the AIDS clinical trials unit experience; nursing care of children with HIV infection; helping people with AIDS live well at home; psychosocial issues of AIDS in the nursing care of homosexual men; risks to health care workers and infection control; a strategy for educating health care providers about AIDS; ethical issues confronting nurses; and hospice care. The articles in the second section cover: bacterial vaginosis; nursing management of the patient with chlamydia; gonorrhea; pelvic inflammatory disease; genital herpes simplex; sexually transmitted diseases in pregnancy; chronic exposure to sexually transmitted diseases; and taking a sexual history and educating clients about safe sex.

Of interest to nurses and other health professionals.

966. HEFFERN, Mary Kate. "While the world waits." *American Journal of Nursing* 87 (1987): 932.

Points out the importance of the role played by nurses in the fight against AIDS.

Editorial

In the absence of a cure, nurses provide a wide range of services to help combat the devastating effect of AIDS. These include comfort and caring, preventive education, dispensing accurate information to help dispel the fear of family and friends, and nonjudgmental emotional support.

Of interest to nursing personnel.

967. KENNEDY, Margaret. "AIDS: Coping with the fear." *Nursing* 17, no. 4 (April 1987): 44-46.

Discusses how nurses can help patients and those around them deal with their AIDS-related fears.

Commentary

Although AIDS patients may respond to their disease in a variety of ways, their underlying emotion is fear. Nurses have an obligation to use their skills and knowledge, not just to prevent transmission of AIDS, but to control the fear it creates. Although they may not always succeed, nurses frequently can help patients and those around them cope with their fears by offering information and support. However, they must first confront their own attitudes and fears and those of the people who are concerned about them. The more health care workers know about the disease, and the more AIDS patients they've cared for, the more likely they are to feel comfortable and to communicate their confidence to others.

Of interest to nurses and other health care workers.

968. KRENER, Penelope G. "Impact of the diagnosis of AIDS on hospital care of an infant." *Clinical Pediatrics* 26 (1987): 30-34.

Reports detailed analysis of caretaker response to the first infant at a university hospital to be diagnosed with AIDS.

Research

Nursing notes were reviewed for the periods before diagnosis of AIDS, after diagnosis, and after psychiatric consultation, during which five consultation questions were posed. It was found that the percentage of time that PRN medication was given dropped after diagnosis of AIDS, but rose above the initial level after consultation. The number of times per shift the nurse touched the baby was not found to be associated with use of PRN medication, but was explained by which nurse was caring for the child. Although the level of care given the baby was consistently high, it was found that certain nurses became attached to her, while others distanced themselves from her, and the infant's behavioral responses varied depending upon the amount of personal attention she received. It is speculated that caretakers of patients with AIDS may normally have feelings considered unacceptable in medical settings, including fear, blaming the patient, or a wish to avoid the patient. Such feelings are especially difficult to tolerate in the care of children or infants.

Of interest to nurses, physicians, and hospital administrators.

969. LESSOR, Roberta. "Fieldwork relationships on an AIDS ward: Verstehen methodology as a source of data." *Clinical Sociology Review* 6 (1988): 101-112.

Examines researcher/respondent relationships in a fieldwork study of a hospital ward for the care of AIDS patients.

Descriptive

The nurses' work was the subject of study. Taking the position that verstehen is a precondition of research, and using Mead's argument that one can be an object to oneself, key aspects of the relationship between the researcher and the nurses are rendered problematic. The investigation illuminates institutional constraints, the ideological position of the nurses, and the social psychology of work on the ward. It is argued that substantive elements of the situation may be discovered through the analysis of personal relationship data.

Of interest to clinical sociologists and social and behavioral scientists.

970. LILLARD, Jenifer, Patricia Lotspeich, Joyce Gurich, Jerilyn Hesse. "Acquired immunodeficiency syndrome (A.I.D.S.) in home care: Maximizing helpfulness and minimizing hysteria." *Home Healthcare Nurse* 2, no. 5 (1984): 11-16.

Uses a case study to illustrate proper home care of persons with AIDS.

Descriptive

Nursing intervention for AIDS patients must focus first on physical problems and then on psychosocial ones. The etiology and treatment interventions for oral candida, edema, fever, diarrhea, herpes, Kaposi's sarcoma, and dyspnea are given, and basic guidelines for protecting patients and caregivers against infections are provided. Home caregivers are challenged to work to maximize the quality of life for AIDS patients, reduce the risk of AIDS transmission, and educate the public.

Of interest to visiting and home care nurses.

971. SALYER, Jeanne, Haidee Waters, Patricia Yow. "AIDS: Holistic home care." *Home Healthcare Nurse* 5, no. 2 (1987): 10-21.

The authors advocate holistic home care for PWAs.

Descriptive

Patients with AIDS can be cared for safely and effectively at home if caregivers have accurate information about AIDS and follow sound principles for managing the problems encountered by PWAs and their families. Information on AIDS, infectious disease guidelines, current treatment for opportunistic diseases, and a model nursing care plan is presented for caregivers. Suggestions are made for helping families to deal with grief.

Of interest to home health care nurses.

972. THOMPSON, Sharon W., and Karen R. Gietz. "Acquired immune deficiency syndrome in infants and children." *Pediatric Nursing* 11 (1985): 278-280.

Written to familiarize pediatric nurse practitioners with AIDS.

Discussion

A brief discussion of the epidemiology, pathophysiology, and diagnostic criteria of AIDS, focusing on the nursing care concerns and issues involved in treating infants and children with AIDS.

Of particular interest to nursing care providers for AIDS patients.

c. Dissertation

973. GERSON, Linda Danielle. "The relationship between providing nursing care to patients with acquired immunodeficiency syndrome and nurses' anxiety, depression, and hostility." Ph.D. dissertation. University of Maryland, College Park, 1987.

A study to investigate the relationship between providing nursing care to patients with AIDS and nurses' anxiety, depression, and hostility.

Research

The findings did not support a relationship between the provision of care to patients with AIDS and nurses' anxiety, depression, and hostility.

Of interest to nurses.

3. PSYCHOSOCIAL INTERVENTIONS

a. Books

974. BAUMGARTNER, Gail Henderson. *AIDS: Psychosocial Factors in the Acquired Immune Deficiency Syndrome.* Springfield, IL: Charles C. Thomas, 1985.

Examines the psychosocial factors affecting individuals at risk for AIDS.

Research/Literature Review

Findings delineate ways in which social workers, working as part of a multidisciplinary team, can help AIDS patients come to terms with their illness, work through their problems, and find support.

Should interest social workers and other members of the helping professions.

975. HELQUIST, Michael (Ed.). *Working with AIDS: A Guide for Mental Health Professionals.* San Francisco: The AIDS Health Project, University of California, San Francisco, 1987.

A training manual and resource guide for all mental health professionals who work with AIDS-related issues.

Guide Book

The 11 chapters focus on people with AIDS and ARC, AIDS antibody testing and the worried well, treatment issues and approaches in the long term care of patients with AIDS, the impact of AIDS on women, AIDS in ethnic communities, AIDS-related suicide, AIDS and substance abuse, youth and AIDS, psychiatric and ethical issues in the care of patients with AIDS. The guide includes a glossary of AIDS-related terms, lists of national and local organizations, a selected bibliography for mental health professionals, and a selected bibliography for clients.

Especially useful for mental health professionals.

976. JÄGER, Hans (Ed.)., and J.L. Francis (Translation Ed.). *AIDS and AIDS Risk Patient Care.* Chichester: Ellis Horwood, 1988.

Papers presented at the Munich AIDS Support Group and AIDS Working Party in February 1986.

Conference Proceedings

The 16 chapter topics include: an overview of the psychosocial aspects of HIV infections; medical bases; homosexuality today; AIDS and drug dependency; anxiety in dealing with AIDS patients; ethical guidelines; self-help groups for HIV-positive patients; experiences in psychosocial and psychiatric practice; AIDS in prison; women and AIDS; pastoral aspects; AIDS and dying; potentials and problems of AIDS help; and potentials for psychopharmacological management.

This book is aimed at physicians, psychologists, nurses, social workers, theologians, lawyers, and public health officials.

977. KELLY, Jeffrey A., and Janet S. St. Lawrence. *The AIDS Health Crisis: Psychological and Social Interventions.* New York: Plenum, 1988.

Provides information about AIDS and its risk behaviors for mental health, social service, and counseling professionals in practice or training; reviews behavior change methods for the primary prevention of HIV infection at the individual, group, and community levels; discusses psychological and social difficulties experienced by persons with AIDS and HIV infection; and outlines clinical interventions that can help to alleviate some of these difficulties.

Textbook

The nine chapters cover: the medical aspects of AIDS; transmission and risk factors for AIDS; risk reduction counseling for individuals and groups; behavioral interventions at a community level; psychosocial consequences of HIV seropositivity; psychosocial interventions for HIV seropositive persons; psychological consequences of AIDS and ARC; psychosocial care needs of persons with AIDS; and effective help providing: knowledge, sensitivity, and ethics.

Written for psychologists, social workers, nurses, counselors, and others who work with AIDS patients.

978.   LEUKEFELD, Carl G., and Manuel Fimbres (Eds.).   *Responding to AIDS: Psychosocial Initiatives.*   Silver Spring, MD: National Association of Social Workers, 1987.

Discusses what is known about the psychosocial issues accompanying AIDS and ARC; the role professionals must play in fulfilling the psychosocial needs of individuals, families, and communities, and the training required to produce such qualified professionals; and which services are needed, how they should be delivered, and the implications for developing social policies.

Book of Readings

The eight chapters cover: the challenge presented by AIDS; current and anticipated trends; research on the psychosocial aspects of AIDS; meeting the psychosocial needs of people with AIDS; the family and AIDS; women and children with AIDS; identifying and meeting the needs of minority clients with AIDS; and social, psychological, and research barriers to the treatment of AIDS.

Intended for social workers, but may be helpful to anyone in the social services.

979.   NICHOLS, Stuart E., and David G. Ostrow (Eds.).   *Psychiatric Implications of Acquired Immune Deficiency Syndrome.*   Washington, DC: American Psychiatric Press, 1984.

A succinct description of AIDS, primarily focusing on the psychiatric and social implications of the disease.

Book of Readings

Divided into three sections--medical aspects, psychiatric treatment, and social responses--and an epilogue.   The first three chapters present an overview of the epidemiologic, medical, and neurological

conditions encountered with AIDS.   Chapters four through seven deal
with therapeutic approaches for persons who are anxious about contracting AIDS, approaches for facilitating coping in patients who have
been diagnosed as having AIDS, psychiatric care of the seriously ill
AIDS patient, and the importance of support networks for victims of
AIDS. The next five chapters consider the medical, psychological, and
social issues presented by AIDS, and the epilogue clarifies the role
of psychiatry when confronted with AIDS-associated mental health
problems and the consequences of prejudice and stigmatization, and
presses for preventive approaches as well as treatment.

Intended for psychiatrists, but should interest other members of the
helping professions.

980. PAINE, Leslie (Ed.).   *AIDS: Psychiatric and Psychosocial*
      Perspectives. London: Croom Helm, 1988.

This position paper sets out what appears to be the outstanding
psychiatric and psychosocial dimensions of AIDS and related disorders
and explains possible directions for further developing the
understanding necessary for appropriate service developments.

Book of Readings

The eight chapters and epilogue cover a variety of topics including:
the biology of AIDS; epidemiology, control of infection, and medical
treatments, psychiatric sequelae of HIV; medical and psychiatric
nursing care; services for people dependent on drugs; young children
at risk; social problems, emotional symptoms, and psychiatric
disorders; and counseling in relation to HIV.

Of interest to a variety of health professionals.

981. RODWAY, Margaret, and Marianne Wright (Eds.).   *Sociopsycho-*
      logical Aspects of Sexually Transmitted Diseases. New York:
      Haworth Press, 1988.

Addresses some of the sociopsychological counseling and educative
dimensions that need to be taken into account if changes in our
approaches to the social problems inherent in STDs are to be made.

Book of Readings

Attention has primarily been focused on herpes and AIDS, but they are
not the only sexually transmitted diseases. The others are curable,
but they too can have devastating results. STDs provide a challenge,
not only for medical clinicians, but for other helping professionals.
The nine chapters in this volume are divided into three sections. The
first provides medical, social, and psychological perspectives on
STDs. The second is directed toward aspects of counseling clients.
The final section is devoted to the education and teaching
professionals and the general public about STDs. The book concludes
with an epilogue on the epidemic.

Of interest to medical and mental health professionals.

b. Articles

982. AMCHIN, Jess, and H. Jonathan Polan. "A longitudinal account
      of staff adaptation to AIDS patients on a psychiatric unit."
      Hospital and Community Psychiatry 37 (1986): 1235-1238.
Describes how the staff of a voluntary acute-stay psychiatric unit
progressed over a two-year period from having difficulty coping with
AIDS patients to directly confronting the issues raised by the disease
among themselves and the patient population.

Descriptive

As more patients with AIDS and AIDS-related syndromes are admitted to
psychiatric units, staff must meet new diagnostic and therapeutic
challenges while adapting to the unique stresses of treating these
patients. The authors discuss several case vignettes to illustrate
how the staff of one such unit developed coping skills. The authors
believe that clinical experience and educational programs were major
contributors to the staff's adaptation, and that the staff's ability
to cope with AIDS patients may have strongly influenced the patient
community's ability to cope. Several recommendations for psychiatric
units beginning to treat AIDS patients are made.

Of interest to health professionals, mental health professionals, and
hospital administrators.

983. BATKI, Steven L., James L. Sorensen, Barbara Faltz, Scott
      Madover. "Psychiatric aspects of treatment of IV drug
      abusers with AIDS." *Hospital and Community Psychiatry* 39
      (1988): 439-441.
Describes selected psychiatric aspects of drug abuse treatment of IV
opiate addicts suffering from AIDS and AIDS-related conditions.

Discussion

Providing substance abuse treatment to AIDS patients can be difficult
because their medical and social problems are frequently exacerbated
by psychiatric problems, particularly depression and anxiety. It has
been suggested that addicts may use drugs to blunt the impact of
anxiety-producing or painful stimuli because of a failure to develop
adequate coping mechanisms. Addicts can be expected to have fewer
psychological resources for coping with the stress of AIDS, ARC, and
associated problems than patients with the same conditions who do not
abuse drugs. Only by acknowledging the special problems of addicts
with AIDS, can substance abuse treatment be made more accessible and
useful to them. Guidelines for practices in treating AIDS patients
are offered to mental health and drug abuse staff.

Of particular interest to drug abuse counselors.

984. BELFER, Myron L., Penelope K. Krener, Frank Black Miller.
      "AIDS in children and adolescents." *Journal of the American
      Academy of Child and Adolescent Psychiatry* 27 (1988):
      147-151.

An understanding of the impact of AIDS on psychological development and the necessity of specialized support services for providers is discussed.

Discussion

Child psychiatrists will need to conceive of themselves as agents for promoting the public health as AIDS increases. Their role must go beyond that of patient care. The irrational use of such defenses as denial and projection, which impede the understanding of AIDS in children and adolescents, must be combatted. Rational knowledge to promote social awareness needs to be promoted.

Of interest to pediatricians and child development specialists.

985. BUCKINGHAM, Stephan L. "The HIV antibody test: Psychosocial issues." *Social Casework* 68 (1987): 387-393.

Identifies the unique, psychologically distressing concerns of persons who are HIV seropositive or have ARC, and offers suggestions for mental health practitioners working with these people.

Commentary

There are no easy answers to the AIDS problem. However, the clinician must be aware that self-awareness, sufficient knowledge, and attention to his/her own needs and limitations are all prerequisites to helping the victims of HIV seropositivity, ARC, and AIDS. Offering specific guidelines for health enhancing behaviors may be particularly helpful to clients who are grasping for control. These include the following: 1) protection from further exposure to the virus, 2) observation of safe sex practices, 3) regular visits to the physician for physical and medical monitoring, and 4) avoiding alcohol and drugs, maintaining good nutrition, and getting sufficient sleep.

Of interest to social workers and other mental health professionals.

986. BURTON, Stephen W. "The psychiatry of HIV infection." *British Medical Journal* 295 (1987): 228-229.

Discusses the psychological impact of AIDS.

Review

An appreciable number of AIDS patients show abnormalities in cognitive function. Although most are minor, HIV may cause a presenile dementia, known as the AIDS dementia complex, that usually causes slow, but steady deterioration which, at its most advanced, can be severe. Patients with AIDS are referred to psychiatrists because of depression, suicidal ideation, treatment refusal, agitation, anxiety, and inability to cope. Adjustment disorders have been found in 60% of individuals with AIDS-related complex, 41% of those with AIDS, and 23% of asymptomatic but infected patients. Many patients from high risk groups--the worried well--present because of the publicity surrounding AIDS, are anxious despite frequent reassurance, and may develop persistent and refractory depressions. More understanding and compassion is needed for those at risk for AIDS.

Useful for physicians, mental health professionals, social workers, and other members of the caring professions.

987. CAPUTO, Larry. "Dual diagnosis: AIDS and addiction." *Social Work* 30 (1985): 361-364.

Establishes a framework for understanding the psychosocial impact of AIDS on intravenous drug abusers, and explores the extent to which biopsychosocial services may be integrated into the health care system.

Discussion

Discusses the impact of AIDS, its demographics, addiction and AIDS, intervention strategies for social workers, support for supporters of persons with AIDS, and what can be done. Strongly suggests that helping professionals take an active role in seeking solutions to the complex problems that AIDS presents to individuals and to our society. Accurate information about AIDS, its treatment, and available medical, financial, and psychosocial resources should be widely disseminated to reduce AIDS phobia and the stigmatization of persons in high risk groups.

Particularly useful to social workers and other social service professionals.

988. CATALAN, Jose. "Psychosocial and neuropsychiatric aspects of HIV infection: Review of their extent and implications for psychiatry." *Journal of Psychosomatic Research* 32 (1988): 237-248.

Considers, in detail, the psychosocial and neuropsychiatric problems that can develop at the various stages of HIV infection and discusses their implications for the mental health services in terms of provision of services, legal and ethical problems, and further research.

Review

The development of AIDS is associated with a further increase in mental health problems, both functional and organic. More work is needed to establish the prevalence of problems and the factors associated with their presentation. Further research is needed to develop diagnostic procedures to clarify the etiology of the various syndromes and to implement effective treatments. Prospective studies of representative samples of patients are needed to establish the frequency and extent of the syndrome, its course, and its significance in relation to the development of other HIV-related problems.

Of interest to mental health professionals and social and behavioral scientists.

989. COCHRAN, Susan D., and Vickie M. Mays. "Women and AIDS-related concerns: Roles for psychologists in helping the worried well." *American Psychologist* 44 (1989): 529-535.

Examines AIDS and HIV-related concerns in women with a focus on the personal dilemmas for the practicing psychologist, problems in health behavior advocacy, and methods and pitfalls in modifying sexual behaviors.

Descriptive

Covers the incidence and prevalence of AIDS in women, dilemmas of the practicing psychologist, AIDS anxiety, ethical perplexities, issues in health behavior advocacy, and problems in modifying behavior. Psychologists have a unique opportunity to contribute to stopping the spread of AIDS by intervening now before the prevalence of AIDS in women escalates.

Of special interest to psychologists and mental health therapists.

990. COOPER, Alison, and M.P. Bender. "AIDS--what should psychologists be doing?" *Bulletin of the British Psychological Society* 40 (1987): 130-133.

Identifies the role of psychologists in the AIDS epidemic.

Descriptive

Psychologists should be responsible for three levels of intervention in the AIDS epidemic. At the level of the individual and his family, the psychologist's role involves helping patients with stress reduction and with dealing with negative emotions, and providing psychological support to relatives of AIDS patients. At the staff level, psychologists can provide training and support for staff members who care for AIDS patients. At the organizational level, psychologists should be involved in setting non-discriminatory policies and in recommending strategies that allay public fear.

Of interest to mental health professionals.

991. DANE, Barbara Oberhofer. "New beginnings for AIDS patients." *Social Casework* 70 (1989): 305-309.

Examines, within the model of Lydia Rapoport's crisis-intervention model, three sets of interrelated factors that can produce a state of crisis.

Descriptive

To work successfully with AIDS patients, practitioners must search out and test old and new treatment methods. New treatment strategies can be built around the crisis-intervention model. Families, including the patient's lover, often need emotional support and counseling as well as assistance in making funeral arrangements, paying bills, etc.

Of interest to social workers and mental health professionals.

992. DAVID, Irene Rosner, Sharon Sageman. "Psychological aspects of AIDS as seen in art therapy." *American Journal of Art Therapy* 26 (August 1987): 3-10.

A discussion of the psychological aspects of AIDS reflected in the artwork of AIDS patients.

Essay

Depression, social isolation, and feelings of inadequacy are common psychological problems of AIDS patients. Art therapy helps patients to release their negative feelings in a safe and supportive environment, and their art reflects their mental status at various stages of their illness. The role of the art therapist and its attendant stresses are discussed and illuminated by two illustrated case studies of AIDS patients, and protective measures to be taken during the performance of the therapist's job are outlined.

Of interest to therapists, mental health professionals, and concerned laypersons.

993. DILLEY, James W., Herbert N. Ochitill, Mark Perl, Paul A. Volberding. "Findings in psychiatric consultations with patients with AIDS." *American Journal of Psychiatry* 142 (1985): 82-85.

Details the psychiatric profiles of 13 AIDS patients who were admitted for psychiatric consultation.

Research

Recurrent psychological themes of the patients were: dealing with a life-threatening illness, uncertainty about the implications of the AIDS diagnosis, social isolation, and guilt over their former life styles. The role of the primary physician and health care professional in the psychological care of AIDS patients is discussed.

Of interest to physicians and mental health professionals.

994. DILLEY, James W., Earl E. Shelp, Steven L. Batki. "Psychiatric and ethical issues in the care of patients with AIDS: An overview." *Psychosomatics* 27 (1986): 562-566.

Highlights issues confronting the consultation-liaison psychiatrist asked to see a patient with AIDS.

Descriptive

Some aspects examined as they confront the consultant are: the high incidence of neurologic complications; the nonspecific nature of psychiatric symptoms; the need for the patient to select a reliable person to make legal and health-care decisions if and when that is necessary; assessment of suicidal ideation; decisions about terminal care and life supports; and the need to decide how rigorously to pursue treatment for drug abuse in the patient who has contracted AIDS intravenously.

Of interest to psychiatrists, psychologists, and social workers.

995. DOHERTY, John P. "AIDS: One psychosocial response." *Quality Review Bulletin* 12 (1986): 295-297.

Discusses the work of the Howard Brown Memorial Clinic.

Descriptive

In 1982, when only 20 cases of AIDS were recognized in the Chicago area, the support services division of the Howard Brown Memorial Clinic began to investigate the needs of people with AIDS and to set up psychosocial services. The clinic, which does not discriminate against anyone on the basis of race, creed, sex, sexual orientation, or past drug use, has served all of the 382 PWAs in the Chicago area, and continues to serve the surviving 120. A paid staff of two, and more than 125 specially trained volunteers, under the direction of the support services director, provide a wide variety of support services for AIDS patients, families, and significant others. The clinic's primary function is to help each client to be as independent as possible for as long as possible. It attempts to provide quality services in a sensitive respectful manner. The clinic's research unit, in collaboration with Northwestern University School of Medicine, is engaged in important research pertaining to AIDS, utilizing a large number of infection-free volunteers who are willing to cooperate in long-term testing and evaluation.

Of particular interest to social service workers and mental health professionals.

996. DUNKEL, Joan, and Shellie Hatfield. "Countertransference issues in working with persons with AIDS." *Social Work* 31 (1986): 114-117.

Examines, within the conceptual framework of countertransference, issues, feelings, biases, and fears that have been identified by the authors in working with gay males with AIDS and with health care providers.

Discussion

The authors highlight eight countertransference issues that workers typically confront, and present strategies for dealing with these issues.

Of special interest to mental health counselors and therapists.

997. FAULSTICH, Michael E. "Psychiatric aspects of AIDS." *American Journal of Psychiatry* 144 (1987): 551-556.

An overview of current knowledge concerning the manifestations and psychiatric aspects of AIDS.

Descriptive

AIDS has neuropsychiatric and psychopathological complications; anxiety, depressive symptoms, and suicidal ideation are common. Patients may express anger toward ineffective medical care and perceived public discrimination, guilt about sexual practices or drug abuse, reactions to social isolation, and uncertainty about the implications of an AIDS diagnosis. CNS dysfunction and subsequent neuropsychiatric impairment are common and are initially characterized by decreased acuity, slowed mentation, and psychomotor retardation that can resemble depression. Marked global cognitive deficits, disorientation, and delusions arise.

Of interest to mental health professionals and counselors.

998.   FERNANDEZ, Francisco, Valerie F. Holmes, Joel K. Levy, Pedro
        Ruiz.   "Consultation-liaison psychiatry and HIV-related
        disorders."   *Hospital and Community Psychiatry* 40 (1989):
        146-153.

The authors describe neuropsychiatric, psychosocial, and ethical-legal problems associated with HIV infection that are commonly encountered in a consultation-liaison psychiatry setting.

Descriptive

Because of HIV's potential for undermining cognitive function, the authors recommend a systematic neurobehavioral assessment for the differential diagnosis of emotional disturbance, including a test battery that also identifies neurotoxic effects of pharmacological agents. Among significant psychosocial and ethical-legal problems are patients' reactions to AIDS, their fears of social abandonment, staff burnout, antibody testing, confidentiality, and the use of life support measures. The consultation-liaison psychiatrist's awareness of the complexities of HIV-related neuropsychiatric symptoms and psychosocial issues can be of enormous benefit to medical caregivers and to patients.

Of interest to mental health professionals, physicians, nurses, and social workers.

999.   FLAVIN, Daniel K., John E. Franklin, Richard J. Frances.
        "The acquired immune deficiency syndrome (AIDS) and
        suicidal behavior in alcohol-dependent homosexual men."
        American Journal of Psychiatry 143 (1986): 1440-1442.

Examines the interrelationship among alcoholism and substance abuse, homosexuality, suicidal behavior, and AIDS.

Case Study

Support groups for AIDS patients, education of high risk groups on means of reducing the spread of AIDS, and early diagnosis and treatment of substance abuse and depression may all reduce the spread of AIDS and improve the quality of life for its victims. Being able to recognize patients at increased risk for suicide can lead to interventions aimed at breaking through destructive defense mechanisms, using family and social support networks, and offering viable alternatives to such behavior.

Of interest to health professionals, especially mental health professionals.

1000. FRIERSON, Robert L., and Steven B. Lippmann. "Psychologic implications of AIDS." *American Family Physician* 35, no. 3 (1987): 109-116.

Eleven patients with AIDS were seen by a psychiatric consultation service over a four year period.

Descriptive

Psychologic issues identified in these patients included changes in body image, feelings of helplessness and isolation, sexual concerns, and the grief process. Management should be aimed toward maintaining a nonjudgmental stance, providing liaison with other caregivers, and securing appropriate information and grief counseling for patients, with provision for the patients' loved ones.

Of special interest to mental health professionals and counselors.

1001. ———. "Suicide and AIDS." *Psychosomatics* 29 (1988): 226-231.

Discusses three cases of attempted suicide in response to AIDS.

Case Histories

The authors delineate 11 recommendations for decreasing AIDS-related suicides. These include: developing an increased sensitivity to depression; providing patients and families with accurate, current information about the disease; soliciting and respecting the wishes of AIDS patients regarding life supports; encouraging support groups for family members of AIDS patients; being aware of the depressant effects of medication; and recognizing the fact that demented and delirious patients are at a risk for self harm.

Of interest to all persons providing care to AIDS patients.

1002. FROLKIS, Joseph P. "'AIDS anxiety': New faces for old fears." *Postgraduate Medicine* 79 (1986): 265-276.

Describes the effects of intense anxiety about AIDS in patients who are not at risk.

Case Studies

"AIDS anxiety" can include symptoms of typical panic attacks combined
with a hypochondriacal conviction of the presence of undiagnosed AIDS.
The author describes three patients, none of whom was at risk for
AIDS, who sought medical attention because of intense fear and an
unshakable certainty that they had the disease. All exhibited
nonspecific "functional" symptoms, somatic preoccupation, persistence
in seeking a confirmatory diagnosis, and failure to find reassurance
in normal physical and laboratory studies. Now that heterosexual
transmission has been documented and the theory advanced that
prostitutes may be a source of the virus, primary care physicians may
soon find themselves dealing with persons who have engaged in casual
or promiscuous heterosexual sex and are in search of reassurance from
their doctors. Some may have concerns about AIDS that represent the
latest in a series of physical preoccupations. This concern may be
typical of the somatoform disorders rather than normal anxiety about a
worrisome symptom.

Of interest to primary care physicians and mental health
professionals.

1003. FURSTENBERG, Anne-Linda, and Miriam Meltzer Olson. "Social
      work and AIDS." *Social Work in Health Care* 9, no. 4
      (1984): 45-62.

Examines individual and societal responses to AIDS and to homosexuality that create issues for social work practice.

Review

General principles of social work practice are applied to the
specifics of dealing with AIDS, and social work tasks with patients,
families and significant others, health care staff, the community, and
policymakers are identified. The need for social workers to examine
their own attitudes, beliefs, and feelings on their responses, to
assure that their interventions are guided by their clients' needs
rather than their own, is pointed out.

Intended for social workers working with AIDS patients and their
families.

1004. GAMBE, Richard, and George S. Getzel. "Group work with gay
      men with AIDS." *Social Casework* 70 (1989): 172-179.

Describes a model for group work practice with gay men who have AIDS.

Descriptive

The emotional, social, economic, and political implications of AIDS
for gay men at diagnosis and during subsequent stages of the disease
process are discussed. The practice approach employed is supported by
concepts from crisis intervention as well as interactionist and
existential psychological theories. Stages of group development are
examined with regard to the changing biopsychosocial condition of
group members. The special skills required for group-work practice
are detailed.

Of interest to mental health professionals and counselors.

1005. GLASS, Richard M. "AIDS and suicide." *Journal of the American Medical Association* 259 (1988): 1369-1370.

Discusses the issues raised by the documentation of an increased suicide rate among AIDS patients.

Editorial

The documentation of an increased suicide risk among AIDS patients raises important issues, which include a complex set of clinical, ethical, and public policy problems. While some individuals and groups have proposed that suicide can be a rational choice for patients with a terminal illness such as AIDS, careful evaluation of suicides almost invariably reveals evidence of a psychiatric disorder rather than a rational choice, and most religious, ethical, and legal traditions have remained firmly opposed to suicide as an appropriate option for the terminally ill. Physicians should be aware of the periods of particularly high risk for suicide and should be highly suspicious of the risk, openly inquire about it, and arrange for psychiatric consultations at the first indication of a depressive syndrome or central nervous system complications. The risk of suicide in persons without AIDS who are informed of a positive test result for HIV antibodies constitutes a serious public health problem, and counseling by appropriately trained persons must be recognized as an essential aspect of HIV testing.

Of interest to health professionals and public health officials.

1006. GOULDEN, Terry, Peter Todd, Robert Hay, Jim Dykes. "AIDS and community supportive services: Understanding and management of psychosocial needs." *Medical Journal of Australia* 141 (1984): 582-586.

Discusses the need for research in the psychosocial aspects of AIDS and for planning for supportive services.

Discussion

As the numbers increase, it will no longer be possible to provide psychological and emotional support to persons with AIDS on an ad hoc, case by case basis. Therefore, it is necessary to plan for the coordination of home help services and for support groups and psychological assistance for persons with AIDS, their partners, and their families. Research in AIDS should go beyond the immunological and virological aspects of the disease to include the psychological and sociological implications of the epidemic. The mere delivery of facts and advice to affected subpopulations will not bring about the changes in sexual activity that are required if the epidemic is to be brought under control.

Of interest to health professionals, mental health professionals, health educators, public health planners, legislators, and policymakers.

1007. GREIF, Geoffrey L., and Edmund Porembski. "Significant others of drug abusers with AIDS: New challenges for drug treatment programs." *Journal of Substance Abuse Treatment* 4 (1987): 151-155.

Provides a case example of what the authors believe to be typical of what happens in a family when a drug abuser who previously had been estranged from the family is diagnosed with AIDS.

Review

A treatment program, which addresses both IV drug abuse and AIDS, is described.

Of special interest to social workers, drug abuse counselors, and mental health professionals.

1008. GRIMSHAW, Jonathan. "ABC of AIDS: Being HIV antibody positive." *British Medical Journal* 295 (1987): 256-257.

A personal account of the experience of being HIV antibody positive.

Essay

Having HIV disease has a demoralizing effect on an individual's emotional equilibrium, social and sexual lifestyle, self-confidence, and self-esteem. Doctors can help their patients come to terms, emotionally, socially, and psychologically, with the diagnosis and direct them into channels where they can find help that is appropriate to their particular needs. It is essential that doctors not only refer patients to counselors and agencies able to assess and meet their needs, but that they encourage them to develop the determination to achieve a sense of well-being through their own actions.

Of interest to physicians and other health professionals and to anyone who is at risk of HIV infection.

1009. GURDIN, Phyllis, and Gary R. Anderson. "Quality care for ill children: AIDS-specialized foster family homes." *Child Welfare* 66 (1987): 291-302.

Describes a special foster care demonstration in behalf of AIDS infants.

Descriptive

A foster care program specializing in serving children with AIDS or ARC, many of whom are abandoned at birth, has been established by the Leake and Watts Children's Home in New York City with the support of the AIDS Institute of New York, New York State Social Services, and New York City Special Services for Children. The project has demonstrated that special foster parents can be recruited and foster homes established to serve children infected with AIDS, although the need, at any one time, will undoubtedly exceed the number of available homes, making continuous recruitment necessary.   For those children too sick to live in foster homes, small agency-operated boarding homes might be a viable alternative to long hospitalizations in acute care facilities.   The child welfare system has the opportunity and the responsibility to provide quality services, including home care, for children infected with HIV.

Of interest to child welfare workers and other members of the helping professions.

1010. HENRY, Keith, Joseph Thurn, Daniel Anderson.   "Testing for human immunodeficiency virus: What to do if the result is positive." *Postgraduate Medicine* 85 (1989): 293-309.

The authors describe several tasks that have different sensitivities, specificities, and implications, and discuss some of the complex ethical and legal issues involved in testing for HIV.

Descriptive

The physician should discuss risks, prognosis, and alternative therapies in an open and candid manner, and educate patients about the disease and behaviors that reduce the risk of transmission.   Patients with HIV infection and AIDS are persons who deserve, expect, and need the same understanding and care given to other patients.

Of interest to health professionals, lawyers, public health professionals, and laypersons.

1011. HOLLAND, Jimmie C., and Susan Tross.   "The psychosocial and neuropsychiatric sequelae of the immunodeficiency syndrome and related disorders."   *Annals of Internal Medicine* 103 (1985): 760-764.

Discusses the psychological and neurologic symptoms of AIDS and the difficulty in differentiating the symptoms by source.

Descriptive

Patients' ability to tolerate the consequences of AIDS depends on their emotional strength and the availability of social support.   The social and psychological impact of AIDS may result in symptoms such as anxiety, depression, and delirium.   Since encephalopathy and dementia occur frequently in patients with AIDS, it is difficult, in the early stages, to separate reactive depression and psychomotor retardation from symptoms of central nervous system complications.

Of interest to physicians, psychologists, nurses, social workers, and counselors.

1012. HOOYMAN, Nancy R., Karen I. Fredriksen, Barbara Perlmutter.   "Shanti: An alternative response to the AIDS crisis." *Social Work* 12, no. 2 (1988): 17-30.

Reviews Shanti's mission and objectives and how these have changed over time; describes the decision-making structure that has evolved from these objectives; identifies the major strengths and limitations of this structure; and suggests implications for those presently engaged in designing and delivering services for persons with AIDS.

Review

Shanti has undergone significant changes since its inception. During its development, it faced a dilemma common to most alternative organizations: the need to achieve a balance between process and task performance. In addition, Shanti experienced the tensions generated by a need to provide sufficient time for conflict resolution and the personal growth of volunteers while devoting tremendous energy to organizational demands. Issues such as long-range planning, program development, and fund-raising are discussed in light of the demands on volunteers' time. Implications of Shanti's organizational structure and administrative tasks for other alternative organizations are discussed.

Of interest to physicians, social and behavioral scientists, clergy, and mental health professionals.

1013. JAMES, Mark E.   "HIV seropositivity diagnosed during pregnancy: Psychosocial characterization of patients and their adaptation." *General Hospital Psychiatry* 10 (1988): 309-316.

Describes and discusses the psychosocial problems encountered in 15 patients referred for psychiatric evaluation following diagnosis of HIV seropositivity during pregnancy.

Research

The diagnosis of HIV infection is uniquely traumatic to the pregnant patient. Her adjustment is complicated by concern for her fetus and by coexisting psychiatric disorders. The 15 obstetric patients described demonstrated significant comorbidity, increasing psychoactive substance abuse or dependence, adjustment and mood disorders, and personality disorders. Treatment should address not only adaptation to HIV infection, but also the psychodynamics of pregnancy, the anticipation of illness in the infant, and the management of drug addiction.

Of interest to obstetricians, family physicians, and mental health professionals.

1014. JOHNSON, Joyce M.   "AIDS-related psychosocial issues for the patient and physician." *Journal of the American Osteopathic Association* 88 (1988): 234-240.

Focuses on three issues—patients' fears and concerns, HIV antibody testing issues, and AIDS-related suicides.

Discussion

Discusses the social and emotional concerns of HIV-infected patients, pre, and post HIV antibody test counseling procedures, and risk factors specific to persons with HIV disease that enhance the risk of suicide.

Of interest to all physicians and health professionals.

1015. KIM, Choong R., and Leland S. Rickman. "Psychological aspects of the acquired immunodeficiency syndrome: A case report and review of the literature." *Military Medicine* 153 (1988): 638-641.

A case of a reservist with HIV infection is presented to highlight some of the potential psychological problems with HIV infection. A review of the medical literature revealed that the most common psychiatric consultations in patients infected with HIV were to evaluate the patients' anxiety and depression.

Review

Often, the psychological impact of AIDS is not considered until the late stages of the syndrome when life-threatening opportunistic infections appear. Patients with AIDS are at high risk for psychological problems that may need to be explored and dealt with carefully. Patients usually go through psychological adjustment processes similar to those of patients with other terminal illnesses. It is often helpful to confirm that the patient's own reactions to AIDS are understandable and normal and to facilitate them with supportive services such as crisis, legal, and financial counseling.

Of interest to mental health professionals.

1016. LAUER-LISTHAUS, Barbara, and John Watterson. "A psychoeducational group for HIV-positive patients on a psychiatric service." *Hospital and Community Psychiatry* 39 (1988): 776-777.

Reports on a pilot study for educating psychiatric patients about their HIV positive status.

Research

The results of six educational sessions, conducted to provide four psychiatric patients with accurate information about their HIV seropositivity, a support system, and an understanding of their responsibility for not infecting others, were investigated. Findings suggest that the psychoeducational group approach is effective.

Of interest to health educators, mental health professionals, and psychiatric nurses.

1017. LEUKEFELD, Carl G. "Psychosocial issues in dealing with AIDS." *Hospital and Community Psychiatry* 40 (1989): 454-455.

An update on the psychosocial aspects of AIDS.

Commentary

Dealing with the psychosocial aspects of AIDS can be as important for persons with AIDS and their families as dealing with the medical aspects. Health care professionals must be prepared to offer substantial help in solving psychosocial problems and obtaining such necessary community resources as housing, income, maintenance, long-term and hospice care, home care, counseling and mental health services, legal assistance, medical care, and health education. Professionals must also be aware of the psychosocial context of their own feelings and anxieties. Suggestions are made for helping social workers to avoid burnout and continue to contribute to the treatment of persons with AIDS and their families.

Of particular interest to social workers.

1018. LOCKHART, Lettie L., and John S. Wodarski. "Facing the unknown: Children and adolescents with AIDS." *Social Work* 34 (1989): 215-221.

An overview of recent trends in pediatric and adolescent AIDS, describing the impact of AIDS on children and recommending roles for social workers.

Descriptive

An increasing number of children and adolescents have been diagnosed with AIDS. Like adults, these youngsters not only must struggle for survival, but must contend with social isolation, rejection, and ostracism. Because of the devastating psychosocial impact of AIDS on children and adolescents and their families, social workers must try several approaches to counseling and treatment. They must consider the legal and ethical issues involved in placing youngsters with AIDS who lack family support in foster care. They also must identify the concerns of specific cultural and minority groups, test methods of intervention, and determine service and practice requirements for staff and programs.

Of interest to social workers and educators.

1019. LOPEZ, Diego, and George S. Getzel. "Group work with teams of volunteers serving people with AIDS." *Social Work with Groups* 10 (1987): 33-48.

Explains the development of volunteer groups related to the special needs of people with AIDS.

Descriptive

Particular attention is given to the kind of activities and issues that arise in volunteer and training groups. Using their insights of small group theory and their understanding of the types of problems faced by victims of AIDS who are trying to support themselves in the community, volunteers are helped to work more effectively with persons afflicted with this disease.

Of interest to mental health professionals, especially social workers.

1020. ———. "Strategies for volunteers caring for persons with AIDS." *Social Casework* (1987): 47-53.

Discusses the volunteer program of the Gay Men's Health Crisis, a New York based volunteer agency that serves gay and non-gay persons with AIDS.

Descriptive

The psychosocial and sociopolitical characteristics of the AIDS epidemic are outlined. Strategies that sustain and support workers and volunteers in their efforts are described.

Of interest to social workers and volunteers.

1021. LOVEJOY, Nancy C., and Theresa A. Moran. "Selected AIDS beliefs, behaviors and informational needs of homosexual/bisexual men with AIDS or ARC." *International Journal of Nursing Studies* 25 (1988): 207-216.

Describes AIDS beliefs, behaviors and informational needs of patients with AIDS or AIDS-related complex seven years into the epidemic.

Research

Study results showed that 90% of outpatients at an internationally recognized AIDS medical center wanted more information about building their immune systems. Surprisingly few patients (10%) wanted explicit information about safe sex. Results suggest that nurses need to take a more active role in monitoring and addressing patients' changing informational needs.

Of interest to nurses and allied health professionals.

1022. MAHORNEY, Steven L., and Jesse O. Cavenar, Jr. "A new and timely delusion: the complaint of having AIDS." *American Journal of Psychiatry* 145 (1988): 1130-1132.

Presents three cases that document the delusion of having AIDS in patients who are not members of high risk groups, but have psychiatric disorders.

Case Reports

These cases illustrate that as the AIDS epidemic becomes a fixture in the public consciousness, it may become increasingly incorporated into the delusional material of patients with psychiatric disorders. The authors think it important that physicians become aware that patients without evidence of compromised immune status and without membership in high risk groups may present with a complaint of having AIDS. Such a presentation should raise the physicians' suspicion of an underlying delusional disorder.

Of interest to mental health professionals.

1023. MALONEY, Bland D. "The legacy of AIDS: Challenge for the next century." *Journal of Marital and Family Therapy* 14 (1988): 143-150.

Presents an organized method of therapy based on a stage-related intervention process for dealing with AIDS.

Descriptive

Suggests a method of response that involves three stages of therapy: dealing with the crisis of disclosure, interacting with larger systems, and working on family relationships and the grieving process. Countertransference issues, which threaten to disrupt this three-stage process, are discussed.

Of particular interest to psychotherapists and counselors.

1024. MILLER, David, John Green, Roger Farmer, and Gillian Carroll. A 'pseudo-AIDS' syndrome following from fear of AIDS." *British Journal of Psychiatry* 146 (1985): 550-551.

Demonstrates how the fear of AIDS can produce symptoms that mimic those of AIDS.

Descriptive

The early symptoms of AIDS are similar to those of anxiety and depression. Two case studies of homosexual males who showed psychiatric symptoms associated with a fear of AIDS, resulting in significant functional impairment, are presented. As the number of AIDS patients increases, more cases of this nature, in which psychiatric symptoms resulting from the fear of AIDS mimic the prodromal stages of AIDS, are likely to appear. Clinicians need to be alerted to the likelihood of psychiatric complications arising from fear of AIDS in their homosexual patients.

Of particular interest to primary care physicians and psychiatrists.

1025. MORIN, Stephen F., and Walter F. Batchelor. "Responding to the psychological crisis of AIDS." *Public Health Reports* 99 (1984): 4-9.

Discusses the broad psychological ramifications of AIDS for individuals, friends and family, health care workers, and society.

Descriptive

Individuals are reacting to the threat of an unknown but deadly epidemic with fear when strength is needed, with denial when awareness is needed, with guilt when understanding is needed, and with withdrawal when caring is needed. The authors believe that it is the responsibility of the health and mental health communities to respond to the psychological needs of persons with AIDS, and to the needs of their lovers and friends.

Of interest to all kinds of health professionals.

1026   NELSON, Marven O., and Kent Jurratt.   "Spiritual and mental
        health care of persons with AIDS."   *Individual Psychology*
        43 (1987): 479-489.

The Metropolitan-Duane United Methodist Church's Center for Mental Health, located in Greenwich Village, undertook a program for persons with AIDS and ARC. The program, persons, therapy, and therapists are discussed.

Descriptive

The authors describe an Adlerian-based program that grew out of one church's response to a crisis within its community. An integral part of the program is the acknowledgment that since a community is made up of personalities, the role of the therapist is to preserve the individual personality and to resist attempts at categorizing persons with AIDS or ARC as victims with stereotyped responses.

Of interest to clergy, counselors, and mental health professionals.

1027. NICHOLS, Stuart E.   "Emotional aspects of AIDS--Implications
        for care providers."   *Journal of Substance Abuse Treatment* 4
        (1987): 137-140.

Addresses the effect of AIDS on the emotions.

Review

A discussion of the care for the emotional concerns of AIDS patients, specific psychiatric entities seen in AIDS, and adjustments to AIDS as a catastrophic reaction.

Of interest to laymen and health professionals.

1028. NICHOLS, Stuart E., Jr.   "Psychiatric aspects of AIDS."
        Psychosomatics 24 (1983): 1083-1089.

The author discusses his experiences with AIDS patients, pointing out their psychosocial needs.

Editorial

Discusses support systems, emotional reactions, and the types of psychiatric assistance needed in treating AIDS patients.

Of interest to mental health professionals.

1029. OLSON, Roberta A., Heather C. Huszti, Patrick J. Mason, Jeffrey M. Seibert. "Pediatric AIDS/HIV infection: An emerging challenge to pediatric psychology." *Journal of Pediatric Psychology* 14 (1989): 1-21.

Examines selected clinical and ethical issues psychologists may encounter in research or psychotherapy with children, adolescents, or parents who are positive for the HIV virus or have AIDS.

Descriptive

Areas of opportunities and problems for psychologists are briefly identified. These areas include prevention, clinical issues, public education, research, neuropsychological effects, psychoneuro-immunological issues, and ethical concerns. Current epidemiological projections and future directions for research are also discussed.

Of special interest to psychologists.

1030. OSTROW, David G., Jill Joseph, Andrew Monjan, *et al.* "Psychosocial aspects of AIDS risk." *Psychopharmacology Bulletin* 22 (1985): 678-683.

An overview of the known psychological and behavioral consequences of AIDS risk.

Review

Profound changes are taking place in the male homosexual population as the result of the health crisis brought about by AIDS. The psychological consequences of the threat of developing AIDS have been coupled with the secondary stresses of behavioral change and the isolation and social stigmatization of the disease. In addition, the effects of central nervous system infection by HIV must be added to the list of factors potentially contributing to the depression and anergy seen by the authors in the Multicenter AIDS Cohort Study population. Carefully designed prospective examinations of psychological, cognitive, and neurological functioning in persons who are HIV infected are necessary to determine the relative contributions of these factors to the overall mental health impact of AIDS.

Of interest to health professionals and mental health professionals.

1031. PERRY, Samuel W., and Susan Tross. "Psychiatric problems of AIDS inpatients at the New York Hospital: Preliminary report." *Public Health Reports* 99 (1984): 200-205.

A retrospective review of the charts of 52 patients with AIDS in the New York Hospital was conducted to determine the prevalence of recorded psychiatric complications and the use of psychiatric consultation.

Research

Although references to neuropsychiatric complications appeared in every patient's chart, neurological complications were seldom explicitly diagnosed and psychiatric consultation was requested for only ten patients because of management problems, for diagnostic assessment, or by self-referral. The results suggest that the neuropsychiatric complications of AIDS are underdiagnosed during acute illness and that psychiatric consultation is underutilized. AIDS patients have a heightened risk of psychological problems. Contributing factors may include the threat to life, severe physical debilitation, central nervous system involvement, fear of contagion, disclosure of homosexuality or drug abuse, and guilt associated with sexual transmission.

Of interest to primary care physicians and mental health professionals.

1032. "PSYCHOLOGY and AIDS." *American Psychologist* 43 (1988): 835-987.

A resource for those interested in the psychological dimensions of AIDS and HIV infection in training, research, and practice settings.

Special Journal Issue

Divided into six major sections, each with an introduction. Provides an overview of the roles of psychology in the AIDS health crisis. Reviews the primary issues that AIDS commands us to examine, such as public health, antibody testing, AIDS and the communities of black and Hispanic men, IV drug use, sexual behavior change, stigma, and psychoneuroimmunology. Covers the contributions of psychology as a science in a series of articles on scientific issues. Reflects clinical and counseling issues in a series of articles about how psychological distress and neuropsychological complications of AIDS affect psychotherapy and about how practitioners need to deal with the ethical and legal aspects of AIDS in their work. Some special issues in education and prevention, including those relating to minorities, are covered, and organizational issues are presented.

Of special interest to social and behavioral scientists.

1033. RENDON, Mario, Phyllis Gurdin, Jorge Bassi, Martha Weston. "Foster care for children with AIDS: A psychosocial perspective." *Child Psychiatry and Human Development* 19 (1989): 256-269.

Chronicles the development of the first foster boarding home program in the United States for babies with AIDS.

Descriptive

The first foster boarding home program for babies with AIDS in the United States was started in 1985 by the Leake and Watts Children's Home in New York. The authors describe the stages of the program, the possible reasons for its success, and some general characteristics of the AIDS epidemic. They also present preliminary findings about the characteristics of the children and foster parents in this group. General psychosocial issues concerning AIDS are discussed.

Of interest to pediatricians, social workers, and other professionals involved in foster care.

1034. RYAN, Caitlin C. "The social and clinical challenges of AIDS."
      Smith College Studies in Social Work 59 (1988): 3-20.

Discusses the tasks of social workers, at each stage of HIV infection, in helping clients and their families maintain control over their illness.

Discussion

The task of the social worker, at the onset of the illness, is to help clients/families deal with their emotions, restructure relationships, and obtain necessary information about HIV infection and about sources of help. During the adaptation stage, the social worker should help patients grieve over the loss of health and changes in appearance, make decisions about informing others of their illness, discuss the issues of suicide and dementia, and help the client understand options for treatment. In the final stage of illness, the social worker's task includes helping patients/families in planning final rites and coping with grief. Social workers should receive AIDS inservice education and support, which will equip them to educate clients/families about their financial entitlements, legal rights, and legal obligations to the clients' sexual partners. The author recommends that professional social work organizations lobby for non-discriminatory legislation and adequate resources for persons infected with HIV.

Of interest to social workers, social work administrators, mental health professionals, and health educators.

1035. SCHINDLER, Victoria J. "Psychosocial occupational therapy intervention with AIDS patients." *American Journal of Occupational Therapy* 42 (1988): 507-512.

The role of psychosocial occupational therapy with AIDS patients is explored.

Descriptive

The clinical picture is defined, information regarding the transmission, incidence, diagnosis, and treatment is presented, and the impact of the illness on the developmental life cycle is described. The occupational behavior framework is used to guide evaluation and intervention, and case examples are provided. Fears and issues affecting therapists working with AIDS patients are explored.

Of special interest to occupational therapists and other allied health professionals.

1036. SEPTIMUS, Anita. "Psychosocial aspects of caring for families of infants infected with human immunodeficiency virus." *Seminars in Perinatology* 13 (1989): 49-54.

Describes an AIDS comprehensive family program, which provides preventive, medical, social, and emotional care for inpatients and outpatients.

Descriptive

In order to keep HIV infected families functional, a synchronized network of hospital and mental health professionals and community resources is needed to reach out to these families and bring them support within their own ethnic, societal, and religious contexts. To respond to the magnitude of this crisis, comprehensive AIDS programs with heavy emphasis on mental health and social services are strongly advocated and supported.

Of interest to family medicine physicians, social workers, and pediatricians.

1037. TEHAN, Claire. "Training volunteers to care for AIDS patients." *Volunteer Leader* 28, no. 2 (1987): 10-13.

Describes a training program to prepare a corp of heterosexual volunteers, already trained and experienced in the care of "traditional" hospice patients, to meet the unique needs of gay AIDS patients.

Descriptive

A training program for volunteers to address the unmet needs of AIDS patients was developed by the volunteer director of the hospice program of Hospital Home Health Care Agency of California. The program appears to have been successful in helping volunteers transcend the barrier of homophobia and accept their gay patients' lifestyles. Because AIDS patients' physical and psychological problems can be overwhelming to those who care for them, volunteers are encouraged to attend hospice team meetings and meet regularly with the nurse and social worker. The volunteers have been enthusiastic about their training and their work with patients. In future versions of the program, the volunteers will serve as faculty and share their first-hand experience of the rewards and difficulties of working with gay AIDS patients with new trainees.

Of interest to hospice staff, hospital administrators, and volunteer directors.

1038. THOMPSON, Leslie M. "Dealing with AIDS and fear: Would you accept cookies from an AIDS patient?" *Southern Medical Journal* 80 (1987): 228-232.

Proposes that health professionals have generally failed to provide adequate support systems to deal with the emotional needs of dying AIDS patients.

Commentary

Health professionals must now move rapidly to develop support systems based on a realistic understanding of the fears and other powerful emotions confronted by AIDS victims. Such systems must permit AIDS patients to give meaning to their adversity.

Of general interest to health professionals.

1039. TSOUKAS, Chris. "AIDS: Future implications for palliative care." *Journal of Palliative Care* 2, no. 1 (1986): 35-38.

Reports on the implications of AIDS for outpatient care.

Discussion

An AIDS service is needed to coordinate inpatient and outpatient care. Social and psychiatric status should be assessed prior to performing a physical examination or requesting laboratory tests.   Counseling should be provided as necessary, and legal issues addressed before the patient becomes incompetent.   A multidisciplinary team, including a primary care physician, psychiatric nurse, home care nurse, social worker, and community volunteer, should care for persons with AIDS.

Of interest to nurses, physicians, counselors, social workers, and volunteers.

1040. WHITEFORD, Harvey A., and John G. Csernansky. "Psychiatric aspects of acquired immune deficiency syndrome (AIDS)." *Australian and New Zealand Journal of Psychiatry* 20 (1986): 399-403.

Suggests that behavioral interventions are needed to provide stress reduction while encouraging behavioral change.

Editorial

Because psychological, social, psychiatric, and neurological complications occur frequently in the course of AIDS, the management of a patient must involve an integrated biopsychosocial treatment plan. Psychological morbidity can be limited by early professional intervention. Marshalling social supports is invaluable for most patients.

Of interest to mental health professionals and health educators.

1041. WIENER, Lori. "Helping clients with AIDS: The Role of the worker." *Public Welfare* 44, no. 4 (1986): 38-41, 47.

Addresses the special needs which human service workers face in helping clients with AIDS, the unique psychosocial needs of this client population, and how workers can deal with their own concerns about this disease and the persons it affects.

Descriptive

Through education and preparation, a worker can develop personal skills and resources to become more effective in dealing with the client who has AIDS. Workers must remember to respond to the client with AIDS with neutrality, not prejudice, and to maintain confidentiality about the case. Human service workers must remain sensitive to the needs of those who are dying from the disease. They must work toward eliminating social bias and discrimination against all minorities. At the same time, they must not ignore the stress that working with this population will place upon them.

Of particular interest to social workers, counselors, and other human service workers.

1042. WOLCOTT, Deane L. "Psychosocial aspects of acquired immune deficiency syndrome and the primary care physician." *Annals of Allergy* 57 (1986): 95-102.

Reviews the psychosocial aspects of AIDS and AIDS-related complex, and the primary physician's role in the care of AIDS and ARC patients.

Review

While the needs and problems of AIDS patients are similar to those of other young adults with chronic life-threatening illness, multiple factors create unique patterns of stress for AIDS patients, members of their social networks, and health care personnel. The primary care physician needs to concern himself with understanding the psychosocial stresses of AIDS and work with a multidisciplinary team to provide support for the patient and his family.

Of interest to primary care physicians.

1043. ——, Fawzy I. Fawzy, John Landsverk, Martin McCombs. "AIDS patients' needs for psychosocial services and their use of community service organizations." *Journal of Psychosocial Oncology* 4 (1986): 135-146.

A study of AIDS-affected individuals in Los Angeles was undertaken to assess the needs of AIDS patients for psychosocial services, the extent of their use of such services, and the level of their satisfaction with services received from community-based service organizations.

Research

Patients expressed the need for many kinds of services, including those that provide medical information, medical referrals, and practical help as well as support groups and individual therapy. Most patients were satisfied with the services they used, but patients were most satisfied with individual therapy and services that provided transportation, food, and clothing. The results of the study made it clear that organizations which serve AIDS patients should provide a wide variety of psychosocial services.

Of interest to administrators, staff, and volunteers working for community-based service organizations.

1044. ———, Fawzy I. Fawzy, Robert O. Pasnau. "Acquired immune deficiency syndrome (AIDS) and consultation-liason psychiatry." *General Hospital Psychiatry* 7 (1985): 280-292.

The psychosocial effects of AIDS for patients, family and friends, and health care professionals are discussed.

Descriptive

An integrated multidisciplinary team, providing coordinated medical and psychiatric care to patients during inpatient and outpatient phases of treatment, should be developed by each institution that treats a significant number of AIDS patients. This approach would greatly facilitate optimal clinical patient care, as well as longitudinal research that is needed to characterize the psychiatric and psychosocial problems of AIDS patients more fully.

Of interest to virologists, psychiatrists, social workers, nurses, and other health professionals caring for AIDS patients.

1045. ZUCKERMAN, Connie, and Lauren Gordon. "Meeting the psychosocial and legal needs of women with AIDS and their families." *New York State Journal of Medicine* 88 (1988): 619-620.

Discusses the need of women with AIDS and their families for more comprehensive assistance than diagnosis and treatment.

Discussion

Women diagnosed with AIDS and their families have special psychosocial and legal needs. They may need help in arranging for child care, dealing with blame and denial, mediating family conflicts, and practicing safer sex. Legal advisors and consultants can help in arranging for durable powers of attorney, drafting wills, and petitioning courts to appoint guardians for children. Coordination and integration of these services with therapeutic interventions in a medical setting are needed.

Of interest to physicians, social workers, attorneys, and educators.

A. COUNSELING

a. Articles

1046. BARRET, Robert L. "Counseling gay men with AIDS: Human dimensions." *Journal of Counseling and Development* 67 (1989): 573-575.

Provides case material that demonstrates emotional responses of gay men to AIDS.

Descriptive

Counselors need to become familiar with the psychological manifestations of AIDS. Denial, anger, rage, guilt, and shame are discussed with an emphasis on the human dimensions of AIDS.

Of interest to mental health professionals and counselors.

1047. BOR, Robert, Riva Miller, Lucy Perry. "AIDS counseling: Clinical application and development of services." *British Journal of Guidance and Counseling* 16 (1988): 11-20.

The role of the counselor, both in medicine and in the field of AIDS/HIV infections, is outlined.

Descriptive

The psychosocial difficulties accompanying AIDS are reviewed. Stress is placed on the need to consider not only the clients, but also their sexual partners, family, friends, colleagues, and other members of the health care team. Further investigations need to be carried out to clarify where AIDS counseling services fit in with other medical and paramedical services.

Of interests to mental health professionals.

1048. ———. "Systemic counseling for patients with AIDS/HIV infections." *Family Systems Medicine* 6 (1988): 21-39.

Describes the impact on various parts of the hospital system of a system counseling service for patients with AIDS/HIV infections.

Descriptive

Conversations between counselors and referrers serve to demonstrate how the counseling task was clarified. Explanations are offered for different views of counseling as a part of the care of patients with AIDS/HIV infections, and the implications of setting up a systemic service are discussed.

Of interest to hospital staff and mental health professionals.

1049. ———. "A systems approach to AIDS counselling." *Journal of Family Therapy* 11 (1989): 77-86.

Describes the initial tasks of a systemic AIDS counselor in accepting a referral.

Descriptive

An AIDS counselor, using a systems approach, must first describe the context of the problem, then obtain a clear definition of the problem, respond to changing views of the problem over time, and identify whom the problem affects. Failure to consider these issues can result in extraneous difficulties in counseling sessions. Two case studies illustrate the changing definition of a problem.

Of interest to AIDS counselors, social workers, nurses, and educators.

1050. BRUHN, John G. "Counseling persons with a fear of AIDS." *Journal of Counseling and Development* 67 (April 1989): 455-457.

Fears accentuated by AIDS are discussed and guidelines for counseling offered.

Descriptive

A background of the roots of public fears about AIDS is given. Types of AIDS fear are presented and discussed in terms of HIV status and risk group membership. Finally, guidelines for counseling persons about the fear of AIDS are offered.

Of interest to counselors, mental health professionals, and social workers.

1051. FRIERSON, Robert L., Steven B. Lippmann, Janet Johnson. "AIDS: Psychological stresses on the family. Recommendations for counseling relatives of the AIDS patient." *Psychosomatics* 28 (1987): 65-68.

Psychological repercussions of AIDS on 50 relatives of 15 AIDS patients were assessed and treated during psychiatric consultations over a period of four and one half years.

Descriptive

The most frequent sources of stress were fears of contracting AIDS, the simultaneous revelations of homosexual or bisexual activity and what could prove to be a terminal disease, notoriety, a sense of helplessness, and grieving, especially among parents. Beneficial interventions for relatives included the provision of accurate information, a non-judgmental approach, grief counseling, and peer support groups, which were particularly helpful in combatting the sense of isolation felt by the family.

Of interest to mental health professionals.

1052. GEIS, Sally B., Ruth L. Fuller, Julian Rush. "Lovers of AIDS victims: Psychosocial stresses and counseling needs." *Death Studies* 10 (1986): 43-53.

Indepth interviews and observations of a small, nonrandom sample were used to identify the major psychosocial stresses of lovers of AIDS patients.

Research

Major areas of psychosocial stress for lovers were identified as disease management problems, including misdiagnosis, protocol changes, and fear of insensitivity on the part of caregivers as well as isolation from such support groups as family, friends, and churches. The authors conclude that stress resulting from stigma and isolation should not be underestimated; AIDS patients, their lovers, and their biological families need counseling.

Of interest to counselors, mental health professionals, and social workers.

1053. GRANT, Duncan and Mark Anns. "Counseling AIDS antibody-positive clients: Reactions and treatment." *American Psychologist* 43 (1988): 72-74.

Describes experiences in counseling antibody-positive clients at the Albion Street Clinic in New South Wales.

Commentary

A description of short and long term reactions to antibody-positive results and their possible outcomes for patients.

Of special interest to health professionals, counselors, and public health officials.

1054. HOLMAN, Susan, Marise Berthaud, Ann Sunderland, Gail Moroso, Frank Cancellieri, Hermann Mendez, Eva Beller, Adrien Marcel. "Women infected with human immunodeficiency virus: Counseling and testing during pregnancy." *Seminars in Perinatology* 13 (1989): 7-15.

Focuses on the appropriate counseling of women found to be HIV positive during pregnancy, and on those issues that the diagnosis of HIV infection raises in their lives.

Descriptive

Describes a counseling program, which is part of an ongoing perinatal HIV transmission study being conducted at SUNY-Health Science Center at Brooklyn, New York. Pregnant women at risk for HIV infection are counseled and offered confidential HIV testing. Those who test positive are assigned two counselors, one to provide information and one to provide emotional support. Written materials are provided for the women to take home. Abortion is discussed with those women who are less than 24 weeks into their pregnancy. Within a week of the initial counseling session, a follow-up session, to provide additional information and identify special needs for support or help in coping, is scheduled. When necessary, role playing is used to help a woman prepare to inform her sexual partner of her HIV status. Psychosocial assessment and support are provided on an ongoing basis, even when the pregnancy is terminated.

Of interest to social workers, counselors, and mental health professionals.

1055. KINNIER, Richard T. "The need for psychosocial research on AIDS and counseling interventions for AIDS victims." *Journal of Counseling and Development* 64 (1986): 472-474.

Suggests what counselors can learn from epidemics of the past and summarizes several of the salient psychological needs of AIDS victims, individuals with "pre-AIDS," and the "worried well."

Descriptive

Practitioners and researchers in the social sciences can contribute to alleviating the pain and suffering associated with the AIDS epidemic. Researchers face the challenge of identifying psychosocial factors that may be associated with the prevention of AIDS and with the health improvement of AIDS victims. Practitioners can help victims to cope and to fight for their lives, high-risk individuals to control their anxiety and to reduce their risks, and everyone else to avoid unhealthy worry and to make decisions rationally and with compassion toward victims.

Of interest to social and behavioral scientists and mental health professionals.

1056. KRIEGER, Irwin. "An approach to coping with anxiety about AIDS." *Social Work* 33 (1988): 263-264.

Describes a stepwise counseling approach for assisting persons with heightened anxiety about AIDS and ways to handle fears about the sexual transmission of AIDS.

Descriptive

The counseling approach presented here provides a framework for addressing anxiety about AIDS and helping others overcome it. In clinical work, anxiety about AIDS may be a client's presenting problem or an issue of secondary importance. It may be a motivating factor in a pattern of self-destructive behavior. The fear of AIDS affects anyone with a risk of exposure to HIV to some degree. When that fear becomes unmanageable, intervention is needed.

Of interest to counselors, mental health professionals, and health educators.

1057. MAGALLON, Dorothy T. "Counseling patients with HIV infections." *Medical Aspects of Human Sexuality* 21, no. 6 (1987): 129-147.

Provides advice for counselors of HIV infected patients.

Descriptive

Management of an ultimately fatal disease for which there is currently no cure, no definitive treatment, and no specific preventive regimen depends primarily on patient education and counseling for maximum effectiveness. Patients who are HIV-positive or have progressed to AIDS require far more than the brief, explanatory counseling that is usually adequate for other complaints. The author offers guidelines to the physician for providing the patient with the information needed to bridge the gap between diagnosis and the point at which referral for specialized services and counseling may become necessary.

Of particular interest to primary care physicians.

1058. NAJI, Simon, Patricia Wilkie, Ivana Markova, Charles Forbes, Judy Watson. "Coping strategies of patients with haemophilia as a risk group for AIDS (Acquired Immune Deficiency Syndrome)." *International Journal of Rehabilitation Research* 9 (1986): 179-180.

Describes a study in which 90 patients and, where possible, their spouses are participating in an attempt to determine what kinds of information patients with hemophilia need to have about AIDS, and how, when, and by whom it should be given.

Research

The authors hope to identify the ways in which patients with hemophilia and their families assimilate, psychologically represent, and interpret information about AIDS, and how they use it in decision making; to explore the attitudes and perceptions of medical, nursing, laboratory, and ancillary staff towards AIDS and risk groups; to use the preceding information to construct a coherent counseling model for high risk groups; and to extend the results to counseling in other medical problems in which a person has to make judgments under uncertainty.

Of interest to hematologists, counselors, and mental health professionals.

1059. PERRY, Samuel W., and John C. Markowitz. "Counseling for HIV testing." *Hospital and Community Psychiatry* 39 (1988): 731-739.

Recommendations are presented for counseling individuals who wish to know if they have been infected by HIV.

Descriptive

Pretest counseling includes explaining the sensitivity and meaning of HIV antibody tests and the limits of confidentiality, assessing the patient's potential strengths, vulnerabilities, coping capacity, and supportive resources, and mutually deciding if the test is advisable.

Populations that have been identified as being at risk for HIV infection are listed, and four case vignettes that illustrate the complexity of the decision to be tested are provided. Post test counseling includes notification of test results, reducing the immediate distress of seropositive patients, educating about how HIV is and is not spread, explaining methods to prevent transmission, advising the patient about who should be told the test results, and arranging follow-up care.

Of interest to physicians, nurses, and mental health professionals.

1060. PRICE, Richard E., Michael M. Omizo, Victoria L. Hammett. "Counseling clients with AIDS." *Journal of Counseling and Development* 65 (1986): 96-97.

The authors discuss issues and suggestions relative to counseling clients with AIDS.

Descriptive

Several psychosocial issues are presented, and a psychoeducational model of treatment to meet the needs of AIDS clients is described.

Of interest to counselors and mental health professionals.

1061. SPENCER, Norman. "Medical anthropology and the AIDS epidemic: A case study in San Francisco." *Urban Anthropology* 12 (1983): 141-159

Describes the contribution of anthropology to developing and implementing a counseling program offered to participants in an "Alternative Test Site Program" sponsored by the Centers for Disease Control.

Descriptive

The decision to take the test for antibodies to the AIDS virus is a complex issue for gay and bisexual men in San Francisco. How test results confirming a potentially life threatening condition are heard, interpreted, and acted upon is a complex psychological and cultural process, even without the social stigma surrounding homosexuality and AIDS. Statements by program participants suggest that the process of confronting critical information, no matter what the result, is a strong catalyst for major shifts in personal and social values. These changes tend to be in the direction of decreased hedonism, increased social responsibility, and an affirmation of gay lifestyle.

Of interest to anthropologists, educators, and mental health professionals.

1062. Van DEVANTER, Nancy L., Jo Ann B. Grisaffi, Melanie Steilen, Mary E. Scarola, Ruth M. Shipton, Catherine Tendler, Johanna Pindyck. "Counseling HIV-antibody positive blood donors." *American Journal of Nursing* 87 (1987): 1026-1030.

Describes a program for detecting, notifying and counseling HIV antibody positive blood donors.

Descriptive

The Greater New York Blood Program offers counseling, information, and support to donors who are found to be seropositive, while maintaining strict confidentiality. This innovative program for helping persons infected with HIV to cope appropriately is described in detail.

Of interest to blood bank nurses, technicians, and administrators as well as mental health professionals.

1063. WILKIE, Patricia A. "Counselling in HIV infection." *Scottish Medical Journal* 32 (1987): 114-116.

A discussion of issues in counseling HIV seropositive patients.

Discussion

An HIV positive diagnosis may seem like a death sentence to some patients. In counseling, it is important to look at the good things in the patient's life, to encourage the patient to pursue interests and hobbies and to carry on with living as full a life as possible. This helps to put the diagnosis in perspective.

Of interest to counselors.

B. PSYCHOTHERAPY

a. Articles

1064. ADLER, Gerald, and Alexandra Beckett. "Psychotherapy of the patient with an HIV infection: Some ethical and therapeutic dilemmas." *Psychosomatics* 30 (1989): 203-208.

Discusses therapeutic and ethical dilemmas and countertransference difficulties that arise in psychotherapeutic work with patients with AIDS-related complex.

Case Report

The psychotherapeutic results with patients with HIV infections can be very gratifying. Not only can the acute issues surrounding the patient's illness be addressed, but long-term personality problems can be modified at a time when the patient is facing a life-threatening and probably fatal disease and struggling with the desire to make creative use of a shortened life span. The therapist's work can be made easier by an understanding of the complex intrapsychic, often conflicting, interpersonal and social issues involved, as well as by the availability of colleagues with whom to share these painful clinical dilemmas.

Of interest to psychotherapists and mental health professionals.

1065. BARROWS, Paul A., and Richard P. Halgin. "Current issues in psychotherapy with gay men: Impact of the AIDS phenomenon." *Professional Psychology: Research and Practice* 19 (1988): 395-402.

Addresses the impact of the AIDS phenomenon on psychotherapy with asymptomatic gay men.

Descriptive

The authors address specific issues pertaining to psychotherapy with gay men and offer suggestions about how professionals might address these issues in the helping context. Discusses ways in which therapists can help gay clients develop a positive gay identity, to reevaluate their patterns of socializing, to learn safe sex techniques and develop positive attitudes toward them, to learn new styles of intimacy, to understand the HIV test and the implications of testing, and to develop coping strategies for dealing with the loss of loved ones and acquaintances.

Of interest to counselors of gay men and mental health professionals.

1066. ISAACS, Gordon.   "Crises psychotherapy with persons experiencing the AIDS related complex." *Crisis Intervention* 14, no. 4 (1985): 115-121.

A discussion of crisis psychotherapy with persons experiencing the AIDS related complex.

Descriptive

Persons with ARC and the "worried well" form a significantly larger population among those directly affected by the wider AIDS scare than do those persons actually diagnosed with AIDS. Crisis psychotherapy can be an effective approach within the existing structures being provided for dealing with AIDS.

Of interest to mental health professionals.

1067. LOMAX, Gary L., and Jeffrey Sandler.   "Psychotherapy and consultation with persons with AIDS." *Psychiatric Annals* 18 (1988): 253-259.

Presents two papers prepared as part of a four-session educational program titled, "A psychosocial AIDS/ARC update: A multidisciplinary symposium," sponsored by the Department of Psychiatry at Pacific Presbyterian Medical Center, San Francisco, which focused on neuropsychiatric complications of AIDS and therapeutic issues relevant to the treatment of inpatients, outpatients, and the "worried well."

Review

Part I outlines the tasks of psychotherapy with an AIDS patient within a framework for understanding the patient's emotional issues and needs throughout the course of the illness. It offers a model consisting of four stages, each of which defines a significant phase of the illness and concomitant psychosocial issues: diagnosis, stabilization, deterioration, and terminal stage. Part II looks at the patient's surrounding social milieu and the mechanics of actually providing a psychiatric consultation. It discusses the need for a systems approach in dealing with all of the members of the team of health professionals who provide care for the AIDS patient, the consultation procedure, and the ongoing therapeutic relationship.

Of interest to all mental health professionals caring for AIDS patients.

1068. McKUSICK, Leon. "The impact of AIDS on practitioner and client." *American Psychologist* 43 (1988): 935-940.

Discusses the dynamics of the psychotherapeutic relationship, using antibody status for HIV as a frame of reference.

Descriptive

The psychological and social ramifications of individuals' knowledge about their HIV status are discussed, as well as their reactions to testing either positive or negative for HIV antibodies. The impact of the combined antibody statuses of therapist and client with the therapeutic interaction are described. Case reports are presented in order to convey a deeper understanding of transference and counter-transference issues in those affected by the AIDS epidemic.

Of interest to mental health professionals and counselors.

1069. PATTEN, John. "AIDS and the gay couple." *Family Therapy Networker* 12 (1988): 37-39.

Discusses the need for therapists to confront their own attitudes about homosexuality so they can offer appropriate help to homosexual couples.

Descriptive

Many therapists harbor attitudes, the most extreme of which is homophobia, that make it difficult for them to respond to the needs of gay clients. Clinicians need to understand that the differences between gay and straight relationships have been enormously exaggerated. From a systems perspective, homosexual and heterosexual relationships share more similarities than differences. The basic task of the therapist remains one of helping two human beings who are struggling with closeness, conflict, family legacies, and unpredictable crises. The author suggests that straight therapists, uncertain how to work with gay couples, consider approaching them as they would a couple from another culture whose relationship differs from mainstream American patterns, appreciating the differences and enlisting the clients' help in learning about them. A case study of a gay couple struggling to cope with one partner's diagnosis of AIDS is presented as an example of how therapists can help such couples live their lives fully and prepare themselves to handle the crises that lie ahead.

Of interest to mental health professionals.

1070. SPECTOR, Ivan C., and Richard Conklin. "AIDS group psycho-
      therapy." *International Journal of Group Psychotherapy*
      37 (1987): 433-439.

Attempts to clarify some of the psychological issues that concern AIDS
patients.

Descriptive

Because the diagnosis of AIDS or ARC is frequently followed by fear,
anxiety, depression, a sense of hopelessness, and a variety of somatic
concerns and the disease, itself, is complicated by many psychiatric
and social problems, AIDS patients are in special need of psychotherapy. Group psychotherapy provides a valuable support system
and a forum in which patients can discuss their concerns with an
accepting group of their peers. Observations of psychotherapy groups
of AIDS and ARC patients and their sexual partners over a period of 10
months are presented together with additional information regarding
families and caretakers derived from personal observations on an AIDS
treatment unit. Suggestions are made for therapists conducting
similar groups.

Of particular interest to mental health professionals.

b. Chapters

1071. KEELING, Richard P. "AIDS." *In* Paul A. Grayson, and Kate
      Cauley (Eds.). *College Psychotherapy.* New York: The
      Guilford Press, 1989.

Presents specific management guidelines for therapists working with
healthy students who fear AIDS, healthy students who are seropositive, students with limited clinical manifestations, students with
full-blown AIDS, and students who are concerned about others.

Descriptive

Students have a great need for information about AIDS and may need
therapy to understand and manage their feelings about AIDS and to cope
with psychological symptoms. However, working with students who are
concerned about AIDS places demands upon therapists and can lead to
problems in treatment. Therapists must face their own feelings and
cope with their own concerns as they deal with students concerned
about AIDS. There is much that is in common in the experience of all
students concerned about AIDS, but certain students (i.e., gay men, IV
drug users, hemophiliacs) have special needs. Students with concerns
about HIV infection and AIDS may present with virtually any psychological symptom. Therapists must, therefore, be prepared to appropriately respond to both the specific issues concerning AIDS and
the more general need for assessment, evaluation, and therapy of
psychological discomfort.

Of particular interest to college therapists.

1072. NICHOLS, Stuart E. "Psychotherapy and AIDS." *In* Terry S. Stein, and Carol J. Cohen (Eds.). *Contemporary Perspectives on Psychotherapy with Lesbians and Gay Men.* New York: Plenum, 1986.

Discusses the preparation that therapists should undertake before working with AIDS, and offers advice about the assessment and treatment of AIDS patients and the "worried well."

Discussion

Therapists are vital to the strong and humane leadership needed to manage the catastrophe of AIDS, and, because of the need for a cooperative response to the epidemic, may be forced to assume unaccustomed roles with patients, colleagues, and the agencies of health care and government. Because AIDS forces society to deal with some hitherto taboo subjects, such as death and sexuality, therapists have an unusual opportunity to participate in genuine social progress. In addition, therapists may be able to assist individuals to achieve greater personal growth because AIDS may allow them to explore, more honestly than before, the meaning of their existence.

Of particular interest to mental health professionals.

C. SUPPORT GROUPS

a. Articles

1073. FULLER, Ruth L., Sally B. Geis, Julian Rush. "Lovers of AIDS victims: A minority group experience." *Death Studies* 12 (1988): 1-7.

Presents a conceptual approach for introducing mental health research and/or consultation to support groups for lovers of AIDS victims.

Theoretical

Describes, in detail, an initial encounter with one support group. Examines stereotyping, depersonalized treatment, isolation, discrimination, and rage as realistic minority group issues. Gives a ten-step outline for minority mental health consultation or research, and suggests that the use of minority mental health concepts by the researcher/consultant facilitates the establishment of mutual credibility between the group members and the newcomer.

Of particular interest to mental health professionals.

1074. GRANT, Duncan. "Support groups for youth with the AIDS virus." *International Journal of Group Psychotherapy* 38 (1988): 237-251.

A description of the Albion Street Center, a screening clinic for the AIDS virus, which provides medical management and psychosocial services to infected youth.

Descriptive

Reviews the literature relating to support groups and suggests why this therapeutic approach is especially useful for youth who have come into contact with the AIDS virus. The nature of the support group is detailed with particular reference to important issues, and suggestions are made for future developments in its operation.

Of interest to mental health professionals, public health officials, and social scientists.

1075. GREIF, Geoffrey L., and Curtis Price. "A community-based support group for HIV positive IV drug abusers: The HERO program." *Journal of Substance Abuse Treatment* 5 (1988): 263-266.

Describes a community-based group, sponsored by Health Education and Resource Organization (HERO), for IV drug abusers who have been diagnosed as HIV positive.

Descriptive

The IV drug abuser who has a history of non-compliance is one of the most difficult to reach among those at risk for contracting AIDS. This article details one approach being attempted at HERO, a Baltimore-based grass roots organization that provides education about HIV infection, referral, and treatment for those infected and for their significant others.

Of interest to health educators, public health professionals, and social scientists.

1076. KLEIN, Sandra Jacoby, and William Fletcher, III. "Gay grief: An examination of its uniqueness brought to light by the AIDS crisis." *Journal of Psychosocial Oncology* 4, no. 3 (1986): 15-25.

A grief recovery group was convened under the auspices of the AIDS Project Los Angeles over an 18-month period and attended by 32 men, most of whom had lost a partner to AIDS.

Descriptive

Although feelings of grief are similar among all people experiencing loss, this population exhibited unique needs. Among the numerous concerns that complicated their grief were social stigma, homophobia, fear of contracting AIDS or of being a carrier, and special re-entry and dating problems. The authors compare traditional and nontraditional grief groups and share experiences from their group.

Of interest to counselors and mental health professionals.

Chapter 6

Coping With AIDS

1. Social, Psychological, and Cultural Issues, 427-465
2. Spiritual and Religious Issues, 465-471
3. Terminal Care/Death and Dying, 471-475

1. SOCIAL, PSYCHOLOGICAL, AND CULTURAL ISSUES

a. Books

1077. BRIDGE, T. Peter, Allan F. Mirsky, Frederick K. Goodwin
(Eds.). *Psychological, Neuropsychiatric, and Substance Abuse
Aspects of AIDS. Volume 44, Advances in Biochemical
Psychopharmacology.* New York: Raven Press, 1988.

Spans relevant research areas ranging from the molecular to the
psychosocial, emphasizing traditional and recently developed research
approaches to AIDS.

Book of Readings

The 23 chapters cover the neuropsychiatric aspects of AIDS, models for
understanding the psychiatric consequences of AIDS, stress response
and AIDS, legal and ethical issues in research, neuroendocrine
properties of the immune system and numerous others dealing with the
immune, virologic, and CNS mediated mechanisms of HIV infection.

Of interest to all AIDS researchers and other health personnel.

1078. DAVIS, Christopher. *Valley of the Shadow.* New York: St.
Martin's Press, 1988.

A tragic love story.

Novel

Tells a touching story of two young men who love each other and must
cope with illness, separation, and death due to AIDS. Provides an
interesting insight into the gay culture in New York City and Fire
Island, both before and after the onset of the AIDS epidemic, and an
appreciation of the impact that AIDS has had on the gay community.

Of general interest.

1079. DREUILHE, Emmanuel. *Mortal Embrace: Living With AIDS.*
Translated by Linda Coverdale. New York: Hill and Wang,
1988.

A medical literary work in which the author describes his personal
battle with AIDS.

Diary

By turns personal and philosophical, Dreuilhe grapples with the full
panoply of human emotions as AIDS invades his body, destroys his
lover, and compels him to confront death. His journal is a refusal to
succumb to pessimism and hostility.

Of general interest.

1080. FELDMAN, Douglas A., and Thomas M. Johnson (Eds.). *The
Social Dimensions of AIDS.* New York: Praeger, 1986.

Concerned with the psychosocial and cultural dimensions of AIDS and
the methodological dilemmas of conducting this type of AIDS research.

Book of Readings

Fifteen chapters by AIDS researchers from highly diverse backgrounds
have been divided into six sections: AIDS social research strategies,
social epidemiology, lifestyles and behavior change, AIDS and the
media, health beliefs and behavior, and the impact of AIDS on health
care delivery. The book's underlying premise is that an interdisciplinary approach to AIDS, including research in the social and
behavioral as well as the biomedical sciences, is necessary for a
comprehensive understanding of the epidemic.

Should interest social and behavioral scientists, psychologists,
psychiatrists, social workers, nurses, and public health
professionals.

1081. FERRO, Robert. *Second Son.* New York: Crown, 1988.

A fictional account of a homosexual man's struggle to achieve personal
fulfillment while coping with AIDS.

Novel

Second Son is basically a story about relationships and about love and
caring. Mark Valerian, the sensitive, artistic hero of the novel, is
ill with a dread disease, obviously AIDS, which the author never
names. He is more fortunate than others in his situation in that he
has a loving family that is generally supportive and accepting,
despite some serious family conflicts. His family members have met
with varying success in their efforts to understand and accept Mark's
homosexuality and cope with their fear of his disease, but all have
made the effort. Because of his illness, Mark has, for some time,
denied himself the intimacy and comfort of physical love; however, he

meets and falls in love with a young man who, like himself, is ill. Together they fulfill one another's need for love, help each other through the difficult stages of their illness, and provide the hope and support that each needs to help him cope with his fears. While the reader is aware, throughout the novel, of the progress of the disease, he is never fully touched by the intensity of its horror.

For general audiences.

1082. GREENLY, Mike. *Chronicle: The Human Side of AIDS.* New York: Irvington, 1986.

A series of interviews interspersed by personal commentary.

Essay

Each of the 36 chapters in this book is based upon one or more personal interviews, many of which were obtained by "computer conference." While the subjects include a wide variety of people from vastly different walks of life, all have been touched, in some way, by the AIDS epidemic. Together, these essays serve to demonstrate the impact of AIDS upon the human community.

Of interest to a general audience.

1083. HAY, Louise L. *The AIDS Book: Creating a Positive Approach.* Santa Monica, CA: Hay House, 1988.

Based on the author's work in her weekly support group, this book contains real life experiences of people with AIDS.

Sourcebook

The 25 chapters are organized into three parts: understanding the disease of AIDS, healing yourself, and finding help. The references, affirmations, and awareness exercises are equally valuable for anyone facing cancer, heart disease, diabetes, or any other life threatening disease.

Of interest to laymen, health professionals, and AIDS patients.

1084 HOFFMAN, Alice. *At Risk.* New York: G.P. Putnam's Sons, 1988.

Tells the story of an 11-year-old girl with transfusion-related AIDS.

Novel

Except for the stigma and fear uniquely connected with AIDS, Amanda, the central character of this novel, might be suffering from any terminal illness. The story of the social and psychological impact of her illness on Amanda, her family, its individual members, and the community in which they live is told with sensitivity and a lack of sentimentality.

Recommended reading for general audiences.

1085. HOWARD, Billy. *Epitaphs for the Living: Words and Images in the Time of AIDS.* Dallas: Southern Methodist University Press, 1989.

A collection of photographs of persons living with AIDS.

Photographic Essay

Each of the 68 portraits in this collection is accompanied by a written comment by its subject, demonstrating the courageous struggle of each of these individuals to understand, cope with, and find meaning in his/her illness.

Of interest to a general audience.

1086. HOYLE, Jay. *Mark: How a Boy's Courage in Facing AIDS Inspired a Town and the Town's Compassion Lit Up a Nation.* South Bend, IN: Langford Books/Diamond Communications, 1988.

Explores the personal and social dimensions which AIDS victims, their families, and their communities must face.

Biography

A father's moving account of his son's 16 month struggle against AIDS. Mark contracted AIDS as a result of treatment for his severe hemophilia. Written in a diary-like form, the book allows the reader to get to know Mark and his family and to experience their daily battle to keep hoping in the face of physical and emotional pain.

Of interest to the general public.

1087. KUKLIN, Susan. *Fighting Back: What Some People are Doing About AIDS.* New York: G.P. Putnam's Sons, 1989.

Reports on the events that occurred during a nine-month period that the author spent with a team of volunteers in New York City who offered support to people with AIDS.

Text

A book about volunteers or buddies who assisted persons with AIDS. The author, to show what it is like to be working with victims of a potentially terminal illness, interviewed and photographed the volunteers associated with a particular team. Noted is a recurrent theme that the clients gave the volunteers much more than was given in return.

Of general interest to the public and to health professionals.

1088. McCARROLL, Tolbert. *Morning Glory Babies: Children With AIDS and the Celebration of Life.* New York: St. Martin's Press, 1988.

A true story of three babies with AIDS and the small lay Catholic community that opened its farm home to care for them.

Chronicle

This is an intensely moving story of the pain of fighting indifferent bureaucrats so that the babies would not be warehoused into hospitals; a courageous story in which the initial hysteria and hostility of rural neighbors are transformed into acts of kindness and charity; a sad story of one baby who dies the day after cutting his first tooth. It is a story of hope, a saga of how good people rally round to guarantee that children do not die among strangers.

Of interest to the general public.

1089. MARTELLI, Leonard J., with Fran D. Peltz, William Messina. *When Someone You Know Has A.I.D.S.: A Practical Guide.* New York: Crown, 1987.

Written by an AIDS "carepartner" and two professional therapists for anyone who cares about a friend, relative, or lover with AIDS or ARC.

Guidebook

This book is filled with practical advice about how to cope, interspersed with stories of loving relationships. It will help friends of people with AIDS better understand the disease and how it affects its victims, helping to support and maintain friendships with persons with AIDS. Contains a bibliography, glossary, and directory of AIDS-related organizations.

Of interest to the general population.

1090. MILLER, David. *Living with AIDS and HIV.* London: Macmillan, 1987.

A practical guide to coping with the problems raised by HIV for HIV-infected persons and their caregivers.

Guidebook

Presents information on the virus and its spread; the clinical manifestations of AIDS; coming to terms with diagnosis and being seropositive; practical, psychological, and relationship adjustments; and religious issues. Offers practical advice for managing HIV infection and AIDS and responding actively to the disease rather than with a reliance on others or a helpless acceptance of the circumstances.

For persons with HIV infection or AIDS and their caregivers.

1091. MOFFATT, Betty Clare. *When Someone You Love Has AIDS: A Book of Hope for Family and Friends.* Santa Monica, CA: IBS Press, 1986.

The mother of a young man who has AIDS draws upon personal experience to offer information and suggestions to help others cope with the disease.

Guidebook

The author provides accurate medical information about AIDS, and shares her thoughts and feelings and her personal struggle to cope with the disease. She offers advice on the practical aspects of living with a person with AIDS, giving and seeking care and support, and, finally, achieving acceptance.

Of interest to anyone concerned about AIDS or touched by the AIDS crisis, including health professionals, therapists, support groups, family members, friends, and co-workers of persons with AIDS.

1092. MONETTE, Paul. *Borrowed Time: An AIDS Memoir.* San Diego: Harcourt Brace Jovanovich, 1988.

The author chronicles the personal battle that he and his "beloved friend," Roger Horwitz, fought against AIDS from the time of diagnosis until Roger's death, two years later.

Biography

A story of desperation, courage, and love, told without sentimentality. The author tells how he and his lover coped with and fought the disease, so that they "never lost the will to win, and thus never lost a minute of the whole twenty months."

Of general interest.

1093. NATIONAL Institute of Mental Health. *Coping with AIDS: Psychological and Social Considerations in Helping People with HTLV-III Infection.* Rockville, MD: U.S. Department of Health and Human Services, Public Health Service, Alcohol, Drug Abuse and Mental Health Administration, 1986.

Intended to familiarize health and mental health professionals and paraprofessionals with the psychological and social problems associated with AIDS.

Pamphlet

Includes sections on the realities of AIDS, the challenge for health care professionals, the neuropsychiatric dimensions of HTLV-III infection, treating patients, the needs of health professionals, recommended reading, AIDS hotline telephone numbers, and AIDS information from State Departments of Health.

Of interest to health and mental health professionals.

1094. NUNGESSER, Lon G. *Epidemic of Courage: Facing AIDS in America.* New York: St. Martin's Press, 1986.

A book of interviews, conducted between February and October 1984, with persons whose lives have been affected by AIDS.

Book of Interviews

Part One consists of interviews of persons with AIDS and Part Two, "Gay Family Network," with members of their support network, including family members, lovers, friends, and therapists. Each person shares his or her personal experiences, thoughts, feelings, and strategies for coping with the AIDS crisis.

Of interest to mental health professionals, members of high risk groups and of their social networks, and concerned laypersons.

1095. ————, with William D. Bullock. *Notes on Living Until We Say Goodbye: A Personal Guide.* New York: St. Martin's Press, 1988.

A person with AIDS talks about the issues and events that arise for people facing a life-threatening illness, focusing on individual self-determination and freedom in medical decision making.

Self Help Manual

The author emphasizes the advantages of having an awareness of one's mortality and an active involvement in promoting one's health, and advocates the patient's right to reject, disagree with, or work with persons in medical authority. He promotes the basic message that one can do more than exist with illness; each individual is challenged to make the most of his/her life. The six chapters deal with: coping with terminal diagnosis; the stigma related to illness; the effects of daily coping methods on health and morale; hope and realism; taking stock of one's life; and managing medical, social, and economic needs.

Of interest to any persons coping with terminal illness, and to their friends, families, and care providers.

1096. PEABODY, Barbara. *The Screaming Room.* San Diego: Oak Tree Publications, 1986.

A mother's journal of her son's struggle with AIDS.

Journal

An emotional daily account of the medical, social, and psychological effects of AIDS on the patient and the family. The journal begins with a son's diagnosis of AIDS and details events over a period of a year and a half, ending with his death.

Of interest to laymen and health professionals.

1097. REED, Paul. *Facing It: A Novel of AIDS.* San Francisco: Gay Sunshine Press, 1984.

The story of a young man diagnosed with AIDS.

Novel

When Andy Stone's health first began to fail, doctors were unable to diagnose his condition. Then the CDC published its initial reports of KS and *Pneumocystis* pneumonia in previously healthy homosexual men. This novel is the story of Andy's struggle to understand, accept, and live with AIDS; to come to terms with his own identity; to appreciate what is good and beautiful in his life while having to cope with his own fear, with homophobia and fear of AIDS among his peers, and with rejection from his family; and to accept the inevitability of his own untimely death. It is told with sensitivity, compassion, and a lack of sentimentality. The book also deals with medical politics and with the struggle, when AIDS was first recognized, to obtain research funds for the "gay disease."

Of interest to a general audience.

1098. ———. *Serenity: Challenging the Fear of AIDS--From Despair to Hope.* Berkeley, CA: Celestial Arts, 1987.

The eight essays in this volume chronicle one man's journey through the crippling fear of AIDS.

Essay

The author discusses the experience of the AIDS epidemic within the gay community--what it's like to live with the stress of the epidemic, the kinds of problems being encountered, and the changes that are taking place; the importance of confronting reality in order to take action; and the pitfalls and dangers of accepting reality (i.e., fatalism, depression) and how to avoid them. He concludes with suggestions and examples of ways to make the best personal decisions for living in the midst of the AIDS epidemic; and provides an annotated list of books that he found to be helpful and the phone numbers of organizations that can provide further guidance for the reader.

Helpful to members of the gay community and to those who care about them.

1099. RIEDER, Ines, and Patricia Ruppelt (Eds.). *AIDS: The Women.* Cleis Press, 1988.

Documents women's roles in the AIDS epidemic.

Book of Readings

This volume deals with women's perspectives on the AIDS epidemic; the contributors are all women who have had their personal or working lives directly affected and changed by AIDS. In telling their stories, they focus on the human aspects of the epidemic. The book is divided into seven sections: family, lovers, and friends; women with AIDS/ARC and HIV-positive women; the professional caregivers; lesbians facing AIDS; prostitution in the age of AIDS; women AIDS educators; and AIDS prevention policies. The appendices include a glossary, a list of resources, and a selected bibliography on women and AIDS.

Of interest to a general audience.

1100. SHANDS, Nancy. *AIDS: The Lonely Voyage.* San Carlos, CA: Wide World/Tetra, 1988.

Tells how AIDS affected the lives of 25 gay men.

Research

This study grew out of the author's interest in hospice care for the terminally ill and in family systems therapy. The research reported is not quantitative, nor is the sample random, but the information provided is intended to provide some understanding of how persons with AIDS confront the disease and the adequacy of their support systems. The book tells the story of 25 men, all of whom felt a sense of isolation and estrangement, but many of whom also experienced heartwarming support.

Of interest to the lay public.

1101. SOLOMON, Rosalind. *Portraits in the Time of AIDS.* New York: Grey Art Gallery and Study Center, New York University, 1988.

An exhibition of 75 portrait photographs of persons living with AIDS.

Photographic Essay

A series of portraits representing the diverse population of individuals who are touched by AIDS. Included are gay men, former drug addicts, women, and children, most of whom were photographed in their homes. The portraits range in format from single full figures to group images, from dramatic close-up facial shots to still-lifes of anatomical details.

An artistic work of general interest.

1102. TATCHELL, Peter. *AIDS: A Guide to Survival.* London: GMP,
       1986.

Intended as a brief and simple guide to understanding, preventing, and
fighting back against AIDS.

Handbook

The author contends that AIDS is not inevitably fatal and those
infected with the virus are not powerless and helpless. Instead of
passively accepting their fate, giving in to despair, and sliding into
the sick role, people with HIV infection and AIDS can choose to
mentally and physically fight the disease by complementing conventional medical treatment with what he calls the "whole person"
approach to health. The five chapters deal with: understanding AIDS,
preventing AIDS, fighting back against AIDS, living with AIDS, and
campaigning to defeat AIDS.

Intended for persons with HIV infection and AIDS, but may also be of
interest to their caretakers and loved ones and to mental health
professionals.

1103. WHITMORE, George. *Someone was Here: Profiles in the AIDS
       Epidemic.* New York: New American Library, 1988.

This book consists primarily of interviews with people who told their
stories to the author in an effort to promote further understanding
about AIDS and the human tragedy it perpetrates.

Text

A factual narrative of conversations and incidents about all aspects
of AIDS: fear, prejudices, hope.

Of interest to the general public.

                              b. Articles

1104. AGLE, David, Henry Gluck, Glenn F. Pierce. "The risk of
       AIDS: Psychologic impact on the hemophilic population."
       General Hospital Psychiatry 9 (1987): 11-17.

A questionnaire to assess the psychologic impact of the risk of AIDS
was administered to 116 hemophiliacs, age 16 or older, and to 48 mates
and 94 parents of hemophiliacs.

Research

The mean group distress ratings indicated a lessening of emotional
discomfort over time, but ongoing distress, as well as interference
with life activities, was reported. Parents indicated more distress
than either hemophiliacs or mates. Health preoccupation, fear of
being contagious, interference with parent-child intimacy and sexual

intimacy between hemophiliacs and mates were noted. A significant decrease in the use of clotting factor concentrates, which have been linked to the transmission of AIDS, for the treatment of bleeding episodes was noted. The overall hemophiliac population is coping effectively with the AIDS risk, although some hemophiliacs are at increased risk for psychiatric morbidity, social isolation, hypochondriasis, and medical noncompliance. Increased parental anxiety is likely to lead to over-protective child rearing practices. The authors describe stress responses likely to be present in other at risk groups besides hemophiliacs, and suggest that specific psychosocial interventions are needed.

Of interest to mental health professionals.

1105. BATCHELOR, Walter. "AIDS: A public health and psychological emergency." *American Psychologist* 39 (1984): 1279-1284.

Summarizes current (1984) knowledge and assumptions about AIDS as a disease entity, the assumptions and findings guiding research, the problems that have hampered research, and the role of psychological factors in these efforts.

Review

Pervasive psychological factors have hampered data collection, clinical research, and medical practice, making AIDS a mental health as well as a public health emergency. Mounting frightening statistics have caused increased fear and depression in society in general as well as in groups at risk. Public education and psychological interventions can assuage some of these problems, but they will not resolve them. Therefore, it is imperative that scientists, in their quest for enlightenment and understanding, expand their investigations to include social and behavioral input.

Of interest to social and behavioral scientists and medical and scientific researchers.

1106. BROTMAN, Andrew W., and Marshall Forstein. "AIDS obsessions in depressed heterosexuals." *Psychosomatics* 29 (1988): 428-431.

Reports the phenomenon of obsessive ruminations about having AIDS in a group of low-risk, depressed heterosexuals.

Case Reports

As the prevalence of HIV infection in the general population increases, it will be increasingly important to carefully distinguish between realistic fears of contracting the infection and the incorporation of such fears into pre-existing depressive and anxiety syndromes and AIDS anxiety.

Of interest to mental health professionals, social workers, and counselors.

1107. CARL, Douglas.   "Acquired immune deficiency syndrome: A
      preliminary examination of the effects on gay couples and
      coupling." *Journal of Marital and Family Therapy* 12 (1986):
      241-247.

Discusses the impact of AIDS on the early stages of gay coupling as
well as the final stage of death.

Discussion

Among gay men, the AIDS epidemic seems to have brought about an
increased consideration about coupling and the nature of coupled
relationships along with parallel struggles around the issues of sex
and intimacy. In addition, large numbers of people have been forced
to deal with death long before the normal time. These issues together
with widespread AIDS anxiety are sending many people to therapists in
the midst of full-blown crises.   Therapists dealing with gay male
clients need to be aware of factors specific to this risk group.   In
addition, they need to have access to resources that deliver accurate
information about the physical aspects of diagnosis and prognosis;
provide contact with others who find themselves in similar situations;
can help to coordinate professionals of different disciplines working
with a patient; and provide some support for the therapist as well as
for other professionals working with persons affected by this disease.

Of interest to social scientists, health professionals and mental
health professionals.

1108. CASSENS, Brett J.   "Social consequences of the acquired
      immunodeficiency syndrome." *Annals of Internal Medicine* 103
      (1985): 768-771.

Discusses the need for understanding the psychosocial stresses of
persons at risk for AIDS and the implications for treatment and
research.

Descriptive

Awareness of the psychosocial dimensions of AIDS provides researchers
and clinicians with an understanding of factors impinging on their
relationships with persons at risk for AIDS. Persons at risk for AIDS
endure the stresses of uncertainty in patient care and prognosis and
loss of confidentiality. "Expert" opinions and media sensationalism
increase fear and prejudice in the community.   Members of all
communities should work together to eliminate social ignorance about
AIDS.

Of interest to physicians, nurses, social workers, and researchers.

1109. COATES, Thomas J., Ron Stall, Jeffrey S. Mandel, Alicia
      Boccellari, James L. Sorensen, Edward F. Morales, Stephen
      F. Morin, James A. Wiley, Leon McKusick. "AIDS: A
      psychosocial research agenda." *Annals of Behavioral
      Medicine* 9, no. 2 (1987): 21-28.

Reviews empirical findings relevant to four major research components of a research agenda for the study of psychosocial factors important to the spread and onset of AIDS.

Review

Identifies psychosocial aspects of the AIDS epidemic that require immediate scientific attention. Psychosocial research is essential to understanding and treating AIDS.

Of interest to social and behavioral scientists, social epidemiologists, and health educators.

1110. COATES, Thomas J., Lydia Temoshok, Jeffrey Mandel. "Psychosocial research is essential to understanding and treating AIDS." *American Psychologist* 39 (1984): 1309-1314.

Describes the necessary research agenda for AIDS.

Descriptive

Points out the importance of research that examines the interface between biological and psychosocial variables, the psychological consequences of AIDS, psychosocial determinants of health-promoting and health-damaging behaviors, and psychosocial factors related to disease incidence and progression.

Of importance to all researchers conducting psychosocial research on the topic of AIDS.

1111. EBBESEN, Peter, Mads Melbye, Jorn Beckmann. "Fear of AIDS: A communication from biologists to psychologists/sociologists." *Scandinavian Journal of Social Medicine* 14 (1986): 113-118.

Draws attention to aspects of the AIDS epidemic that may be relevant to psychologic and sociologic research.

Discussion

The fear caused by AIDS appears to justify an expanded research capacity for psychology and sociology. The authors make the following recommendations: a cost/benefit study of the consequences of informing persons about their seropositivity and the implied possibility that they may develop AIDS; a detailed study of early AIDS research in the U.S. and Africa to discover which social factors promote the early detection of new diseases; a comparative study of strategies used by various health authorities, concentrating on the feasibility of establishing information systems that can utilize instant feedback from the target groups; contingency plans for the social and psychological treatment of the development of AIDS in a high percentage of heterosexual males and females; a study to describe life circumstances of non-infected people, infected people who do not have AIDS, and infected people who are ill with AIDS; and a study to clarify and refine the most appropriate psychotherapeutic methods available for dying AIDS patients.

Of interest to social and behavioral scientists.

1112. FEINBLUM, Sandi. "Pinning down the psychosocial dimensions of AIDS." *Nursing and Health Care* 7 (1986): 254-257.

Identifies the psychosocial problems faced by caregivers of patients with AIDS.

Descriptive

Caregivers of persons with AIDS face many psychosocial problems similar to those faced by their clients. These include social stigma, anger, denial, isolation, and loss. Support from formal or informal groups within the workplace can help caregivers reach a balance between feelings of empathy for their clients and professional burnout.

Of interest to nurses and social workers.

1113. FERRARA, Anthony J. "My personal experience with AIDS." *American Psychologist* 39, no. 11 (1984): 1285-1287.

A brief description of an AIDS patient's personal experience with the disease.

Commentary

The patient describes his feelings and experiences from initial diagnosis throughout treatment and concludes with a plea for public acceptance of AIDS patients as sick people.

Of general interest to laymen and health professionals.

1114. FORSTEIN, Marshall. "The psychosocial impact of the acquired immunodeficiency syndrome." *Seminars in Oncology* 11 (1984): 77-82.

Psychosocial issues related to persons with AIDS, those who are at high risk for AIDS, and those who are not at risk are presented.

Discussion

Presents four stages of response to a diagnosis of AIDS, clinical symptoms and treatment, and the impact of AIDS on the general public.

Of interest to health professionals and laymen.

1115. FRANK, J.W., R.A. Coates, B.J. Harvey, V. Goel, V. Schiralli. "A critical look at HIV-antibody tests: 2. Benefits, risks and clinical use." *Canadian Family Physician* 33 (1987): 2229-2235.

Focuses on the benefits and risks that may result from the use of HIV-antibody tests.

Theoretical

Significant social and psychiatric risks may outweigh any medical benefit of testing, especially for persons at high risk of HIV infection. A detailed protocol is suggested for managing both patient requests and physician-perceived indications for HIV-antibody testing, and an approach to obtaining informed consent before ordering the tests is outlined.

Of interest to physicians, public health professionals, and mental health professionals.

1116. FRIEDLANDER, Arthur H., and Ransom J. Arthur.   "A diagnosis of AIDS: Understanding the psychosocial impact." *Oral Surgery, Oral Medicine and Oral Pathology* 65 (1988): 680-684.

Focuses on the psychosocial aspects of AIDS as they relate to dental care.

Descriptive

Two cases of patients who came for dental care and were HIV positive are presented to illustrate how dentists are involved in the HIV epidemic. Oral disease in persons with or at high risk for AIDS is abundant. Unfortunately, dentists are uncomfortable about providing services to patients with AIDS or to those at high risk. Some have refused to provide treatment or have provided abrupt, inadequate treatment. This article attempts to help dentists understand the psychosocial aspects of HIV and appeals for their compassion, rationality, and professionalism.

Of special interest to dentists and dental hygienists.

1117. GEIS, Sally, and Ruth L. Fuller.   "The impact of the first gay AIDS patient on hospice staff." *Hospice Journal* 1, no. 3 (1985): 17-36.

Reports on the experience of caregivers in hospice settings that have received only a few AIDS patients, all of whom were young, gay males.

Research

The psychosocial impact of AIDS patient care on hospice staff must be addressed if the experience is going to be a positive one for both the hospice and the patient/patient family. Data gathered by the authors through structured interviews and observations at four different hospices revealed that the issues that most affected hospice staff were fear of contagion, unresolved feelings about sexuality, and embarrassment about irrational responses to AIDS patients.

Recommendations are made that institutional and personal fear and anxiety be acknowledged, that adequate inservice training be provided, and that strong support networks be developed. Hospice staff should participate in policy setting and educational programs well before the first AIDS patient is admitted. After admission, personal and institutional support should be provided for caregivers to enable them to deal with their own psychological concerns.

Of interest to hospice staff and administrators and mental health professionals.

1118. GIACQUINTA, Barbara Stewart. "Researching the effects of AIDS on families." *American Journal of Hospice Care* 6, no. 3 (1989): 31-36.

A study of how family members of AIDS patients cope with the illness.

Research

Provides readers with a brief chronicle of the first year of fieldwork with the families of persons with AIDS. Excerpts from interviews with family members reveal the emotional exile of PWA families from their friends and relatives; their stifled communications within the immediate family; the multiple and intense stressful life events preceding or occurring along with the AIDS crisis; and the emotional havoc caused by these and other AIDS-related factors atypical of other life tragedies.

Of special interest to providers of care to AIDS patients, nurses, physicians, and mental health professionals.

1119. GREIF, Geoffrey L., and Edmund Porembski. "AIDS and significant others: Findings from a preliminary exploration of needs." *Health and Social Work* 13 (1988): 259-265.

Discusses the findings from interviews with 11 significant others of AIDS patients.

Research

Although based on a small sample, the data indicate that significant others of persons with AIDS experience trauma and difficulty after their loved one has been diagnosed with AIDS. Significant others have many needs, such as the need for social support and the need for more information about AIDS, as well as referral sources.

Of interest to social workers and mental health professionals.

1120. HANEY, Patrick. "Providing empowerment to the person with AIDS." *Social Work* 33 (1988): 251-253.

A person with AIDS discusses his experiences and feelings since diagnosis.

Essay

An appeal for advocacy for the needs and rights of AIDS patients and to break down the fear, oppression, and ignorance that surrounds the disease.

Of general interest to the lay public.

1121. HAROWSKI, Kathy J.   "The worried well: Maximizing coping in the face of AIDS."   *Journal of Homosexuality* 14 (1984): 299-306.

The AIDS epidemic is discussed in terms of its impact on the psychology of individuals and their relationships.

Descriptive

Special emphasis is given to treatment strategies that therapists may find useful in working with the worried well presenting with psychological and sexual difficulties resulting from AIDS anxiety. Issues of denial, control, and compliance are presented as central to working with this population.

Of interest to health professionals and social and behavioral scientists.

1122. JACOBS, Troy A., and Michael S. Wilkes.   "Cremation patterns for patients dying of AIDS in New York City."   *New York State Journal of Medicine* 88 (1988): 628-632.

Reports on the cremation rates of persons dying of AIDS in New York City.

Research

Blacks and Hispanics, aged 25 to 44, dying between 1982 and 1986 in New York City, were more likely to be cremated if they died of infectious diseases, and whites who died in non-private hospitals, were more frequently cremated than were white patients in private hospitals. Patients who died of AIDS were cremated more frequently then their counterparts who died of other causes, regardless of race or location of death. It is suggested that funeral directors, because of their fear of contagious diseases, especially AIDS, may influence families to request cremation as an alternative to embalming and burial.

Of interest to social and behavioral scientists, AIDS activists, public policymakers, funeral directors, and attorneys.

1123. JACOBSEN, Paul B., Samuel W. Perry, Dan Alan Hirsch, Donna Scavuzzo, Richard B. Roberts.   "Psychological reactions of individuals at risk for AIDS during an experimental drug trial."   *Psychosomatics* 29 (1988): 182-187.

In an attempt to examine the impact of experimental drug testing on psychological distress in individuals at risk for AIDS, 26 asymptomatic homosexual and bisexual men, seropositive for HIV, were assessed at the opening and closing phases of a 12-week trial of the antiviral agent, ribavirin.

Research

Drug study participants reported significantly more emotional stress than did a comparison group of seropositive men who were not receiving experimental treatment. The high level of distress evidenced by the sample at the beginning of the experimental trial did not impede adherence, decrease over the period of the study, or relate to subjects' beliefs that they were receiving a placebo; however, distress did relate to subjects' perceptions of how HIV test results were communicated prior to entry into the study. These findings suggest the feasibility of placebo-controlled studies in this distressed population and provide a focus for psychosocial counseling.

Of interest to research physicians, mental health professionals, and counselors working with persons who are HIV positive.

1124. JOSEPH, Jill G., Carol-Ann Emmons, Ronald C. Kessler, Camille B. Wortman, Kerth O'Brien, William T. Hocker, Catherine Schaefer. "Coping with the threat of AIDS: An approach to psychosocial assessment." *American Psychologist* 39 (1984): 1297-1302.

Describes an attempt to develop psychosocial inventories for the study of the response of gay men to the threat of AIDS.

Research

A full appreciation of the strains created by AIDS, which extend well beyond the perceived risk of contracting the disease, requires an understanding of the medical aspects of AIDS, the ways in which core characteristics of the gay lifestyle are affected by the illness, and the climate of public concern that AIDS has created.

Of interest to social and behavioral scientists.

1125. KELLY, Jeffrey A., Janet S. St. Lawrence, Steve Smith, Jr., Harold V. Hood, Donna J. Cook. "Medical students' attitudes toward AIDS and homosexual patients." *Journal of Medical Education* 62 (1987): 549-556.

Medical students, after being given one of four vignettes to read, which were identical in content except for the fact that the patient was identified as having either AIDS or leukemia and being either heterosexual or homosexual, completed a set of objective measures that assessed their attitudes toward the patient.

Research

Analyses of the students' responses revealed negative and prejudiced attitudes towards both the AIDS and homosexual patients. Medical educators need to recognize the stigmatizing, negative attitudes of many students toward homosexuals and AIDS patients and make an effort to promote greater sensitivity, knowledge, and understanding among medical students toward those at risk for AIDS and AIDS patients.

Of interest to medical educators.

1126. KESSLER, Ronald C., Kerth O'Brien, Jill G. Joseph, David G. Ostrow, John P. Phair, Joan S. Chmiel, Camille B. Wortman, Carol-Ann Emmons. "Effects of HIV infection, perceived health and clinical status on a cohort at risk for AIDS." *Social Science and Medicine* 27 (1988): 569-578.

Reports on a study to determine the social and emotional effects of HIV status, clinical signs, and perceived symptoms among healthy homosexual men.

Research

Although the emotional and social function of the participants was affected by their perception of symptoms, independent of their HIV status, the perception of symptoms could not be attributed solely to the high level of distress in the cohort; it could, partially, be attributed to problems at work, in the community, and with families faced by members at risk for AIDS. Physicians should be aware of the psychological toll imposed on gay men who develop health problems.

Of interest to physicians, mental health workers, and counselors of homosexual men.

1127. KING, Michael B. "Psychosocial status of 192 out-patients with HIV infection and AIDS." *British Journal of Psychiatry* 154 (1989): 237-242.

Investigates the psychological and social status of a consecutive series of 192 outpatients with HIV infection.

Research

Thirty-one percent of the subjects had significant psychiatric problems, about half of whom reported emotional problems before HIV infection. Twenty-two percent complained of difficulties with memory or concentration. Excessive health ruminations were an important indicator of more extensive psychological problems. Patients appeared to have adapted well, despite the stigma and poor prognosis of their condition.

Of interest to mental health professionals and health professionals caring for AIDS patients.

1128. KOWALEWSKI, Mark R. "Double stigma and boundary maintenance: How gay men deal with AIDS." *Journal of Contemporary Ethnography* 17 (1988): 211-228.

Concerned with the responses of "normal" members of stigmatized groups to others who possess a second discredited characteristic--a double stigma.

Research

Examines the strategies gay men use to limit or avoid contact with persons with AIDS. Data were collected through interviews and a focus group with gay men who did not have AIDS.

Of interest to social and behavioral scientists and mental health professionals.

1129. LINN, Ruth. "When an AIDS child enters the classroom: Moral-psychological research questions." *Psychological Reports* 61 (1987): 191-197.

Raises questions regarding the rights of the child with AIDS within the educational setting.

Theoretical

Discusses the moral dilemmas involved in the decision-making process regarding such questions as whether the AIDS child should be allowed to enroll in school, whether his name should be made public, what the school should do about parents who object to his presence in the classroom and vice versa, the status of the infected teacher or food service worker, and what should be done about the healthy teacher who refuses to teach an AIDS child. Examines the issues within the framework of Kohlberg's moral psychological theory, which focuses on our moral effectiveness in deriving the most just and fair solution.

Of interest to educators, school administrators, psychologists, and concerned parents and teachers.

1130. LYTER, David W., Ronald O. Valdiserri, Lawrence A. Kingsley, William P. Amoroso, Charles R. Rinaldo, Jr. "The HIV antibody test. Why gay and bisexual men want or do not want to know their results." *Public Health Reports* 102 (1987): 468-474.

Gay and bisexual men who were enrolled in the Pitt Men's Study, the Pittsburgh cohort of the Multicenter AIDS Cohort Study, were offered the results of their antibody test and asked to fill out a question-naire designed to assess the factors influencing their decision.

Research

Of the 2,047 men contacted, 1,251 (61%) accepted, 188 (9%) declined, and 608 (30%) failed to respond. Fifty-four percent learned their results. No significant differences in demographic, behavioral, and attitudinal characteristics or HIV seroprevalence were noted between the men who accepted and those who declined, but the group that did not respond was composed of a greater proportion of younger, non-white, less educated men. The most frequently cited reason for wanting test results (90%) was to determine if the participant had been infected with HIV. Of those who declined, 30% listed concerns about the psychological impact of a positive result, 48% believed the test not to be predictive of the development of AIDS, and 48% were concerned about the worry of a positive result.

Of interest to social and behavioral scientists.

1131. MARTIN, John, and Carole S. Vance. "Behavioral and psychosocial factors in AIDS: Methodological and substantive issues." *American Psychologist* 39 (1984): 1303-1308.

Reviews and critiques methodological and substantive issues in conducting research on behavioral and psychosocial factors in AIDS.

Critique

Investigators should design research based on what is known about disease processes in general; competing hypotheses can be contrasted with one another within the same study. Critical review of initial studies on AIDS suggests the need for prophetic designs with healthy, but at-risk subjects, in order to reduce several biases and increase the quality of inference.

Of interest to social and behavioral scientists doing research on AIDS.

1132. MARTIN, John L. "Psychological consequences of AIDS-related bereavement among gay men." *Journal of Consulting and Clinical Psychology* 56 (1988): 856-862.

In 1985, a community sample of 745 gay men in New York City were interviewed to determine the relation between AIDS-related bereavement and psychological distress.

Research

The loss of a lover or close friend was experienced by 27% of the sample, one-third of whom had experienced multiple losses. A direct relation was found between the number of bereavements and symptoms of traumatic stress response, demoralization, sleep problems, sedative use, recreational drug use, and the use of psychological services because of AIDS concerns. The relations remained strong after controlling for the appraised threat of AIDS, the knowledge of a positive HIV antibody status, the presence of ARC symptoms, and sexual behavior history. Symptoms of distress increased directly with the number of bereavements, suggesting that gay men are not adapting psychologically to repeated experiences with AIDS-related bereavements.

Of interest to mental health professionals and behavioral scientists.

1133. MARZUK, Peter M., Helen Tierney, Kenneth Tardiff, Elliot M.
      Gross, Edward B. Morgan, Ming-Ann Hsu, J. John Mann.
      "Increased risk of suicide in persons with AIDS." *Journal of
      the American Medical Association* 259 (1988): 1333-1337.

The rate of suicide in New York City residents diagnosed with AIDS was
studied.

Research

The relative risk of suicide in men with AIDS, aged 20 to 59, was
found to be 36.30 times that of men in the same age group without this
diagnosis and 66.15 times that of the general population.   AIDS
represents a significant risk factor for suicide.

Of interest to all health professionals and the general public.

1134. MORIN, Stephen F, Kenneth A. Charles, Alan K. Malyon.
      "The psychological impact of AIDS on gay men." *American
      Psychologist* 39 (1984): 1288-1293.

An overview of the numerous psychological factors that impact on gay
men as a result of AIDS.

Descriptive

Discusses a variety of issues that arise among gay men as a result of
the AIDS epidemic, such as anxiety, depression, isolation, need for
social support, and concern about sexual expression.

Of particular interest to persons counseling homosexual patients.

1135. MOULTON, Jeffrey M., David M. Sweet, Lydia Temoshok,
      Jeffrey S. Mandel. "Attributions of blame and responsibility
      in relation to distress and health behavior change in people
      with AIDS and AIDS-related complex." *Journal of Applied
      Social Psychology* 17 (1987): 493-506.

Examines the impact of attributions of blame and responsibility for
the cause and course of disease in 103 persons with AIDS and ARC.

Research

Blaming one's self for disease was significantly positively correlated with dysphoria (combined depression, anxiety, and negative mood)
in persons with AIDS, whereas self attributed improvement was
significantly negatively correlated with dysphoria in the ARC group.
Persons with AIDS who attributed more responsibility for improvement
to themselves also made more behavior changes, but health behavior
change was not associated with attribution of responsibility for
improvement in the ARC group.   No relationship was found between
self-blame and any distress or behavior change measures.   The
differences in the pattern of association between attribution of

responsibility in persons with AIDS and in those with ARC underscores the need to examine psychological processes within the context of particular conditions of health. The results also suggest that attributing responsibility for improvement to the self lacks the negative psychological effects associated with blaming the self for AIDS.

Of particular interest to behavioral scientists.

1136. NELKIN, Dorothy. "AIDS and the social sciences: Review of useful knowledge and research needs." *Reviews of Infectious Diseases* 9 (1987): 980-986.

Reviews several areas of social science research that are relevant to the critical social dimensions of the AIDS crisis.

Review

Suggests useful avenues for research that could provide the understanding necessary to develop effective ways of approaching the problems presented by AIDS.

Of interest to social and behavioral scientists.

1137. NICHOLS, Stuart E. "Psychosocial reactions of persons with the acquired immunodeficiency syndrome." *Annals of Internal Medicine* 103 (1985): 765-767.

The psychosocial impact of AIDS on patients follows the situational distress model of crisis, transitional state, and deficiency state.

Descriptive

Additional psychosocial problems are caused by the intensified prejudice against homosexual men and drug addicts. Society, itself, has been disrupted by the new information about sexual behavior that has been brought to light by AIDS, indicating that primitive sexual taboos still influence modern society. Understanding the various psychosocial reactions to AIDS offers opportunities for social progress and personal growth.

Of interest to health professionals, especially mental health professionals and behavioral scientists.

1138. OSTROW, David G., Jill G. Joseph, Ronald Kessler, Jerome Soucy, Margalit Tal, Michael Eller, Joan Chmiel, John P. Phair. "Disclosure of HIV antibody status: Behavioral and mental health correlates." *AIDS Education and Prevention* 1, no. 1 (1989): 1-11.

Contrasts the pre- and postdisclosure characteristics (behavioral and psychological) of two groups of participants in the Multicenter AIDS Cohort Study who obtained their HIV test results and two groups who did not.

Research

Identical psychological and behavioral assessments were administered to all four groups. Mental health functioning improved over time for seropositives who did not wish to know their HIV status, for seronegatives who did wish to know, and for seronegatives who did not wish to know; it decreased on all dimensions measured for those who learned of their seropositive status. They reported more obsessive-compulsive behavior, anxiety, and distress. All groups, regardless of whether they chose to learn their antibody status, showed consistent reduction in HIV risky sexual behaviors; however, disclosed seropositive and seronegative men who had had fewer sexual partners increased the number of partners. In terms of public health policy, this study suggests that caution be exercised in the use of routine HIV testing as a motivation for behavior change.

Of interest to public health professionals, AIDS educators and counselors, legislators, and public policymakers.

1139. OSTROW, David G., Andrew Monjan, Jill Joseph, Mark Van Raden, Robin Fox, Lawrence Kingsley, Janice Dudley, John Phair. "HIV related symptoms and psychological functioning in a cohort of homosexual men." *American Journal of Psychiatry* 146 (1989): 737-742.

The authors administered the Center for Epidemiological Studies Depression Scale (CES-D) to 4,954 homosexual men in the Multicenter AIDS Cohort Study.

Research

HIV antibody status at enrollment was a less important predictor of psychological stress than were reported physical symptoms. Multivariate analysis showed an association between a high score on each CES-D Scale component and the number of self-reported possible AIDS or HIV-related symptoms, perceived lymphadenopathy, and absence of someone to talk to about serious problems. This relationship between self-reported physical symptoms and psychological distress suggests a possible etiologic relationship between perceived AIDS risk and psychological symptoms in men at risk of AIDS.

Of interest to mental health counselors and social and behavioral scientists.

1140. SCHAFFNER, Bertram. "Reactions of medical personnel and intimates to persons with AIDS." *The Psychotherapy Patient* 2, no. 4 (1986): 67-80.

An overview of some of the reactions to AIDS observed among his colleagues by the author.

Descriptive

The author concludes, "I have had to learn new aspects and dimensions of the practice of medicine and psychiatry, and to change some of the methods I had been taught. Above all I have learned that one has to have courage, and that one must find a new way in therapy, a judicious mixture of both psychotherapy and friendship. Still, it is necessary to be on guard not to incorporate the fears and emotional reactions of the patient to the point that one's own stability is overturned."

Of interest to health professionals.

1141. SOLOMON, George F., and Lydia Temoshok. "A psychoneuro-immunologic perspective on AIDS research: Questions, preliminary findings, and suggestions." *Journal of Applied Social Psychology* 17 (1987): 286-308.

Starting with the premise that research questions emanating from the fields of psychoneuroimmunology and behavioral medicine may provide critical information for understanding and treating AIDS, the authors provide a background on psychoneuroimmunology and AIDS.

Review/Critique

A set of 12 questions to be addressed in research on AIDS is presented. Evidence and illustrations from studies in the literature, from the authors' research, and from clinical examples are discussed for each question. Suggestions addressing some of the problems in conducting psychoneurologic research are offered.

Of interest to social and behavioral scientists, virologists, neuropsychologists, and others engaged in AIDS research.

1142. SPREADBURY, Connie. "Variables related to the fear of contracting AIDS." *Journal of College Student Development* 29 (1988): 556-557.

Summarizes a study designed to investigate what makes some people worry about contracting AIDS and others not.

Research

Findings suggest that as young people become more aware that AIDS is a sexual and not a homosexual disease, they are apt to become more worried. Worried college students will probably turn to college personnel for help, and universities should prepare for that event. If university personnel have not already begun to develop policies about AIDS, they should begin to do so now.

Of special interest to university and college administrators and teachers and health educators.

1143. STEVENS, Laurie A. "Techniques for reversing the failure of empathy towards AIDS patients." *Journal of the American Academy of Psychoanalysis* 15 (1987): 539-551.

Offers a psychodynamic explanation of the origins of the irrational fear and anxieties surrounding AIDS patients and the reasons why information alone doesn't allay the anxieties of hospital workers.

Theoretical

Hypothesizes that the underlying dynamics of the panic related to AIDS relate to primitive, unconscious fears, which are so profound and terrifying that they prevent the emergence of normal compassion and empathy towards AIDS victims. Outlines a training program using group process and videotape techniques, which addresses the underlying fears and concerns of hospital staff and can help them deliver more empathetic care to AIDS patients.

Should interest physicians, nurses, hospital administrators, and mental health professionals.

1144. STULBERG, Ian, and Margaret Smith. "Psychosocial impact of the AIDS epidemic on the lives of gay men." *Social Work* 33 (1988): 277-281.

A study was conducted to assess the psychosocial impact of the AIDS epidemic on the lives of gay men who have not been diagnosed with AIDS or ARC.

Descriptive

It was found that volunteering in an AIDS organization was a helpful way of coping with AIDS-related stress, and that relationships, especially monogamous relationships, have become more important, a positive consequence of the AIDS epidemic. The beneficial aspects of community involvement suggest that support groups may be effective, that volunteer work should be encouraged, and that intervention should focus on strengthening or constructing a meaningful social network.

Of interest to social workers and other mental health professionals.

1145. TEMOSHOK, Lydia (Ed.). "Special issue on acquired immune deficiency syndrome (AIDS)." *Journal of Applied Social Psychology* 17, no. 3 (1987): Entire Issue.

A collection of papers reflecting the current state of application of psychological principles and methods to the study, treatment, and prevention of AIDS.

Special Journal Issue

Three significant dimensions of the biopsychosocial research on AIDS provide a context for the articles in this issue: risk or target groups, investigatory perspective and specific topic of investigation, and level of potential application. The papers deal with the relationships among social support, distress, and psychological "hardiness" in gay men with AIDS and ARC; the association of gender, ethnicity, and length of residence in the bay area to adolescents' knowledge and attitudes about AIDS; the behavioral and psychosocial consequences of perceived risk of AIDS in a cohort of gay men; target groups for preventing AIDS among IV drug users; psychosocial responses of hospital workers to AIDS; a psychoneuroimmunologic perspective on AIDS research; coping methods and strategies of gay men with AIDS; and misperception among gay men of the risk for AIDS associated with their sexual behavior.

Of particular interest to social and behavioral researchers and clinicians.

1146. ———, Jane Zich, John Green. "Psychosocial aspects of AIDS." *Psychology and Health* 1 (1987): 39-42.

A discussion of the need for the rapid publication and examination of psychosocial impressions and research on AIDS.

Editorial

The investigation of international data on cultural moderators of the experience and expression of AIDS may tell us how best to intervene with drug-users and persons sexually at risk, how to deal with the ethical dilemmas of transfusion recipients who may have received contaminated blood, and how to address the problems of babies and school-age children with AIDS.

Should interest health professionals, health educators, mental health professionals, social workers, and social and behavioral scientists.

1147. THOMPSON, Chris, and Massimo Riccio. "AIDS phobia." *British Journal of Hospital Medicine* 38 (September 1987): 165.

A discussion of the pathological fear of AIDS.

Editorial

Pathological fear of AIDS exists on several levels: that prevalent in society as a whole; that in high-risk groups who do not have symptoms and may have undergone recent behavior changes; that in low-risk groups who suffer from a pathological degree of anxiety; and a rare level in persons with delusional hypochondriasis who are convinced that they have AIDS. AIDS may be part of any psychopathology, and pseudo-AIDS, in which patients genuinely present and suffer symptoms that mimic the disease, is related to AIDS phobia. Fear of AIDS is so widespread that the point at which a diagnosis of AIDS phobia can be made is problematical, and those patients who genuinely may be called AIDS phobic are at the extreme end of the spectrum of anxiety. The term, AIDS phobia, is usually a misnomer since the "worried well," to whom it is most often applied, show little or no tendency irrationally to avoid AIDS.

Of general interest.

1148. TRICE, Ashton D. "Posttraumatic stress syndrome-like symptoms among AIDS caregivers." *Psychological Reports* 63 (1988): 656-658.

Reports on symptoms usually associated with posttraumatic stress disorder (PTSD) among caregiving mothers of adult AIDS fatalities.

Research

Interviews were conducted with 43 mothers of AIDS fatalities two or three years following their sons' deaths. A cluster of symptoms normally associated with PTSD was shown by 84% of the mothers who devoted full-time care to their sons for substantial periods of time, while only eight percent of the mothers who did not engage in extended care experienced three or more of these symptoms. Further research is needed to investigate the possible role of the father/husband in making decisions about caregiving as well as differences in outcomes between caregiving mothers who brought their sons into their homes and those who moved into their sons' environments. The mitigating effects of support groups also need to be examined.

Of interest to mental health professionals.

1149. VINEY, Linda L., Rachael Henry, Beverly M. Walker, Levinia Crooks. "The emotional reactions of HIV antibody positive men." *British Journal of Medical Psychology* 62 (1989): 153-161.

Concerned with the emotional reaction of HIV positive men and with whether their expressed enjoyment was the result of a defensive or coping mechanism.

Research

One hundred and five men in three age-matched groups were surveyed to determine the extent and source of their emotional reactions. Enjoyment, anxiety, depression, and hopelessness were expressed more freely by the HIV seropositive men and by those with major illnesses than by healthy college men serving as controls. Seropositives expressed more anger, and yet more competence, than the other patients. The enjoyment appeared to be the result of effective coping with illness; depressive emotions seemed to be reduced when some enjoyment of life was apparent. The implications of these findings for health professionals working with HIV positive people are discussed.

Of interest to mental health professionals.

1150. WEITZ, Rose. "The interview as legacy: A social scientist confronts AIDS." *Hastings Center Report* 17, no. 3 (1987): 21-23.

Describes the experience of conducting social science research on AIDS.

Essay

In a study designed to flesh out the quantitative data collected by other researchers and investigate how the experience of having AIDS may differ for individuals in Arizona from that of persons living in the more liberal communities where most AIDS research has been conducted, the author interviewed 27 persons with AIDS about their experiences and feelings. She discusses the unusual stresses and ethical dilemmas of AIDS research, and the effect it had on her personal attitudes, feelings, and beliefs.

Of particular interest to social science researchers.

1151. WILLIAMS, Michael J. "Gay men as 'buddies' to persons living with AIDS and ARC." *Smith College Studies in Social Work* 59 (1988): 38-52.

Reports on a study examining how gay men, as members of a high-risk group for HIV infection, experience the inherent stress of being a buddy to someone with AIDS or ARC.

Research

A questionnaire designed to determine psychological distress generated by the experience, degree of social support, "coming out," and buddy vulnerability was answered by 54 gay men who had been trained by the Support Services Team of the Boston AIDS Action Committee to serve as buddies to people living with a diagnosis of AIDS or ARC. Results show that, in addition to satisfying a desire to help, volunteering provides some gay men with a sense of mastery over what is happening. Some volunteer in the hope that others will help them if they should develop AIDS; others appear to believe that volunteering may provide them with immunity to AIDS. For many, being a buddy provides opportunities to consolidate their connection with the gay community. Since awareness of one's motives for volunteering can cushion the impact of disappointments and lessen the potential for burnout, organizations should help volunteers to clarify their motivations and expectations.

Of interest to trainers of volunteers in programs providing services to the HIV infected and to mental health professionals.

1152. WOLCOTT, Deane L., Sheila Namir, Fawzy I. Fawzy, Michael S. Gottlieb, Ronald T. Mitsuyasu. "Illness concerns, attitudes towards homosexuality, and social support in gay men with AIDS." *General Hospital Psychiatry* 8 (1986: 395-403.

A study of 50 gay men, recently diagnosed as having AIDS, to document health status, psychologic status, and aspects of social support in patients with life-threatening illness.

Research

Subjects reported levels of illness-related concerns comparable to those of previously studied cancer patients, attitudes towards homosexuality similar to those of previously studied healthy homosexual males, variable social support needs, variable satisfaction with specific types of social support, and moderately small social networks. In this AIDS subject group, illness concerns, attitudes towards homosexuality, and social support satisfaction were significantly correlated with each other and with previously reported levels of psychologic distress and subjective (but not objective) measures of health status.

Of interest to social scientists and physicians caring for AIDS patients.

c. Dissertations

1153. ALUMBAUGH, Mary Jane. "Social support, coping and auto immune deficiency syndrome (AIDS): An exploratory study." Ph.D. dissertation, California School of Professional Psychology, Los Angeles, 1985.

Examines the social support and coping of individuals with AIDS.

Research

A model was tested, which examined environmental, personal, and social factors' influence on physical health and psychological well-being. The model was predictive of psychological outcomes, but not of physical health measures. Variables related to good physical outcomes included self-esteem, satisfaction with support, instrumental support, emotional support, and active coping responses. Results conflict with previous research in that worsened physical condition was not associated with satisfaction with support, was not associated with increased quantitative support, and was negatively associated with instrumental support. Measures of satisfaction with support, instrumental support, and emotional support were quite high, although network size was small.

Of interest to psychologists and mental health professionals.

1154. BECHTEL, Gregory A. "Purpose-in-life and social support in gay men with the acquired immunodeficiency syndrome." Ph.D. dissertation, Texas Women's University, Denton, Texas, 1986.

Investigates the relationship between purpose-in-life and social support in gay men with AIDS and gay men who may be at risk for developing AIDS.

Research

Results demonstrated a significant difference between purpose-in-life scores in the two groups of gay men, although there was no significant difference in their social support scores. Income was found to be the only variable consistently related to social support.

Of interest to social science researchers, public health professionals, health educators, nurses, social workers, and members of gay organizations.

1155. BRIDGE, Michael James. "A phenomenological study of being a homosexual male who has been diagnosed with AIDS." Ph.D. dissertation, California School of Professional Psychology, Fresno, 1986.

An in-depth study of the experience of having AIDS, using a phenomenological approach, was conducted within the homosexual male community.

Research

Extensive open-ended interviews of ten homosexual males who had been diagnosed with AIDS for over six months were conducted, and three phenomenological reductions of the transcribed protocols were performed. Major findings produced a description of the impact of AIDS. Once the individual stabilized, the effect of his diagnosis on his social and family network was assessed. The author chronicles the impact of AIDS on all aspects of the individual's existence, the coping strategies employed, and the insights gained by persons with AIDS. For some, AIDS was ultimately seen as a catalyst to bring about needed change on a societal level, if only among the homosexual community.

Of interest to mental health professionals and social and behavioral scientists.

1156. CLEVELAND, Peggy Hall. "Description of the experiences of AIDS patients with a comparison to terminal cancer patients." Ph.D. dissertation, University of Georgia, 1987.

Examines psychosocial variables in the process of AIDS in order to describe the experience of AIDS patients and analyze differences in state anxiety, trait anxiety, and life events two years before diagnosis in cancer patients and AIDS patients.

Research

There was a significant relationship between trait anxiety and state anxiety in this sample of AIDS patients. It was found that AIDS patients have more trait anxiety and state anxiety than do cancer patients. A multiple regression equation was calculated to examine the relation of the progress of the disease to a linear combination of state anxiety, patient's living arrangement, the number of people in the social network system, and the patient's perception of the attitudes of professionals who work with the patients. The combination of these variables was not significantly related to the progress of disease scores of AIDS patients. A significant negative relation was found to exist between loneliness and perception of support, a positive relation between loneliness and state anxiety, and a positive relation between perceived affective response and affected involvement with the family of origin.

Of interest to mental health professionals and social and behavioral scientists.

1157. DUFFY, Pam Reid.   "Surviving survival: A theory of living
      with the threat of AIDS."   Ph.D. dissertation, The University
      of Arizona, 1987.

A grounded theory, explaining the social and psychological processes
employed by gay men in living with the threat of AIDS, is developed.

Research

Increasingly structured interviews of healthy gay men and an ongoing,
progressive literature and media search were the two major collection
procedures utilized to gather data, which were sampled theoretically
and analyzed in order to identify the elements and structure of the
theory.   Surviving survival, the continuous basic social process used
by gay men to ensure mortal survival as well as outlive the extremity
of the AIDS threat, was identified as the core category of the theory.
The process is comprised of three subcategories: vigilance (the work
of monitoring the threat of AIDS), safeguarding (the behavior of
protecting self and others from the AIDS threat), and balancing
(efforts to conserve the energy required to sustain affirmation of
life despite the threat of AIDS).   In continuous interaction, the
subcategories of surviving survival are interwoven into multiple
aspects of gay living.   This theory explains the profound impact AIDS
has on the mental health of gay men, who daily survive and perceive
the extremity of the AIDS threat.

Of interest to social and behavioral scientists.

1158. EDGAR, Timothy Mark.   "The disclosure process of the stigma-
      tized: Strategies to minimize rejection."   Ph.D. dissertation,
      Purdue University, 1986.

A survey of 148 gay men to determine the process of the disclosure of
stigmatizing information.

Research

The type of communicative strategy used to minimize the chances of
rejection had little impact on the outcome of the disclosure.
However, persons using the most complex strategies experienced high
levels of stress during the disclosure.   A significant number of gay
men have altered their disclosure behavior since the advent of the
AIDS crisis.

Of interest to communications specialists and mental health
professionals.

1159. FRANKLIN, Michael Dean.   "Psychological functioning in people
      with early stage human immunodeficiency virus (HIV)
      infection."   Ph.D. dissertation, California School of
      Professional Psychology, Berkeley, 1988.

Psychological functioning among men infected with HIV was examined.

The findings confirm clinical reports that some, but not all, people
with HIV infection experience distress. During the first month after
diagnosis, people infected with HIV may effectively deny the impact of
their diagnosis and minimize distress. After at least four months,
however, time and the presence of symptoms may reduce denial,
resulting in increased distress. These findings are discussed and
implications drawn for the psychological treatment of HIV infected
people.

Of interest to mental health professionals.

1160. HIRSCH, Dan Alan. "Psychological aspects of the acquired
      immune deficiency syndrome (AIDS)." Ph.D. dissertation,
      Yeshiva University, 1985.

Patterns of psychological symptomatology were assessed in 67 gay men
diagnosed with AIDS and 150 asymptomatic gay men to examine psychological adjustment to AIDS.

Research

Significantly greater psychological distress was observed in the AIDS
patients, with respect to the asymptomatic comparison group on the
following variables: somatization, depression, anxiety, obsessive-compulsive symptoms, phobic anxiety, psychoticism, and global
distress. For the AIDS patient sample only, analyses of the
relationships between coping strategies and three indices of
psychological distress (depression, anxiety, and global distress) were
performed. Two coping strategies, active relaxation and positive
comparison, were found to be significantly negatively associated with
anxiety. No significant associations were obtained between any coping
strategy and depression.

Of interest to psychologists and other mental health professionals.

1161. IRISH, Thomas Mark. "Emotions and fantasy in the discrimina-
      tion and prognosis of patients with acquired immunodeficiency
      and related conditions." Ph.D dissertation. Pacific Gradu-
      ate School of Psychology, 1987.

Assessed whether the levels of self-reported emotional distress or use
of fantasy differentiated between men with AIDS and ARC.

Research

Self-reported measures of psychological distress and use of fantasy
indicated minimal to no differences between groups. ARC patients
differed from AIDS patients only in their greater level of anxiety at
baseline. Except for a greater level of fatigue for AIDS patients who
subsequently died, no differences were reported between groups when
longitudinal medical factors were assessed.

Of interest to psychiatrists and psychologists.

1162. JACKSON, Robert Neil.   "Coping with the reality of AIDS: A
      rhetorical analysis of Kokomo, Indiana's response to the Ryan
      White-Western Schools Corporation controversy."   Ph.D.
      dissertation, The University of Nebraska, Lincoln, 1988.

Focuses on how the citizens of the Kokomo area reacted to the news of
Ryan White's illness and to his subsequent fight to go to school,
exploring how the townspeople named and gave meaning to the problem,
its causes, and the people involved in the dispute, and how this
naming affected the people's ability to communicate with one another.

Research

Five focus groups, two of which supported Ryan's attendance in school,
two of which opposed his presence in the classroom, and one which
acted as a control, were formed and interviewed. How the groups moved
toward symbolic convergence to create three distinct visions of the
drama was explored. The varying visions contain similarities, which
provide areas for possible agreement and communication between the
factions and are expressed through the use of an "insider/outsider"
theme by all the groups.   The study concludes by exploring the
rhetorical possibilities in the three visions.

Of interest to social scientists.

1163. KAISCH, Kenneth Burton.   "The psychology and social conse-
      quences of HTLV-III infection: Homosexuals in Orange
      County, California."   Ph.D. dissertation.   Utah State
      University, 1986.

A study to identify the psychological and social consequences
experienced by homosexual men upon learning that they are HIV positive although they have not, as yet, developed ARC or AIDS.

Research

Results indicate that HIV positive men show considerable disorgani-
zation after hearing test results, and have clinically high levels of
anxiety and of depression. Positives were also quite guarded about
sharing the results of their testing, experienced negative effects in
social and occupational functioning, and reported pervasive changes in
their sexual activity.

Of interest to social and behavioral scientists and mental health
professionals.

1164. LAWTON, Florice Angela.   "The psychosocial impact of the
      AIDS risk on school age children and adolescents with
      hemophilia."   Ph.D. dissertation.   California School of
      Professional Psychology, Los Angeles, 1986.

The level of AIDS-related anxiety reported by pediatric hemophilia patients, and the relationship of AIDS anxiety to AIDS information and psychosocial functioning, were examined.

Research

Results did not indicate that pediatric hemophilia patients are experiencing greater AIDS anxiety than comparison age-mates. However, younger hemophilia patients possessed levels of AIDS information similar to that of both older groups, and older comparison subjects possessed significantly more AIDS information than younger comparison subjects. AIDS anxiety and AIDS information were correlated negatively for the older comparison subjects and the combined hemophilia groups.

Of interest to pediatricians.

1165. MOULTON, Jeffrey Mark. "Adjustment to a diagnosis of acquired immune deficiency syndrome and related conditions: A cognitive and behavioral perspective." Ph.D. dissertation, California School of Professional Psychology, Berkeley, 1988.

The psychological adjustment to a diagnosis of AIDS and related conditions was examined in 37 gay men.

Research

Seventy-eight percent of the subjects attributed the cause of their health problems to themselves. This is a higher rate of self-attribution than was found in a study of women with breast cancer. The use of particular attributions at diagnosis remained relatively stable over time. Compared with attributions involving other sources, self-attributions were associated with greater psychological distress in AIDS and ARC subjects. Attributions to external factors appeared psychologically protective for persons with ARC, who were more likely than those with AIDS to attribute causes to factors other than themselves.

Of interest to social and behavioral scientists and mental health professionals.

1166. O'BRIEN, Caroleen Kerth. "Primary relationships and mental health in a cohort at risk for AIDS." Ph.D. dissertation. University of Michigan, 1987.

The effects of AIDS-related stress and primary relationships on the mental health of homosexually active men at risk for AIDS were examined.

Research

Men who knew someone with AIDS showed increased distress, regardless of whether the infected person was an acquaintance, friend, or sexual partner. Effects of past stress in the personal network were not significant, but current stress was related to an increase in psychological problems. Relationship status was not associated with changes in psychological health. The stress of knowing someone with AIDS did not affect the mental health of men who were consistently out of relationships or of those who were consistently in them. However, stress did affect the mental health of men whose relationship status had changed during the previous year.

Of interest to social and behavioral scientists.

1167. SCAPPATICCIO, James Salvatore. "AIDS risk as psychological threat: The experience of anxiety in gay men at risk for AIDS as a function of anxiety proneness, defense mechanisms, and self-assessment of AIDS risk." Ph.D. dissertation, Columbia University, 1985.

A study of the effects of self-assessment of AIDS risks on gay males, aged 30-39, in New York City.

Research

Anxiety was not increased by the self-assessment of AIDS risk. Strong correlations with certain defense mechanisms were found for some psychological clusters. Lack of anxiety appeared to be related to the high levels of education, volunteering activities, and previous changes in risky behaviors among the participants.

Of interest to mental health professionals.

1168. SCHOTT, Jacqueline Ruth. "Psychosocial reactions to acquired immune deficiency syndrome (AIDS) in two populations at risk: Healthy homosexual men and men with persistent generalized lymphadenopathy (PGL)." Ph.D. dissertation. California School of Professional Psychology, Los Angeles, 1986.

This study employed a self-administered questionnaire that evaluated behavior change, frequency of engagement in self-protective behaviors, and factors associated with behavior change and compliance with health recommendations.

Research

Results indicated that the patients with generalized lymphadenopathy (PGL) engaged in high-risk behaviors before the AIDS outbreak more often than the control subjects. The PGL patients were found to be experiencing significantly more negative mood states compared with controls. Perceived efficacy significantly predicted engagement in self-protective behaviors.

Of interest to social and behavioral scientists and health educators.

1169. SEIRUP, Jon Frederic. "Dreams as the mirror image of AIDS: A study of dream symbols in male homosexuals at risk for AIDS." Ph.D. dissertation. The Wright Institute, Berkeley, California, 1986.

This study, which focused on dream symbols and their relationships to the process of individuation, was designed to determine whether there are differences in the manifest and latent content of the dreams of people at risk for AIDS who seem to be in denial of this risk and those who are not in denial.

Research

There were distinct differences in the manifest content of the dreams of the two groups. The denying group showed more ambiguity, sexual activity, mother characters, misfortune, passive physical activity, preoccupation with the external body, and unconscious compensation symbols. The dreams of the non-denying showed more uncertainty, individuation symbols, and symbols of the self, adulthood, interest in the internal body, aggression by others, mutual friendly interactions, apprehension, and recreational and functional implements.

Of interest to psychiatrists and psychologists.

1170. SICARD, R.A.   "A proposal for measuring the association between stress and the development of opportunistic infections in HIV-1 seropositive individuals." M.P.H. thesis, University of Texas School of Public Health, Houston, May 1988.

Presents a research design seeking to respond to the question, "What is the association between opportunistic infections and stress in HIV seropositive men?"

Research Proposal

Men who present themselves to be tested for the HIV virus would be asked to participate in the measurement of levels of stress. The Holmes/Rahe Schedule of Recent Events Questionnaire would be administered during three yearly intervals along with a continuous medical history and monthly personal counseling. During data analysis, a control group with low stress levels would be compared with a cohort group with high levels of stress.

Of interest to all health professionals, public health officials, and social and behavioral scientists.

1171. THOMPSON, Bruce J.   "The experience of distress and adaptation in response to the threat of AIDS in healthy gay men: An exploratory study." Ph.D. dissertation, Smith College School for Social Work, 1987.

Changes in measures of ego functioning and distress in healthy gay men that might be attributable to the threat of AIDS were examined.

Research

Twenty-four asymptomatic gay men from Boston, MA were enrolled in the study in 1983. Ego functioning of the subjects was inferred from assessments of their adult interpersonal relationships. Narcissistic strengths and vulnerabilities were obtained through two semi-structured clinical interviews, spaced one year apart, and quantified through the use of nine rating scales.   Self-report measures of distress were obtained by using the Beck Depression Index and the Symptom Checklist-90.   The sample was rated slightly above mid-range on ego functioning.   Its distress scores indicated more distress than non-patient normals, but less than psychiatric outpatients. There was no statistically significant association between ego functioning and the level of distress, and there were no significant changes between the 1983 and 1984 measures of ego functioning and distress.   There was no uniform pattern of success in adaptation, but the majority of the sample exhibited adaptive responses.

Of interest to mental health professionals.

1172. WIENER-BRAWERMAN, Lori Sue.   "An attitudinal study of social
      worker's responses to the acquired immune deficiency
      syndrome (AIDS) patient population."   Ph.D. dissertation,
      New York University, 1988.

A mail survey of social workers and social work students examined the extent to which they expressed comfort in working with AIDS patients and their significant others.

Research

Questionnaires were anonymously completed by 264 respondents at 12 hospitals, a 65% response rate.   Support was obtained for all of the research hypotheses.   Level of comfort was positively associated with knowledge about AIDS, knowledge about resources available to this patient population, and job satisfaction, but negatively associated with homophobia, fear of contagion, and negative moral attitudes towards persons with AIDS.   Other variables associated with greater comfort included: length of experience working with AIDS patients, support from the social worker's family and friends, and having gay family members and friends.   Respondents were found to feel more sympathetic, nonjudgmental, helpless, and angry when providing counseling to a hemophiliac with AIDS than a gay man with AIDS.

Of interest to social workers and social work educators.

1173. WOODS, William Joseph.   "A comparison study of the psycho-
      logical status of AIDS-associated Kaposi's sarcoma patients,
      acute leukemia patients, and healthy gay and heterosexual
      men."   Ph.D. dissertation, Ohio State University, 1985.

Compared the self-esteem, locus of control, depression, anxiety, and distress of four groups: gay men with Kaposi's sarcoma, heterosexual men with acute leukemia, healthy gay men, and healthy heterosexual men.

Research

No differences in self-esteem and locus of control were found between the four groups. The two patient groups had significantly higher levels of depression, anxiety, and distress than did the healthy controls. However, the healthy gay men scored in the clinical range of depression, anxiety, and distress, suggesting an overall effect of the AIDS epidemic on gay men.

Of interest to mental health professionals.

2. SPIRITUAL AND RELIGIOUS ISSUES

a. Books

1174. ADMINISTRATIVE Board, United States Catholic Conference. *The Many Faces of AIDS: A Gospel Response.* Washington, DC: United States Catholic Conference, November 1987.

A statement and discussion about AIDS from the United States Catholic Conference, November 1987.

Booklet

Discusses the prevention of AIDS, the care for persons with AIDS, and the Catholic Church's view on AIDS.

Of special interest to clergy and counselors.

1175. ALBERS, Gregg. *Plague in Our Midst.* Lafayette, LA: Huntington House, 1988.

The author, a physician, writes this book for Christian young people and their families.

Text

Chapter topics include: the church in a sexual world; the plague of AIDS; the biblical perspective of sexuality; the world's sexuality; sex education and scriptural principles; teaching children about sexual attitudes; adolescent sexual attitudes; sexual maturation and function; sexual problems and issues; and design for revival.

Of interest to the general public.

1176. AMOS, William E., Jr. *When AIDS Comes to Church.* Philadelphia: Westminister Press, 1988.

An odyssey of a pastor's relationships in the First Baptist Church of Plantation, Florida.

Chronicle

This book describes what happened to one pastor, his congregation, the AIDS patients, and the members of their families in the circumstances of AIDS.

Of interest to clergy, counselors, and the general public.

1177. FORTUNATO, John E.   *AIDS, The Spiritual Dilemma.*   San Francisco: Harper & Row, 1987.

Deals with the spiritual consequences and meaning of AIDS from the gay perspective.

Monograph

Discusses the psychologic pain and spiritual growth experienced by the victims of incurable disease, especially when it is complicated by homophobia. Points out the social, moral, and theological dilemmas that face the church in the midst of the AIDS epidemic, and discusses how the afflicted may be helped through the nourishment of their inherent spirituality and religiosity.

Of interest to clergymen, church members, persons with AIDS, and concerned laypersons.

1178. GALLAGHER, Joseph.   *Voices of Strength and Hope for a Friend with AIDS.*   Kansas City, MO: Sheed & Ward, 1987.

The "letter" contains quotes and encouraging words for persons who have AIDS.

Booklet

A priest who has had a heart attack and coronary bypass operation shares with persons with AIDS his experience with death and his own fragility. He shares some "road-tested" attitudes toward adversity that have fortified him and others. A sensitive, thoughtful, hopeful booklet.

Of interest to the general public.

1179. KAVAR, Louis F.   *Pastoral Ministry in the AIDS Era: Focus on Families and Friends of Persons with AIDS.*   Wayzata, MN: Woodland, 1988.

The author shares what he has found to be important and helpful in ministering to the family and friends of persons with AIDS.

Monograph

Includes chapters on: misconceptions about AIDS; pastoral ministry with families; the family in crisis; living the long haul; and living through death.

Of interest to clergy, counselors, and mental health professionals.

1180. PEARSON, Carol Lynn. *Good-Bye, I Love You.* New York: Random House, 1986.

The true story of a woman whose homosexual husband developed and succumbed to AIDS.

Autobiography

The author tells of her struggle to understand and accept her husband's homosexuality, to preserve their friendship despite the dissolution of their marriage, to maintain a loving family relationship, and, finally, to help her husband through his final illness. Her story illustrates how religious faith and involvement in a supportive community can provide the strength to endure and cope successfully with extremely painful life events.

Of interest to general audiences.

1181. SERINUS, Jason (Ed.). *Psychoimmunity & the Healing Process: To Immunity and AIDS.* Berkeley, CA: Celestial Arts, 1986.

Offers a holistic approach to understanding and treating immune dysfunction and AIDS.

Book of Readings

The book is divided into three sections. Part one offers an overall perspective on the phenomenon of healing life-threatening illness, and the alignment of mind, body, and spirit, which is the essence of the healing process. The second part, while concentrating on the specific case history of AIDS, contains information that is applicable to all healing. The third part is dedicated to the trance channelings of Kevin Ryerson, Mediator, offering insight into the nature of the healing process and information on human anatomy, biology, and mental functioning.

Of interest to persons concerned with the holistic approach to healing and to spiritualists.

1182. SHELP, Earl E., and Ronald H. Sunderland. *AIDS and the Church.* Philadelphia: Westminster Press, 1987.

A compassionate, insightful, and practical guide and call for the church's response to AIDS.

Text

The authors take a sensitive look at how the church, clergy, and laity should respond to AIDS. They first provide a medical review of the current situation. Then they consider the responsibility that God's people have for the care of the sick, regardless of the illness, and look at AIDS victims as the "poor" for whom there should be a special mission.   Turning from interpretation to application, they describe various ways of ministering to those with AIDS and show how the church should set the example for all of society.

Of interest to clergy and counselors.

1183. ———, Peter W.A. Mansell.   *AIDS: Personal Stories in Pastoral*
        Perspective. New York: Pilgrim Press, 1986.

This descriptive book provides information about AIDS, its effect on people, the response of society, and the obligation of the church. The stories it contains are true.

Text

The church is called upon to meet its obligation to provide compassionate ministries in the crises generated by AIDS. Stories of people with AIDS or ARC, family members, lovers, nurses, social workers, and physicians are told as a means to illustrate the suffering associated with AIDS.   The authors hypothesize that the response to AIDS by the church and society reflects the varied fears that the disease evokes and a disregard for the populations associated with it.   The stories illustrate the need for ministry, and a pastoral commentary suggests ways in which these needs might be met by pastors and congregations.

Of interest to the general public, and especially clergy.

1184. SUNDERLAND, Ronald H., and Earl E. Shelp.   *AIDS: A Manual*
        for Pastoral Care.   Philadelphia: The Westminster Press,
        1987.

A brief manual to help pastors, chaplains, and other caregivers who are called upon to minister to AIDS patients.

Manual

The six chapters cover the medical facts, the fears that grip people, grief recognition and response, and ethical issues. Also provided are three case studies and a bibliography of additional resource materials.

Of special interest to clergy and counselors.

1185. TAPIA, Andrés.   *The AIDS Crisis: The Facts and Myths about*
        a Modern Plague.   Downers Grove, IL: IntyerVarsity Press,
        1988.

Provides some background on the facts about AIDS, and offers guidelines for a "Christian response."

Booklet

Discusses who gets AIDS, what AIDS is, how it is transmitted, the origin of the disease, and various theological viewpoints regarding AIDS. Uses a series of vignettes to illustrate concrete ways in which some churches, communities, and individuals have responded to persons with AIDS, and offers guidelines for meeting the needs of persons with AIDS.

Of interest to laypersons and clergy.

b. Articles

1186. "AIDS: Responding to the crisis." *Health Progress* 67, no. 4 (May 1986): 29-56.

A collection of articles showing how some Christian caregivers have begun to respond to the challenges and dilemmas presented by AIDS.

Special Journal Section

Contains articles on a public policy agenda; justice and compassion in treating AIDS patients; pastoral counseling; pastoral care; legal implications for health care providers; and meeting the needs of AIDS patients.

Of interest to caregivers, clergy, and concerned laypersons.

1187. KAYAL, Philip M. "Morals, medicine, and the AIDS epidemic." *Journal of Religion and Health* 24 (1985): 218-238.

Argues that medical and health care are related to the perceived causality of illness and to the social status of those who are ill.

Analytical

The role of religion in the definition and interpretation of AIDS, as well as its effects on gay people and gay life, is emphasized. A political analysis of AIDS and its assumed causes is also given. These homophobic explanations are viewed as attempts to disenfranchise and discredit gay life further. Responsibility for containing AIDS is discussed in the context of "brokenness" between and among gay people. "Healing" is given as a necessary solution.

Of interest to clergy, social scientists, philosophers, and historians.

1188. MEISENBACH, Albert E., III. "Reflections on the moral dimensions of the AIDS epidemic." *Journal of American College Health* 35 (1987): 279-281.

Examines some probing questions raised by the AIDS epidemic concerning the purpose of sexual intercourse and how sexual activity either facilitates or thwarts the individual's internal drive towards self-fulfillment.

Essay

The author attempts to underscore the importance of individual
morality as a determining and historical factor in sexual expression.
He argues that without the protection of a mutual bond of fidelity,
the chance of obtaining gratification from sexual activity is reduced.
Morality protects and nurtures the expression of sexuality, which
involves the deepest core of a person's spirit, and mutual faith-
fulness is the practical recognition of an evolutionary imperative for
survival.   Educational acknowledgment of these factors may complement
and strengthen public health education in its efforts to gain control
over the AIDS epidemic.

Of interest to educators, counselors, and public health officials.

1189. MURPHY, Timothy F. "Is AIDS a just punishment?" *Journal of
      Medical Ethics* 14 (1988): 154-160.

There are religious and philosophical versions of the thesis that AIDS
is a punishment for homosexual behavior.   It is argued that the
religious version is seriously incomplete.

Discussion

Possible rationales for establishing the immorality of homosexual
behavior are reviewed.   The author claims that the premise that
homosexuality is a sin and is immoral is not well established and that
the religious argument for seeing AIDS as a punishment of
homosexuality is incomplete.

Of interest to philosophers, theologians, and ethicists.

1190. PALMER, Susan J.   "AIDS as metaphor."   *Society* 26, no. 2
      (1989): 44-50.

This study attempts to account for differences in various religious
groups' attitudes towards AIDS.   It is postulated that, in each group,
AIDS is used as a symbol to reference its own particular standards of
sexual behavior and ideal of family life.

Research

The primary method of data collection was the perusal of literature
sent to the author by fundamentalist and evangelical churches,
Christian sects, and cults.   A secondary method was to interview
members of those churches that practiced healing rituals, body rituals
to ward off disease, or instituted obligatory AIDS testing.   Five of
these groups have issued official, well-defined policies concerning
AIDS and AIDS victims, two groups insist on AIDS tests for their
congregations, and one group has not yet published a statement on the
topic.   The author discusses religious responses to AIDS in the
various religious groups.

Of interest to philosophers, clergy, and social and behavioral
scientists.

1191. WENDLER, Klaus. "Ministry to patients with acquired immuno-deficiency syndrome: A spiritual challenge." *Journal of Pastoral Care* 41 (1987): 4-16.

Identifies the psychosocial problems of AIDS patients and offers guidelines for spiritual caregivers in responding to them.

Discussion

Psychosocial problems stem from the effect that AIDS has on the sexual and social life of persons with AIDS and the feelings of alienation, fear of disfigurement, and loss of control. As patients pass through the psychological stages of impact, regression, acknowledgment, and reconstruction, spiritual caregivers can provide patients with their presence, affirmation of self-worth, and reflective listening. The church is challenged to go beyond society's negativism and offer the reconciliation described in the scriptures.

Of interest to pastors, counselors, educators, caregivers, and the lay public.

3. TERMINAL CARE/DEATH AND DYING

a. Books

1192. KUBLER-ROSS, Elizabeth. *AIDS: The Ultimate Challenge.* New York: Macmillan, 1987.

The author describes her experiences.in working with and on behalf of patients with AIDS, their families, and their loved ones.

Descriptive/Philosophical

AIDS has become our biggest sociopolitical issue, and its victims have had to face hostility and discrimination from every direction. Like any terminally ill patients, they must go through the difficult "stages of dying," but are often forced to do so within a society that cruelly discriminates against, judges, and blames them for their "unhealthy lifestyles." The magnitude of the AIDS epidemic is threatening to reach staggering proportions, and unless we approach it in an appropriate fashion, we will find ourselves without the resources that are needed to combat this disease. AIDS challenges all of us to accept its victims as the sick people they are and to provide them with the love, nurturing, and support they need.

Should interest all health care providers and concerned individuals.

1193. SNOW, John. *Mortal Fear: Meditations on Death and AIDS.* Cambridge, MA: Cowley Publications, 1987.

Contains five meditations on AIDS.

Monograph

A brief, readable volume that contains meditations useful to those
ministering to AIDS patients as well as material useful in talks about
AIDS.

Of interest to clergy and counselors.

b. Articles

1194. DOWNING, G. Michael.   "Palliative AIDS care: To be or not to
      be." *Journal of Palliative Care* 1, no. 2 (1986): 32-34.

A discussion of how to be active in the investigation and treatment of
AIDS patients.

Descriptive

The acceleration of the incidence of AIDS poses many questions for
hospice and palliative care programs. Consideration must be given to
many factors, such as active versus palliative treatment, timing of
palliative involvement, the management of fear and anxiety and the
protection of staff and other patients, the role of palliative care in
the societal implications of the disease, and discussions about the
allocation of health care resources.

Of interest to counselors and hospice volunteers and administrators.

1195. "FACING the AIDS epidemic." *American Journal of Hospice
      Care* 3, no. 2 (1986): Entire Issue.

The lack of information about terminal care for AIDS patients motivated the staff of this journal to bridge the gap.

Special Journal Issue

The eight original articles cover: psychosocial aspects of hospice
care for AIDS patients; pastoral care; volunteer aspects; nursing
care; medical care; and two case studies, one of which reports a
personal experience with AIDS, and the other, a community approach to
AIDS through hospice.

Of interest to all health professionals.

1196. GALAZKA, Michal.   "Hospice for AIDS patients: Interesting
      times ahead." *American Journal of Hospice Care* 4, no. 6
      (1987): 11-14.

Discusses how individual hospices and the hospice community as a whole
can best prepare to care for the increasing number of AIDS patients.

Essay

Hospice care for AIDS patients requires significant adaptation of clinical practices, while retaining hospice principles. It requires that hospice professionals explore their personal and professional capacity for change and challenge. It requires the fostering of new professional and community alliances, while honoring all pre-existing commitments. It requires both national and local efforts to ensure that good terminal care for AIDS patients, adequately funded and readily available, becomes the minimum acceptable standard.

Of general interest to the lay public.

1197. McLEOD, W. Alistair, Jaime Smith, Brian Willoughby. "Hospice care of AIDS patients." *Journal of Palliative Care* 2, no. 1 (1986): 33-34.

Discusses the roles of palliative care teams in caring for AIDS patients.

Descriptive

Palliative care teams in hospices can help AIDS patients to re-establish family relationships, provide periodic patient care to relieve family caregivers, and counsel professional and family caregivers. The financial constraints faced by most AIDS patients in their final months must be considered in hospice planning.

Of interest to health professionals and administrators working in hospices.

1198. MURPHY, Sister Patrice. "Experiences in a hospice: The AIDS patient." *Loss, Grief & Care* 1 (1986-1987): 87-91.

Discusses the role of the hospice in ministering to AIDS patients.

Essay

Hospice comes in when all efforts at cure are no longer effective and when care is aimed at providing physical, emotional, and spiritual comfort. Since 1984, St. Vincent's Hospice in New York City has been called upon to minister to patients with AIDS. AIDS patients, many of whom are homosexuals, are particularly vulnerable to psychological as well as physical suffering. In order to comprehend their suffering, one must be aware of the facts surrounding homosexuality--the rejection, isolation, haranguing, ostracism, and blame that homosexuals suffer for a condition they cannot change. Hospice provides comfort in the face of sorrow and despair and tries, in conjunction with other agencies, to discover and respond to financial stresses. Hospice extends compassionate understanding of sorrow and pain to patients and to families and expresses to the dying patient, in actions as well as words, its underlying philosophy that every patient matters because of who he/she is.

Of interest to health care providers, mental health professionals, and concerned laypersons.

1199. POLLATSEK, Judy. "Hospice for AIDS patients: Break down barriers and accept AIDS patients." *American Journal of Hospice Care* 4, no. 6 (1987): 9-10.

Examines the questions raised regarding the appropriateness of hospice care for people with AIDS.

Essay

Three major barriers toward admission of persons with AIDS to hospice are identified: lack of staff skills, fear, and lack of resources. AIDS education, which addresses itself to medical needs, infection control, and psychosocial needs of patients, families, and significant others can effectively overcome two of the barriers. Long term planning should take into account the need for specialized hospices for AIDS patients as well as cancer patients.

Of general interest to the lay public.

1200. SAUNDERS, Dame Cicely. "Hospice for AIDS patients: New teams should be developed for AIDS care." *American Journal of Hospice Care* 4, no. 6 (1987): 7-8.

Discusses the premise that the principles of the hospice movement should not only apply to patients with far advanced cancer, but should be the basis of the care and treatment of patients with any terminal illness.

Essay

Proposes that new teams be developed to care for AIDS patients. Any team can and should set limits of its operation, even if they are flexible. Otherwise, the skills that can be learned, researched, and taught by the specialist will not be developed and hospice care could be a "soft option."

Of interest to the lay public.

1201. SCHIETINGER, Helen. "Hospice care needs of the person with AIDS." *Journal of Palliative Care* 2, no. 1 (1986): 31-32.

Discusses the psychosocial needs of persons in the terminal stages of AIDS.

Discussion

Persons with AIDS need emotional support in coping with the losses and grief associated with the disease. They also need information which will enable them to make informed decisions on the termination of treatment. Health care workers need to be educated about AIDS in order to meet the needs of dying people and to serve as role models for families and friends of persons with AIDS.

Of interest to hospice workers, hospital staff, and volunteers.

1202. SCHOFFERMAN, Jerome. "Hospice care of the patient with AIDS." *Hospice Journal* 3, no. 4 (1987): 51-74.

Discusses those aspects of the biological, psychological, social, and spiritual realms that differentiate hospice care of the patient with AIDS from traditional hospice care.

Descriptive

The biological aspects of AIDS are presented along with psychosocial issues. Although the psychosocial issues surrounding the patient and caregivers of the dying AIDS patient share features common to all dying patients, some are distinct; these psychosocial issues must be recognized and addressed to provide quality palliative care for the AIDS patient.

Of interest to physicians, hospice workers, mental health professionals, and clergy.

1203. STEINBROOK, Robert, Bernard Lo, Jeffrey Moulton, Glenn Saika, Harry Hollander, Paul A. Volberding. "Preferences of homosexual men with AIDS for life-sustaining treatment." *New England Journal of Medicine* 314 (1986): 457-460.

One hundred and eighteen homosexual outpatients with AIDS were surveyed to determine their preferences for life-sustaining treatment and their use of advance directives.

Research

Results of the study suggest that most patients with AIDS have thought about life-sustaining treatment, have preferences about their care, and want to discuss life-sustaining treatment with their physicians. However, many have not provided advance directives, including some who might benefit from the durable power of attorney for health care. Many also have misconceptions about the effectiveness of life-sustaining treatment, even though they are well educated and live in San Francisco where their illness is well publicized. Physicians who care for patients with AIDS and other serious chronic illnesses should take an active role in educating patients about life-sustaining treatment and encouraging them to provide advance directives.

Should interest all primary care physicians.

GLOSSARY

AIDS   Acquired immune deficiency syndrome: The complete collapse of the body's immune system in an individual infected by HIV. Indicated when an associated illness, such as Kaposi's sarcoma, presents and there is a lack of any other underlying cause.

ARC   AIDS-related complex: Developed by some people who are HIV antibody positive. Symptoms can be debilitating. They may include night sweats, weight loss, malaise, and repeated infections.

AZT   Azidothimidine (Generic name, Zidovudine): An inhibitor of the in vitro replication of some retroviruses, including HIV. Used to suppress the AIDS virus.

CDC   Center for Disease Control: National public health agency, located in Atlanta, Georgia.

CMV   Cytomegalovirus: A herpes virus that often produces asymptomatic infection, but can cause serious infections, such as interstitial pneumonitis, in immunosuppressed individuals. Also causes serious birth defects.

DNA   Deoxyribose nucleic acid: Genetic material found inside living cells or viruses.

EAP   Employee Assistance Program: Program offering professional counseling services for employees with a variety of emotional as well as addictive problems. Provides support and referral services for infected persons, support and educational information for co-workers, and interpretation and implementation of pertinent litigation for managers.

ELISA   Enzyme linked immunosorbent assay: A technique used in testing blood for the presence of antibodies to HIV, indicating whether an individual has been exposed to the AIDS virus.

477

HBV   Hepatitis B virus: Causes serious infection of the
                 liver. Transmitted by contact with infected blood or
                 sexual contact. Infected persons may continue to carry
                 and transmit the virus after recovery.

HIV   Human immunodeficiency virus: The retrovirus that
                 causes AIDS, ARC, and PGL. Sometimes called HTLV-III,
                 LAV, or HTLV-III/LAV. People who are HIV antibody
                 positive have been infected with the virus, but may not
                 have any symptoms. However, they are presently
                 regarded to be infectious.

HIV-Ag   HIV antigen: An enzyme that interacts with T-cell
                 lymphocytes to produce antibodies to HIV. Its presence
                 in the body may be the earliest indication of HIV
                 infection.

HIV-2   Human immunodeficiency virus, type 2: A second strain
                 of the HIV, discovered in Africa.

HSV-1   Herpes simplex virus, type 1: Causes cold sores or
                 fever blisters on the mouth or around the eyes. May
                 flare up, after lying dormant in nerve tissue for
                 months or years, under stress, trauma, infection, or
                 immunosuppression.

HSV-2   Herpes simplex virus, type 2: Causes genital and neo-
                 natal herpes and has been implicated as a cause of
                 cervical carcinoma. Transmitted by direct bodily
                 contact.

HTLV   Human T-cell lymphotropic virus: One of a group or
                 family of viruses that, upon invading the body, seek
                 out and attack lymphocytes. HTLV-I and HTLV-II cause
                 rare forms of human leukemia.

HTLV-III   Human T-cell lymphotropic virus III: Now known to be
                 virtually identical to HIV, this virus causes AIDS,
                 ARC, and PGL.

HTLV-III/LAV   The AIDS virus, now commonly referred to as HIV.

KS   Kaposi's sarcoma: A cancer of blood vessels in the skin
                 that is ordinarily rare, appearing only among elderly
                 men, but affects young men with AIDS.

LAS   Lymphadenopathy syndrome: A group of symptoms that are believed to be an early manifestation of HIV infection. Includes fever, weight loss, and swelling of lymph glands over a prolonged period of time.

LAV   Lymphadenopathy-associated virus: A virus that was isolated in France at about the same time HTLV-III was first identified in people with AIDS. HTLV-III and LAV were later found to be virtually identical.

Lymphocytes   White blood cells formed in the bone marrow and lymph nodes: The basis of the body's protective immune system.

PCP   *Pneumocystis carinii* pneumonia: A lung infection caused by an airborne protozoan that is present almost everywhere, but is normally destroyed by the healthy immune system. Seen only in immune-suppressed people, who are susceptible to recurrence, and often fatal.

PGL   Persistent generalized lymphadenopathy: A swelling of the lymph glands that persists for more than three months, which is sometimes developed by persons infected with HIV. May be accompanied by chronic fatigue.

PWA   Person(s) with AIDS.

RNA   Ribose nucleic acid: Genetic material found inside living cells or viruses.

RIPA   Radioimmunoprecipitation assay: Test for the detection of antibodies directed against the human immunodeficiency virus.

STDs   Sexually transmitted diseases: Any diseases that are transmitted by sexual contact. These include syphilis, gonorrhea, herpes simplex type 2, hepatitis B, and AIDS.

T-cells   Lymphocytes: White blood cells (helper/suppressor) that are formed in the marrow and migrate to the thymus gland where they are acted on by hormones before reaching the bloodstream. A part of the immune system that is found to be abnormal in AIDS patients.

T-helper   T-helper lymphocytes: T-cells that help speed up the
                    production of antibodies. Normally outnumber T-sup-
                    pressor cells by about 2:1. This ratio is inverted
                    in AIDS patients.

T-suppressor   T-suppressor lymphocytes: T-cells that slow down the
                    production of antibodies.

Western blot   A test to detect the presence of antibodies to specific
                    proteins or peptides including those of retroviruses:
                    Used to detect antibodies to HIV.

WHO   World Health Organization: An arm of the United
                    Nations, dedicated to international health promotion
                    and disease control.

AUTHOR INDEX

SUBJECT INDEX

Social support (Continued)
  1192. *Also see:* Emotional
    support; Psychological support;
    Psychosocial support; Support.
Social values 444
Social welfare 420
Social welfare programming 294
Social work interventions 368
Social workers 324, 430, 974,
  987, 1003, 1017, 1018
    comfort in working with
      clients with AIDS 1172
    inservice education and
      support 1034
    response to caring for AIDS
      patients 837
    response to persons with AIDS
      and their significant others
      1172
    role 445, 1034
    training 1003, 1034
Societal issues 65
Societal reactions 23
Societal responses to AIDS 374,
  1003, 1183
Societal responses to homsexuality
  1003
Society of Hospital Epidemiolo-
  gists 838
Socioeconomic impact 679
Sociological aspects 931
Sociological factors 242
Sociological issues 179
Sociological perspective 93, 102,
  303
Sociopolitical issues 1020
Socio-psychological needs 60
Sound underwriting 538
Sources of help 1, 43, 115, 127,
  448, 450, 1008
South Africa 680
South America 152, 697
Southland, New Zealand 316
Southwest Baptist Convention of
  Texas 862
Spanish language materials 777
Spatial diffusion of HIV 156, 186
Special interest groups 339
Spectrum House 757
Spermicides 632
Spiritual consequences of AIDS
  1177
Spiritual growth 1177
Spiritual guidance 1178
Spiritual issues 60, 1174-1191
Spiritual meaning of AIDS 1177
Spiritualism 1181

Spirituality 1177
Spread of AIDS 20, 22, 51, 60,
  65, 75, 102, 107, 118, 152, 161,
  174, 175, 177, 201, 287, 370,
  483, 638, 697, 779, 783, 792,
  795, 810, 859, 897, 1090
Spread of HIV 7, 65, 73, 99, 161,
  196, 217, 273
Spread of HIV and AIDS in the
  United States 143
Stabilization 1067
Stages of dying 1192
State activities 117
State agencies' response to AIDS
  68, 104
State departments of correction
  503. *Also see:* Prison(s).
State departments of health 1093
State departments of mental health
  503
State isolation and quarantine
  laws 569
State legislation related to AIDS
  578
State Medicaid policies 523
State policies on AIDS 480
State regulations 578
State tort claims 601
State University of New York
  Health Science Center at
  Brooklyn 1054
Statistical analysis of AIDS
  incidence data 85
Statistical modelling of the AIDS
  epidemic 85
Statistical update, surveys, and
  projections 448
Status of the AIDS epidemic 107,
  705
Statutes and regulations, U.S.
  public health 484. *Also see:*
  Public health law.
Statutory claims 601
Stereotyping 1073
Sterile needles 68, 104. *Also
  see:* Injection equipment,
  sterile; Syringe exchange
  programs.
    issuance to prisoners 807
Sterilization 848
Stigma of AIDS 1084, 1128, 1136,
  1158
Stigmatization 12, 286, 300, 309,
  328, 364, 395, 413, 422, 566,
  686, 926, 931, 979, 987, 1125
    by physicians 413